Herb Toxicities &
Drug Interactions:
A Formula Approach

By Fred Jennes
with Bob Flaws

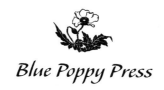

Blue Poppy Press

Published by:
BLUE POPPY PRESS
A Division of Blue Poppy Enterprises, Inc.
5441 Western Ave., Suite 2
Boulder, CO 80301
www.bluepoppy.com

First Edition, July 2004
Second printing, June 2006
Third printing, October 2007
Fourth printing, August 2008

ISBN 1-891845-26-8
ISBN 978-1-891845-26-0
LC #2004093399

DISCLAIMER: The information in this book is given in good faith. However, the author and the publishers cannot be held responsible for any error or omission. The publishers will not accept liabilities for any injuries or damages caused to the reader that may result from the reader's acting upon or using the content contained in this book. The publishers make this information available to English language readers for research and scholarly purposes only.

The publishers do not advocate nor endorse self-medication by laypersons. Chinese medicine is a professional medicine. Laypersons interested in availing themselves of the treatments described in this book should seek out a qualified professional practitioner of Chinese medicine.

Cover & Page Design: Eric J. Brearton

COMP Designation: Original work

10 9 8 7 6 5 4

Printed at Edwards Brothers Digital, Ann Arbor, MI

TABLE OF CONTENTS

This book is dedicated to my first herb teachers: George Kitchie, Christine Harrison, Yan Yun, Jian-Shu Chen, Caylor Wadlington, and Shi Cheng. Their enthusiasm in teaching their subject matter inspired me to enter and explore the exciting world of Chinese medicinals and to successfully incorporate these substances into my practice. To this day, I admire their skills and abilities as healers and herbalists and deeply appreciate what they shared with me.

ACKNOWLEDGEMENTS

This book would not have been possible without a number of people whose belief in its importance and in me brought it to fruition. I would like to thank my colleagues and publishers, Bob Flaws and Honora Wolfe, as well as their stellar employees for their support during this project. Their patience and enthusiasm was much appreciated throughout the long process of conception to publication. I would also like to acknowledge and thank my friend and mentor, Caylor Wadlington, for his timely reminder that our Chinese medicinal pharmacy is, after all, a valuable and safe addition to the tradition of healing. When I was overwhelmed by the inherent dangers in every medicinal I encountered, his was the voice of balance which kept me from becoming an alarmist. And finally, I would like to acknowledge the support and patience of my wife, Helen, and son, Alex. Again they permitted me to lock myself away from them for days at a time while I delved through piles of texts and clicked away relentlessly at the keys of my laptop. They suffered my bouts of fatigue and frustration with their usual grace and love, and for this I am truly grateful.

Fred Jennes, March 2004

I have been a practitioner of modern Western medicine for nearly 30 years, having jumped through all of the standard educational and certification hoops and practiced my craft on thousands of patients. Still, I'm neither so naïve nor so arrogant as to believe that Western science has a corner on what's true and what works, especially not when it comes to healing. When I run out (and sometimes before I run out) of ideas about how to treat a particular patient, I'm more than happy to refer that person to a practitioner who comes at the patient from a totally different perspective than mine. Though I've availed myself of Fred Jennes's healing skills for several of my own ailments and have also referred a number of my patients to him, Oriental medicine remains a mystery to me. It is built on a different foundation than the Western science that I've spent decades learning and practicing. (For one small example, compare the physiologic role of the gall-bladder in Oriental versus Western medicine.) I like some of the alternatives to the type of healing that I know how to practice exactly because I don't understand them.

The medical literature is of little help in integrating what I do, as a modern Western physician, with what the Oriental medicine practitioner does for my patient. When I check the usual reputable sources, I rarely find information that gives a credible objective answer to a question I might have about a diagnosis or treatment that falls outside of the standard medicine that I know. The studies of Oriental medicine that do exist mostly aren't very well done. It is extremely expensive and time-consuming to meet the gold-standard of prospective, double-blind research design that rigorous clinical science demands. Furthermore, there are deep philosophical and methodological debates that question the universal applicability of the tools of modern science to some of the practices of what we call alternative medicine for lack of a better handle.

On the other hand, it is estimated that only about 30% of what I do as a Western physician is backed by hard science. The rest is based on tradition, reasoning from basic principles, and common sense. Much of Oriental medicine is likewise based on tradition and basic principles, albeit different ones than Western medicine embraces. Common sense is the one thing we all share. *Chinese Herbal Toxicities and Drug Interactions* is rife with common sense. The business of Oriental medicine does not have the hugely deep pockets that the manufacturers of Western pharmaceuticals do, nor, fortunately, do Chinese herbs require the hundreds of millions of dollars that must be devoted to research, patenting, and regulation before a new allopathic drug can be brought to market. So, let's face it, most of the Chinese herbs and formulations will never be tested by Western medicine. On the other hand, neither will everything we practitioners of Western medicine do ever be backed by rigorous science. Certainly we should strive to get the sorts of objective evidence that the scientific method can offer about what really works and what doesn't. In the future, when the computerized medical record is a reality, we will be able to ascertain more objectively the validity of some Oriental medical practices via concurrent research. We will have the means to measure outcomes side-by side for example, celecoxib against *Juan Bi Tang* (Assuage Impediment Decoction) by simply mining the clear, comprehensive data contained in the medical records of a large population of patients with joint pain. In the meantime, let's get on with the project of understanding as best we can who we are, what we do, and how we can do it together. *Chinese Herbal Toxicities and Drug Interactions* is a great resource for such a project.

Marc Ringel, MD
Greeley, Colorado

In the mid-1990s, word came from Europe that a number of women who had attended a weight loss clinic in Belgium suffered kidney failure after consuming Chinese medicinal substances.[1] Although the formula which these unfortunate women consumed contained other dangerous pharmaceutical agents, including acetazolamide and belladonna extract, the blame was laid on the incorporation of a Chinese medicinal that contained aristolochic acid (AA), a strongly nephrotoxic substance. Further investigation revealed that the weight loss center clinicians had apparently added the wrong species of herb to their miracle cure, that the herbal product had not been prepared properly, and that just as the amateur mushroom-hunter can inadvertently choose the wrong fungus to feed to his unwitting dinner guests, the clinicians' ignorance had been the cause of their patients' suffering. This incident later caught the attention of practitioners and researchers around the world, and centuries of safe and effective presciption and use of Chinese herbal medicinals suddenly came under suspicion.

Since the Belgian incident, the safety of Chinese medicinal substances has been the focus of many groups, including the Food & Drug Administration (FDA), the American Herbal Products Association (AHPA), and the German "E" Commission. Reasons for this increased scrutiny of the safety of Chinese medicinals is due to several factors:

1. An increasingly risk averse population

2. An aging population therefore using more medical services and taking more medication

3. An increasing dissatisfaction with standard Western medical care

4. An increasing use of complementary and alternative medicine (CAM)

5. Competition in the health care marketplace

Many practitioners of Oriental medicine have made the claim that centuries of careful practice by trained clinicians is proof that these medicinal products, when used appropriately, are as safe and are, in most cases, *safer* than the pharmaceutical agents prescribed by Western physicians. But many watchdog groups, consisting primarily of Western-trained pharmacologists and physicians, have replied with the scientific retort, "Prove it!" So now practitioners of Oriental medicine are being forced to take a closer look at their medicinals and, based on modern pharmacological research, determine their safety.

This book came out of my own [FJ] closer self-examination of Chinese herbal medicine. Two years ago, out of curiosity about the pharmacological safety of the products I have prescribed for years without incident, I attended a seminar on the topic of "Herbal Toxicities & Drug Interactions" offered by my friend and colleague, Bob Flaws. As Bob discussed many of the medicinals I commonly prescribed and considered safe, I was surprised at the number of potential problems that could have arisen from my routine use of these medicinals. As I myself began to perform further research on the medicinal substances in these many formulas, the difficulty I encountered was that, although the safety information was present and accessible via various publications and on the Internet, it was not in one place. In addition, since formulas often contain many medicinal substances, the time needed to determine the safety of the formula's total contents was often long and impractical. What Bob and I decided was needed was a source that contained this information in a convenient, easy-to-consult format. And so the idea for this book was born.

This book is intended for anyone interested in the topic of Oriental herbology whether you are a practitioner, pharmacologist, student, or researcher. But it will be of most use to practitioners of medicine, both Western and Oriental. For our colleagues who practice Oriental medicine, this work will enable you to more precisely and safely prescribe for your patients. Our hope is that, when a pregnant woman asks you, "Will this medicine hurt my baby?" you will be able to answer forthrightly and with certainty instead of guessing and relying solely on your good luck in the past. For our Western medical colleagues, this book will enable you to better understand the nature of the herbal products that many of your patients take. Instead of feeling forced to tell your patients to halt a medication which is benign and appropriate for their condition, you now can prescribe with the knowledge of how your pharmaceutical agent will potentially augment or conflict with the Oriental medical substance your patient is taking.

This book consists of four chapters, several appendices, several indexes, and a companion searchable CD-ROM. Following this Introduction, Chapter 1 discusses the potential for toxicity in the prescription of Chinese medicinals and the factors that can lead to it, notions that we as practitioners must struggle with and understand, if in the Hippocratic ideal, we are to help our patients as much as possible and avoid doing them harm. Chapter 2 focuses in on three major types of toxicity and lists some of the specific medicinals that have been singled out for their toxicity. Chapter 3 suggests how practitioners can most effectively use this book. Chapter 4 lists 100 formulas and their medicinal components. Each medicinal ingredient in each formula is accompanied by its potential toxicity to patients and potential interactions with other Chinese herbs and Western pharmaceuticals. In addition, we have included toxicities and interactions of the formulas themselves, since the additive effect of all the medicinals in a formula may create a toxic or potentially interactive situation with other formulas or drugs. The appendices consist of the American Herbal Products Association (AHPA) categorization of Chinese medicinals, the suspected drug interactions of certain, commonly used Chinese medicinals, and Western pharmaceuticals that can commonly cause certain adverse reactions. Next comes an annotated bibliography followed by a general index, a formula index in Pinyin, a formula index in English, and a Chinese medicinal index in both Pinyin and Latin pharmacological nomenclature.

Our hope is that you, the reader, will find this book useful in your study and application of Chinese medicine, and, as result of using this book, you will practice more safely and effectively.

ENDNOTE

[1] Richard Blackwell, "Cases of Herb Toxicity: Adverse Events Involving Certain Chinese Herbal Medicines and the Response of the Profession," http://acupuncture.com/Herbology/Toxic.htm, 1996, p. 1-3.

CHAPTER 1

THE POTENTIAL FOR TOXICITY

According to *Taber's Cyclopedic Medical Dictionary*, toxicity refers to the extent, quality, or degree of being poisonous,[1] and there is an old saying that goes, *"Ut quod ali cibus est aliis fuat acre venenum."* This can be freely translated as, "One man's meat is another man's poison."[2] Although some people erroneously think that herbs, being "natural," are somehow inherently safe, this is simply not true. Too much of anything taken by the wrong individual under the wrong circumstances can result in illness and death. For instance, water, oxygen, and salt, while necessary to the maintenance of life, can all be lethally toxic when taken in excess. A single peanut or a bite of shrimp may put a susceptible individual into anaphylactic shock, while the rest of us may gorge on these foods to our heart's content. While the substance itself may be benign, its ingestion by a susceptible individual may not be only inappropriate and unwise but also potentially lethal.

Such is also the case with Chinese herbal medicinals.[3] When administered appropriately according to professional standards of care, their effect is beneficial, resulting in the elimination of disease and the restoration and preservation of health. However, when taken ignorantly or carelessly, the result can be unexpected and potentially lethal. So what should one be aware of when prescribing these substances to insure that patients will benefit from them? There are five primary areas of concern *vis á vis* toxicity that need to be considered when prescribing Chinese herbal medicinals safely and effectively. These are diagnosis, preparation, dosage, interaction, and inherent toxicity.

DIAGNOSIS

Professionally trained Oriental medical practitioners prescribe on the basis of two diagnoses (*liang zhen*). The first is a disease diagnosis (*bing zhen*). This may be either a modern Western medical disease diagnosis or a traditional Chinese medical disease diagnosis. From here, the practitioner discriminates the pattern of signs and symptoms which the individual patient is presenting at the time of examination. While the disease diagnosis may be made using modern laboratory tests and imagining techniques, this pattern discrimination (*bian zheng*) is arrived at using only the so-called four examinations. These are inspection, listening/smelling, inquiry, and palpation. By observing the patient's tongue and facial complexion, listening to the sound of the patient's breathing and detecting any odors coming from the patient's body, asking the patient to describe his or her symptoms and the course of their disease, and by feeling the pulse of the radial arteries at both wrists, the trained Oriental medical practitioner is able to identify the pattern of disease the specific patient is currently presenting. Then an effective herbal remedy can be prescribed that precisely matches both the patient's disease diagnosis *and* their personal pattern. In fact, it is an axiom of truth in standard professional Chinese medicine that treatment is primarily based on the patient's pattern discrimination and only secondarily on their disease diagnosis.

For example, a patient presents with a common cold accompanied by a low fever, a red complexion, slight sweating, a prominent sore throat, a red tongue with thin, yellow fur, and a floating, rapid pulse. While the patient's disease diagnosis is an upper respiratory tract infection, based on their particular signs and symptoms, the patient is exhibiting a specific pattern of common cold called a wind heat external contraction. In this case, the treatment principles are to resolve the exterior, clear heat, and disinhibit the throat. Practically, this means the use of a Chinese medicinal formula that primarily contains acrid, cool, exterior-resolving medicinals, such as *Jin Yin Hua* (Flos Lonicerae Japonicae) and *Lian Qiao* (Fructus Forsythiae Suspensae). Because these medicinals' therapeutic actions match the patient's personally presenting pattern, they lower the fever and relieve the sore throat. However, if the practitioner makes a faulty pattern discrimination and prescribes a formula that contains interior-warming medicinals, such as *Gan Jiang* (dry Rhizoma Zingiberis Officinalis) and *Rou Gui* (Cortex Cinnamomi Cassiae), the patient's fever and sore throat may very well worsen and their infection become more severe. Thus these erroneously prescribed medicinals themselves would be toxic to the patient even though, by themselves, they are not considered toxic.

It is Oriental medicine's prescriptive methodology of primarily basing treatment on each patient's personally presenting pattern that makes this system of medicine generally so safe and effective. Medicines in and of themselves are neither good nor bad. The issue is getting the right medicinals to the right patient at the right time, and this is what treatment based on pattern discrimination excels at. Therefore, when prescribing Chinese medicinals, it is extremely important that the practitioner's disease diagnosis *and* pattern discrimination be precise and take into account all the patient's signs and symptoms. Otherwise, even benign medicinals commonly eaten as foods may have toxic effects on a patient's condition.

PREPARATION

One of the most common mistakes leading to toxicity in the prescription of Chinese medicinals is improper processing or preparation. In Chinese, the preparation of medicinals prior to their final cooking or manufacture for administration is called *pao zhi.* This is an ancient art with a literature stretching back over 1,500 years. Many Chinese medicinals need to be prepared in some way before they are infused, decocted, powdered, or pilled. These methods of preparation traditionally include soaking, dry stir-frying, stir-frying in some liquid, such as saltwater, vinegar, alcohol, ginger juice, or honey, steaming, blast-frying, baking, calcining, and carbonizing. These methods of preparation are meant to do either of two things: 1) increase their intended therapeutic effect, or 2) decrease their toxicity. After such preparation, the medicinals are then either boiled or infused in water, powdered, or made into pills for oral administration.

For example, *Ban Xia* (Rhizoma Pinelliae Ternatae*)* is toxic in its unprocessed state, but, when stir-fried with ginger or vinegar, *Ban Xia* becomes a safe medicinal that can be added to a decoction for the effective treatment of many types of phlegm and damp conditions. Similarly, a potentially lethal decoction containing one of the most toxic herbs in the Chinese medicinal pharmacy, *Fu Zi* (Radix Lateralis Praeparatus Aconiti Carmichaeli), becomes safe and useful for treating cold conditions when cooked in combination for a relatively long time with *Gan Cao* (Radix Glycyrrhizae Uralensis) and *Gan Jiang* (dry Rhizoma Zingiberis Officinalis).

While less and less patients both in China and the West are being given bags of bulk-dispensed Chinese medicinals with instructions for making a water-based decoction at home, nevertheless, the issue of preparation is still an important one. Even in the case of ready-made medicines, it is important that companies manufacturing these medicines follow the traditional methods of processing in order to reduce potential toxicity. Practitioners and their patients should ask their suppliers of ready-made Chinese medicines if the medicinals in these products have been prepared correctly to reduce or eliminate potential toxicity.

For more information on the traditional Chinese science of processing medicinals prior to use, readers are referred to Philippe Sionneau's *Pao Zhi: An*

Introduction to the Use of Processed Chinese Medicinals also published by Blue Poppy Press (Boulder, 1995).

DOSAGE

The amount of a medicinal substance prescribed and the duration of its continued administration are important factors in that medicinal's safe and effective use. In standard professional Chinese medicine, there are well established guidelines for the dosage and administration of individual medicinals. These guidelines are presented in such standard materia medica as Bensky and Gamble's *Chinese Herbal Medicine: Materia Medica*[4] and Hong-yen Hsu's *Oriental Materia Medica: A Concise Guide*.[5] As long as one stays within these standard acceptable parameters, there should be little concern about toxicity. For instance, the standard daily dose in decoction of most commonly used Chinese medicinals is 9-10 grams. However, due to known toxicity, the dose of *Chuan Jiao* (Pericarpium Zanthoxyli Bungeani) is only 1.5-6 grams. Conversely, the standard daily dose of *Pu Gong Ying* (Herba Taraxaci Mongolici Cum Radice) begins at nine grams but goes as high as 30 grams due to its low potential for toxicity and the fact that it achieves better therapeutic effects at higher doses. These dosage parameters have been established based on the clinical experience of a hundred or more generations of Asian medical practitioners.

An example of the importance of dosage is the prescription of the medicinal *Ma Huang* (Herba Ephedrae). In the small dosages characteristic of its use in decoctions or Chinese ready-made medicines, *Ma Huang* has been proven to be safe and effective for treating a variety of lung disorders ranging from the common cold to severe asthma. In recent years, this useful medicinal has come under fire due to its misapplication by athletes in the West who have employed it as a performance-enhancing drug. These users ingest dosages many times higher than the amount used in a decoction in order to stimulate cardiopulmonary function, and, as a result, a number of them have died, including several prominent professional athletes.

Another example of the importance of proper dosage is in the prescription of *Chuan Xiong* (Radix Ligustici Wallichii) and *Bai Zhi* (Radix Angelicae Dahuricae). These two medicinals are both powerful pain-stopping herbs, and, because pain is so uncomfortable, there is a tendency to prescribe them at higher than standard doses. However, at doses exceeding 15 grams per day in decoction, *Chuan Xiong* may cause nausea. Short-term, such nausea may be acceptable to a patient suffering from really severe body pain. This is the kind of judgement call practitioners are frequently required to make, but need to make on the basis of sound knowledge.

Symptoms of overdose are mainly those of an exaggerated response to the medicinal. These symptoms may not only be due to true overdose of the medicinal but non-metabolism or non-excretion of or hypersensitivity to the medicinal in particular individuals. The effects of overdosage can usually be controlled by reducing dosage and/or increasing intervals between administration. Because of differences in metabolism, infants, children, the elderly, and the debilitated often require smaller than standard daily adult doses of both Western and Chinese medications.

INTERACTION

Drug interactions (DI) are phenomena during drug therapy when the pharmacological or therapeutic actions of a drug are altered by the co-administration of other drugs or substances. The consequences can either be an exaggeration of pharmacological or toxic effects or a diminished efficacy of drug treatment. In both cases, such interactions may lead to therapeutic failure and endanger the patient's condition. The relevance of DIs depends on how clinically significant is the therapeutic outcome. Drug interactions are commonly categorized in Western medicine in terms of significance as follows:

Early Chinese medical practitioners were well aware of the potential problems their medicinals could cause when mixed together. Bensky and Gamble list many of these potentially toxic interactions in their discussion of the classic 19 antagonisms and 18 incompatibilities.[6] Early practitioners found that seemingly innocuous substances like cloves (*Ding Xiang*, Flos Caryophylli) and turmeric (*Yu Jin*, Tuber Curcumae) will "antagonize," *i.e.*, neutralize, each other, thus cancelling out the beneficial effects of either medicinal. Similarly early practitioners recognized a condition called "mutual incompatibility" which occurs when two toxic substances such as *Wu Tou* (Radix Aconiti) and *Ban Xia* (Rhizoma Pinelliae Ternatae) are mixed together, further enhancing the toxicity of each. Every professionally trained practitioner of Oriental medicine prescribing Chinese medicinals is taught the above 18 incompatibilities and 19 antagonisms, and most Chinese medicinal formulas avoid these antagonisms and incompatibilities. Thus, it is only through inexperience or ignorance that a modern practitioner would create a toxic Chinese medicinal formula through unanticipated interactions.

However, similar antagonisms and incompatibilities between Chinese medicinals and modern Western pharmaceuticals are possible and not so easily known. Many practitioners may unwittingly create a similar toxic situation as what occurred in Belgium due to ignorance of what other medicinal substances the patient may be taking, whether they be Chinese medicinals or Western pharmaceuticals. An example of this is the ubiquitous medicinal licorice root (*Gan Cao*, Radix Glycyrrizae Uralensis). Licorice root is used in many Chinese medicinal formulas as a "harmonizing" agent. This means it moderates the harsh, attacking, damaging, *i.e.*, toxic, effects of other medicinals in the formula, especially those that may cause digestive side effects. In Chinese medicine, licorice is considered a safe herb, but, in a patient taking a cardiac glycoside, such as digitalis (Digoxin®), it may increase the toxicity of the digitalis. Thus a well-intended Oriental medical practitioner may unwittingly create a toxic condition in a patient through ignorance of what that patient is taking for a, perhaps unrelated, cardiac condition.

INHERENT TOXICITY

As stated above, in a large enough dose, anything can be toxic, *i.e.*, harmful to human life. The potential for toxicity depends on the amount of toxins in a given medicinal and the dosage in which it is administered. To keep this issue in perspective, let's first look at some commonly eaten foods and the toxins they contain. For instance, spinach contains oxalates which can cause hypocalcemia and may act as nephrotoxins and coagulants. However, as long as one eats a moderate amount of spinach, one does not have to worry about these toxins. Tea contains tannins which are potentially carcinogenic and are gastric irritants. Again, as long as one does not overdo it, tea does not usually cause either cancer or stomach upset. Potatoes contain solanacia alkaloids which are both hepatotoxins and neurotoxins, but unless one eats way too many potatoes, they are harmless to the average individual. And finally, mushrooms contain hydrazines, known carcinogens. But mushrooms are also touted by the health food industry to help prevent cancer. The issue is the amount of potential toxins a substance contains and the amount one ingests. Over 2,000 years of recorded history, the Chinese have become acutely aware of the major medicinals within their materia medica which inherently contain toxins, and, as stated above, every professionally trained Oriental medical practitioner is taught the dosage ranges, combinations, and processing methods for using these medicinals safely and effectively.

However, when it comes to ready-made medicinal preparations, there are three other sources of potential toxicity. These are contamination, adulteration, and mislabeling. Since the majority of patients in the West using Chinese medicinals do so in the form of ready-made medicines, it is important to discuss each of these three sources of potential toxicity.

CONTAMINATION

Contamination of ready-made Chinese medicinals can be due to heavy metals, pesticides, and microbes. While heavy metal contamination potentially affects all commercially grown Chinese herbal medicinals, both bulk and ready-made, due to the concentration processes by which most ready-made Chinese medicines are made, these processes can also concentrate heavy metals in the finished product. As part of their "feeding" on the soil in which they live, plants take up heavy metals from the ground in which they are grown and from the water which they "drink." Some soils, due to use of certain pesticides and fertilizers contain more heavy metals than others. Likewise, certain bodies of water contain higher concentrations of heavy metals due to their proximity to manufacturing facilities which release heavy metals into the air and thence enter the water. In addition, heavy metals can enter a ready-made medicine in the manufacturing process itself, for instance if the factory uses lead solder in its manufacturing equipment or plumbing.

The heavy metals that are especially of concern in terms of human toxicity are copper, lead, cadmium, arsenic, and mercury. While it is very difficult to completely and absolutely eliminate all traces of these heavy metals from Chinese medicinals, through proper manufacturing processes, they can be rendered so small (in terms of parts per million) that their impact on the human body is virtually inconsequential. Therefore, our suggestion is to only buy ready-made Chinese medicinals from companies who test their medicines for heavy metal contamination and are willing to share with their customers and the public the results of those tests.

When vegetable crops, including medicinal herbs, are grown commercially, pesticides may be picked up by these herbs, pesticides which are harmful to human health. There are two main types of pesticides which may be harmful to human health. These are called organopesticides and chlorinated pesticides. Some well-known toxic organopesticides include Dursban®, Guthion®, Roneet®, Co Ral®, Naled®, Nemacur®, Phosmet®, and Rubitox®. Examples of well-known but potentially harmful chlorinated pesticides include 4,4 DDD, 4,4 DDT, 4,4 DDE, BHC-A, BHC-B, BHC-D, BHC-G, Captan®, Chlordane®, Endrin®, Pyrethrum®, Dylox®, and Mavrik®. One way to avoid contamination by pesticides is to use organically grown Chinese herbs. However, this industry is in its infancy in China and other countries supplying Chinese medicinal herbs. It is also possible to reduce the amounts of pesticides through "washing" processes during manufacture. Therefore, we also recommend that you ask your Chinese herbal suppliers for copies of tests analyzing the concentrations of both organopesticides and chlorinated pesticides in their products. Testing should be done for approximately 200 pesticides known to be harmful to humans.

The third type of contamination of ready-made Chinese medicinals is microbial. Microbial contamination describes potential human toxicity due to the presence of unacceptably high numbers of pathogenic organisms in the medicinal. The two main classes of microbes which may contaminate ready-made

Chinese medicinals are bacteria and yeast and molds. The main pathogenic bacteria that should be routinely tested for by manufacturers of ready-made Chinese medicinals are *Salmonella, Escherichia coli, Klebsiella, Serratia, Stpahylococcus aureus,* and *Bacillus sp.* as well as the total of all species of bacteria present in the finished product. The main types of pathogenic yeast and molds which should be tested for are *Aspergillus niger* and *Candida albicans.*

ADULTERATION

Adulteration in the manufacture of Chinese ready-made medicinals means the addition of Western pharmaceuticals to a traditional Chinese herbal formula in order to make it more powerful and effective. The following is a list of some adulterants that have been found in certain Chinese ready-made, supposedly herbal medicines: acetaminophen, aminopyrine, chlorpheniramine, chlorzoxazone, phenacetin, and phenylbutazone. Some of these are over-the-counter medications in the West and some are by-prescription-only. Some have been taken off the market in the U.S. due to reports of toxicity, including death. While the Ministry of Health in the People's Republic of China have made it illegal to manufacture Chinese herbal medicines adulterated by Western pharmaceuticals, companies operating outside the PRC are still engaging in this practice. Therefore, it is important to buy ready-made Chinese medicinals only from well-established, reputable, and transparent companies. Customers should feel free to ask their suppliers for certificates of analysis (COA) documenting exactly what is in each and every medicine.

MISLABELING

While not as much of a problem as in the past, mislabeling can also cause toxic reactions. Mislabeling here refers to the incomplete disclosure of ingredients, improper listing of ingredients, and/or the misidentification of ingredients. In the past, many Asian firms sought to keep their proprietary formulas secret by failing to completely disclose all the ingredients in a product. Without knowing all the ingredients in a product, there is no way for a practitioner to rationally assess the probabilities of a toxic reaction in a particular individual. It has also been common for Asians to misidentify the ingredients in their products simply through ignorance of either Pinyin or Western pharmacognosy and Latin pharmacological nomenclature. This sometimes means that the ingredients are correctly identified in Chinese (in Chinese characters) but incorrectly identified in either Pinyin or Latin. Just as it is impossible to rationally judge the probability of a toxic reaction if one does not know all the ingredients, neither can one make such a determination if the ingredients contained are not the ones that are listed.

Over the past several years, there have been great improvements in the labeling of ready-made Chinese medicinals for sale in the U.S. Basically, all companies selling herbal supplements in the U.S. must follow the Food & Drug Administration (FDA)'s food labeling rules. This means that all ingredients must be disclosed, beginning with the ingredient in largest proportion by weight to the ingredient in smallest proportion by weight. There must be a nutritional fact panel as well as a serving size. And finally, there must also be instructions as to use.

Unfortunately, when it comes to instructions for use, the FDA does not allow a dosage range but requires a specific daily dose. Because companies are commonly worried about litigation from persons who either accidentally or purposefully take too much, they tend to print low-end doses on their labels. This means that practitioners must commonly increase the stated dosages on the packaging in order for their patients to achieve the expected therapeutic effects in a timely manner. We will talk more about the issue of dosages in Chapter 3, How To Use This Book.

TYPES OF TOXIC REACTIONS TO MEDICINALS, EASTERN OR WESTERN

There are several types or classes of toxic reactions to medicinals no matter what their source or provenance. These include drug poisoning, allergic reactions, and idiosyncratic reactions. Drug poisoning is due to accidental or intentional overdose. It may also occur if a patient is excessively susceptible to the drug or unable to eliminate the drug at the normal rate due to liver or kidney damage. Drug poisoning may lead to collapse or death if the drug is not withdrawn and adequate treatment is not administered. Hypersensitivity or allergic reactions occur either immediately or as a delayed reaction to the ingestion of a medicinal substance. In mild cases, such allergic reactions may result in rash, edema, itching, or flushing of the skin. In severe cases, it may result in anaphalactic shock characterized by collapse or asphyxia. This is an extreme emergency. Idiosyncratic reactions may occur in patients who are genetically predisposed to have a reaction to a particular substance. These kinds of drug reactions are unpredictable. They are similar to hypersensitivity or allergic reactions.

In terms of systems affected, types of adverse medicinal reactions can include changes in mental function, Parkinson-like symptoms, gastrointestinal complaints, urinary tract problems, visual disturbances, respiratory difficulty, and/or the arising of any new symptoms. Changes in mental function may include hallucinations, confusion, delirium, impaired memory, impaired thinking, persistent drowsiness, or persistent wakefulness and excitability. Parkinson-like symptoms are also referred to as extrapyramidal symptoms.

They consist of uncontrolled movement of the face, arms, and/or legs, orthostatic dizziness, and a tendency to falling. Gastrointestinal complaints include nausea, vomiting, abdominal pain, diarrhea, constipation, and/or bleeding. Urinary tract problems mostly consist of difficulty voiding or incontinence. The most common visual disturbances as a medicinal reaction are blurred vision or absence of vision in one or both eyes, while respiratory reactions mostly include shortness of breath, asthma, and/or cough. In particular, the new symptoms that the patient and practitioner should be on the lookout for are fever, headache, pruritus, and skin rashes. Because most medications are orally ingested, gastrointestinal complaints are typically the first adverse reactions to a medicinal.

So, ARE CHINESE HERBAL MEDICINALS SAFE?

A search of the FDA[7] databases which document reports of medicinal toxicity, both from Chinese medicinals and Western pharmaceuticals, shows that there have been very few incidents of poisoning from Chinese medicinals. The few incidents documented are the results of A) abuse, as described in the case of *Ma Huang,*[8] B) improper administration and preparation of aristolochic acid-containing medicinals[9] (a topic to be discussed in more detail in the next chapter), or C) poor diagnosis and improper prescription, often by a layperson taking a medicinal without the supervision of a trained practitioner.[10] Therefore, I believe the answer to the above question is, "Yes, Chinese herbal medicinals are safe *when takien correctly.*" Providing a proper diagnosis (including pattern discrimination) has been made, the medicinals have been properly prepared, the dosage is correct, and potential interactions have been taken into consideration, the Chinese medicinal substances included in this reference guide have minimal chance for toxicity.

FOUR QUESTIONS TO ASK BEFORE TAKING/ ADMINISTERING A CHINESE HERBAL MEDICINAL:

1. Is this herb indicated by both the disease diagnosis *and* the patient's personally presenting Chinese medical pattern discrimination?

2. Has this herb been prepared and/or manufactured properly?

3. Is its dosage within standard parameters?

4. Are there any potential toxic interactions between this medicinal and any other medicinals taken concurrently?

REGISTRY OF CHINESE HERBAL MEDICINE RECOMMENDATIONS FOR THE PRESCRIPTION OF CHINESE MEDICINALS

The Register of Chinese Herbal Medicine (RCHM) is a professional association of practitioners of Chinese herbal medicine in the United Kingdom. The RCHM is very concerned about medicinal toxicities and interactions. We believe the following guidelines should be adopted in all countries where Chinese herbal medicine is practiced.

1. Chinese medicinals should only be prescribed by fully trained practitioners of Chinese herbal medicine in accordance with a traditional individualized diagnosis.

2. Training of practitioners should include the ability to monitor for and recognize adverse effects. Professional bodies will increasingly need to be able to guarantee minimum standards of practice and to enforce codes of ethics and practice.

3. Chinese medicinals should be prescribed in the traditional manner, according to an individualized diagnosis based on the theory and practice of Chinese medicine.

4. The medicinals should be used according to their traditional indications and in established combinations.

5. Whenever it is proposed to use herbs in novel ways, for example in the form of chemical extracts or for symptomatic treatment, then careful and thorough clinical research and monitoring must be undertaken. A similar caution should be applied to the prescribing of obscure or unusual herbs.

6. Proper identification and quality control of medicinals by manufacturers and suppliers is a key ingredient in enabling the safe practice of Chinese herbal medicine.

7. Suppliers should not make available patent medicines whose ingredients are not certain, and practitioners should not prescribe them.

8. Practitioners should maintain good communication with patients.

9. Patients should be regularly monitored.

ENDNOTES

[1] *Taber's Cyclopedic Medical Dictionary*, 19th edition, ed. by Donald Venes, F.A. Davis Co., Philadelphia, 2001, p. 2213

[2] Lucretius, *De Rerum Natura (On the Nature of Things)*, Book 1, Invocation.

[3] In fact, the term "herbal" is at least partially a misnomer. While most Chinese medicinals are vegetable or "herbal" in nature, many come from the animal and mineral realms. Therefore, Chinese medicinals are not all herbs.

[4] Bensky, D. & Gamble, A., *Chinese Herbal Medicine: Materia Medica*, Eastland Press, Seattle, 1993

[5] Hsu, Hong-Yen, *Oriental Materia Medica: A Concise Guide*, Oriental Healing Arts Institute, Long Beach, CA, 1986

[6] Bensky & Gamble, *op. cit.*, Cautions and Contraindications, p. 10-11

[7] www.fda.gov

[8] http://www.fda.gov/oc/initiatives/ephedra/february2004/

[9] http://www.cfsan.fda.gov/~acrobat/lib4212.pdf

[10] http://www.cfsan.fda.gov/~dms/ds-ill.html

CHAPTER 2

THREE IMPORTANT TYPES OF POTENTIAL MEDICINAL TOXICITY

In the past decade, three types of toxicity have received attention and driven concern over the safety of Chinese medicinal substances. These are nephrotoxicity, hepatoxicity, and fetotoxicity.

NEPHROTOXICITY

The greatest concern over the toxicity of Chinese medicinal products remains the potential for nephrotoxicity. This concern was driven by the Belgium incident mentioned in the Introduction.[1] The cause of the nephropathy experienced by the women who took the dangerous "slimming formula" was thought to be aristolochic acid, a known nephrotoxin. The medicinal singled out for the nephrotoxicity was *Han Fang Ji* (Radix Stephaniae Tetandrae) which was alleged to be in the capsules consumed by the women.[2] However, subsequent chromatographic examination of the capsules showed that they did not contain the compound tetandrine which is a major component of *Han Fang Ji* and is used as a chemical marker for this medicinal. Later research suggested that the aristolochic acid intoxication might have come from a different source, such as the medicinal *Guang Fang Ji* (Radix Aristolochia Fangji) which does contain aristolochic acid and may have been included in the capsules due to a purchasing and identification error by the practitioners prescribing it. Or else the toxicity originated from a combination of other causes, such as the low carbohydrate diet the patients were on which might have accelerated and enhanced the effect of all the pharmaceutical products in the formula. It may have also been due to the fact that the Chinese medicinals were not prepared in a decoction but ground up raw, thus greatly increasing their individual potency. Another possibility is that the toxicity resulted from the strange combination of medicinals which included Western appetite inhibitors, including the now banned pharmaceutical, fenfluramine.

Regardless of the cause, upon hearing of the reports from Belgium, the FDA branded all Chinese medicinals containing even trace amounts of aristolochic acid before cooking as being toxic and began moving to prohibit their sale and prescription by 2001.[3] In addition to *Guang Fang Ji* and *Han Fang Ji*, these substances included *Mu Tong* (Caulis Mutong), *Wei Ling Xian* (Radix Clematidis), and *Xi Xin* (Herba Asari Cum Radice), popular and effective medicinals which appear in many formulas.[4] Despite little evidence that these medicinals, when prepared and dosed properly, can cause nephropathy, they remain banned today. Fortunately, a number of respected American pharmaceutical companies who manufacture Chinese medicinal formulas have found a way to process these forbidden herbs so that the trace amounts of aristolochic acid they contain are removed prior to decoction, a measure that should solve the potential toxicity problem. In the meantime, most Oriental medical practitioners are either eliminating these medicinals from their formulas or substituting other medicinals with similar actions to take their place.

HEPATOXICITY

In general, the advantage of most Chinese medicinals is that they are quickly processed and passed out of the liver with no hepatoxic effects. However there are some exceptions which should be noted. *Cang Er Zi* (Fructus Xanthii Sibirici), a commonly used herb for many nasal symptoms, can be both hepa- and nephrotoxic if not decocted properly with other medicinals. This is an example of "mutual counteraction,"[5] wherein the toxic medicinal's potentially toxic effects are eliminated by one or more other substances. As discussed in Chapter 1, the potentially toxic effects of many herbs can be eliminated by appropriate herbal preparation.

Another example is the unfortunate result that may occur when some Chinese herbal medicinals interact with orthodox Western drugs in the liver. Just as the combination of acetaminophen (Tylenol®) and alcohol can create a potentially fatal hepatoxicity, so too can the medicinals *He Zi* (Fructus Terminalia Chebulae), *Wu Bei Zi* (Galla Rhois Chinensis), or *Di Yu* (Radix Sanguisorbae Officinialis) create a hepatoxic combination when processed in the liver with isoniazid, tetracyclines, rafampcin, chlorpromazine, or erythromycin.[6] Patients taking any of these Western pharmaceuticals should be monitored carefully to guard against accidental poisoning due to the combination effects of these substances.

A third example of hepatoxicity due to Chinese medicinals came as the result of the liver damage caused by a ready-made medicine called *Jin Bu Huan*

(More Precious Than Gold), a once-popular remedy for insomnia and pain. In 1993-94, seven adults taking the brand of this formula manufactured by the Kwangsi Pai Se Company developed symptoms of hepatitis consistent with a drug reaction. Although the mechanism that caused the hepatitis in this small number of individuals is still unclear, investigators at the time concluded that it was due to an immunoallergic reaction because of the eosinophilia found in the liver biopsies of two of the patients. At first, it was thought this was perhaps due to a reaction to its supposed primary ingredient, *Yuan Zhi* (Radix Polygalae Tenuifoliae). However, further investigation found that the alkaloids in the remedy did not match those of the *Polygala* family but rather that of the blood-quickening herb *Yan Hu Suo* (Rhizoma Corydalis Yanhusuo). So it remains uncertain whether the remedy contained the wrong medicinal or was adulterated by some other substance which caused the actual hepatotoxicity.[7] In either case, the result was that *Jin Bu Huan* was banned in the United States and the United Kingdom. Curiously, this is still a popular remedy in Far and Southeast Asia with no reports of hepatoxicity from its use in those regions. In any case, these immunoallergic reactions in the U.S. were instrumental in focusing attention on the issue of toxicity and Chinese medicinals with subsequent efforts on the part of manufacturers and distributors to substantially increase quality control.

Risk factors predisposing one to hepatotoxicity include previous notable adverse reactions to drugs or herbs or a history of a number of different allergies, a history of chronic skin rashes, and pre-existing liver disease.
Stop signs when using herbs include:

1. Development of a substantial skin rash

2. Nausea, bloating, fatigue, and/or aching in the area of the liver, yellowing of the eyes or skin, reduction in coloration of the feces

Medicinal-induced hepatitis is defined as inflammation of the liver resulting in loss of integrity of the cell membranes causing leakage of cells' contents into blood plasma. Therefore, there is elevation of the liver enzymes AST (a.k.a. SGOP) and ALT (a.k.a. SGOT).

FETOTOXICITY

Perhaps the most difficult type of toxicity facing the practitioner of either Western or Oriental medicinal products is the potential for causing fetotoxicity. The developing embryo is so vulnerable to damage caused by foreign substances in the mother's blood stream that many Western and Oriental medicinal products, while quite safe for an adult, are considered problematic and potentially lethal for the fetus, either by direct poisoning or by causing spontaneous abortion.

While it is obvious that highly potent and/or toxic substances, such as *Ma Huang* (Herba Ephedrae) or *Fu Zi* (Radix Lateralis Praeparatus Aconiti Carmichaeli), would be harmful to a fetus, an entire class of Chinese herbs known as blood-quickeners are generally forbidden for prescription during pregnancy. These medicinals, which include herbs such as *San Qi* (Radix Notoginseng), *Dan Shen* (Radix Salviae Miltiorrhizae), and the ancient herbs frankincense and myrrh (*Mo Yao*, Resina Myrrhae, and *Ru Xiang*, Resina Olibanui), have the actions of stopping bleeding and/or dispelling blood stasis. They are very effective in treating various forms of bleeding, including external conditions such as traumas and internal issues such as hematuria. They also treat various internal clotting-related symptoms, such as angina due to coronary artery disease. Unfortunately, when these medicinals are used inappropriately in pregnant women, they can potentially interfere with uterine blood flow to the fetus and cause it to be expelled as a clot. Most Oriental medicine practitioners avoid giving this class of herbs to a pregnant patient unless there is a cogent reason.[8]

One more note on this class of Chinese medicinals. It is believed that they can create problems for patients on Western anticoagulant medications. If prescribed to a patient taking a warfarin-based Western pharmaceutical, they can dramatically alter prothrombin times. As a result, this group of Oriental medicinals are generally not prescribed to patients taking these Western drugs.[9]

ENDNOTES

[1] Blackwell, *op. cit.,* p. 1-3.
[2] It should be noted that *Han Fang Ji*, while having diuretic qualities, is not commonly used by trained Oriental medicine practitioners for weight loss. It is generally decocted with medicinals such as *Fu Ling* (Sclerotium Poriae Cocos) and *Gui Zhi* (Ramulus Cinnamomi Cassiae) to treat lower body edema due to fluid accumulation.
[3] FDA Consumer Advisory, http://www.cfsan.fda.gov/~dms/addsbot.html
[4] Chen, J., "Aristolochic Acid and ChineseHerbs,"(http://acupuncture.com/Herbology/aristo.htm), p. 1-3
[5] Bensky & Gamble, *op. cit.,* p. 9
[6] Chan, K. & Cheung, L., *Interactions Between Chinese Herbal Medicinal Products and Orthodox Drugs*, Taylor and Francis, London, 2003, p. 72
[7] Blackwell, *op. cit.,* p. 3-4
[8] In actual point of fact, blood-quickening medicinals are not absolutely forbidden during pregnancy to trained and experienced gynecological specialists. When blood stasis is one of the causes of threatened abortion, they are positively indicated, and

failure to prescribe them may result in a failure to forestall the abortion. However, when used in such circumstances, they should be prescribed in the smallest effective dose and their use should be suspended as soon as they are no longer indicated.

[9] Unfortunately, this is also a complex situation. In China, where integrated Chinese-Western medicine is more advanced and there are senior practitioners specializing in cardiovascular disease with decades of experience, such prohibitions are also not regarded as absolute.

CHAPTER 3

HOW TO USE THIS BOOK

This book has been written as a reference guide specifically on Chinese medicinal toxicity and drug interactions for both Western and Oriental medical practitioners. As such, it does not contain all the information on these medicinals that either Western or Oriental medical practitioners may be accustomed to or want. For more detailed Chinese medical information on the medicinals included in this book, readers are referred to Bensky and Gamble's *Chinese Herbal Medicine: Materia Medica,*[1] Bensky and Barolet's *Chinese Herbal Medicine: Formulas & Strategies,*[2] and/or Flaws's *260 Essential Chinese Medicinals* and *70 Essential Chinese Herbal Formulas.*[3] Similarly, for Western medical practitioners, this book is not designed to replace the *PDR for Herbal Medicines,*[4] a valuable resource that I have utilized throughout this book. Western medical practitioners who wish to gather more complex pharmacological information about the medicinals listed in this book should either consult the *PDR for Herbal Medicines* or Huang's *Pharmacology of Chinese Herbs.*[5]

What this book will enable both Western and Oriental medical practitioners to do is to quickly and accurately assess the potential toxicity that a particular formula and its medicinal components can present. To accomplish this, each formula listing contains the following information:

FORMULA NAME

The formula name is given in both Chinese (in Pinyin romanization) and English. The English translation is primarily based on Wiseman's *English-Chinese Chinese-English Dictionary of Chinese Medicine*[6] supplemented by Bensky and Barolet's *Chinese Herbal Medicine: Formulas & Strategies* and Hong-yen Hsu's *Commonly Used Chinese Herb Formulas with Illustrations*[7]

(*i.e.*, *Si Jun Zi Tang*, Four Gentlemen Decoction a.k.a. Four Major Herb Combination)

CATEGORY

The formula category is taken from the classifications determined by Bensky and Barolet and Flaws. This will be of more relevance to Oriental medicine practitioners but may prove useful to Western medical practitioners as well in determining the kind of diseases and/or patterns for which the formula may be indicated.

FUNCTIONS

This section presents the Chinese medical functions of the formula. These are correlated to the standard treatment principles found as the intermediary step between the disease and patterns diagnoses and the treatment plan in the patient's Oriental medical chart. While some Western practitioners may find these useful, they were primarily included for use by Oriental medical practitioners. These functions were taken from Bensky and Barolet's *Formulas & Strategies* and/or Flaws's *70 Essential Chinese Herbal Formulas* or written by Bob Flaws specifically for this book.

CHINESE MEDICAL INDICATIONS

In this section, we present the main pattern and traditional Chinese medical disease indications for the formula along with a precis of the defining signs and symptoms of that pattern, including in most cases tongue and pulse signs. The use of pulse images is based on the definitions found in Bob Flaws's *The Secret of Chinese Pulse Diagnosis*.[8]

CONTRAINDICATIONS

These are the contraindications for each formula in terms of Chinese medical patterns and traditional Chinese medical disease categories. They are primarily based on Bensky and Barolet's *Formulas & Strategies* and Flaws's *70 Essential Chinese Herbal Formulas*. In a few cases, Bob Flaws has written Chinese medical contraindications specifically for this book. Many of these contraindications underscore the fact that Chinese medicinal formulas are meant to be prescribed primarily on the basis of Chinese medical pattern discrimination and only secondarily on the basis of disease diagnosis, be that traditional Chinese or modern Western medical disease diagnosis.

WESTERN MEDICAL INDICATIONS

Just as the previous sections were provided for primarily Oriental medicine practitioners, this section is primarily for Western medical practitioners. The indications were taken from Bensky and Barolet's *Formulas & Strategies* and Flaws's *70 Essential Chinese Herbal Formulas* and include the most common Western disease applications for each formula. Because Chinese medicinal formulas are prescribed primarily on the basis of pattern discrimination, these Western medical disease indications are only indicative of a formulas scope of application and are not necessarily categorically complete. A popular genre in the contemporary Chinese medical literature is the so-called New Uses article. These articles begin with the words "New Uses of" followed by a standard, well-known formula's name. Thereafter, the author pre- sents several case histories of using this formula for the treatment of new Western medical diseases previously not considered within the standard scope of that formula. In these cases, the rationale for the use of the formula is primarily based on the patient's presenting pattern(s) which does/do conform to the formula's standard pattern indications.

POTENTIAL FORMULA TOXICITIES AND INTERACTIONS

This section is a listing of cautions taken from Bensky and Barolet's *Formulas & Strategies* and Flaws's *70 Essential Chinese Herbal Formulas*. The cautions apply to the formula as a whole. These cautions are often due to some of the individual medicinals in the formula. Occasionally, the sources I employed may disagree or, in some cases, may list additional concerns. To clarify the agreements and disagreements, I have used an abbreviated coding system. "FL" or "B&B" by itself means that the information came solely from the single work. "B&B/FL" indicates that both works agree on the stated cautions. In many cases, the listing for this section is "None listed." In that case, the reader should not assume that, just because neither work listed a formula caution, the formula is entirely safe. Indeed, if no cautions are listed, one should then consult the next section to determine the relative safety of the formula.

POTENTIAL MEDICINAL TOXICITIES AND INTERACTIONS

This section comprises the bulk of each formula's listing. It is divided into three parts: 1) each medicinal's name, 2) standard daily dosage, and 3) the advisories associated with each medicinal based on the sources used.

MEDICINAL NAME

Each medicinal is listed by its most common Chinese names (in Pinyin romanization) followed by its Latin pharmacological name in parentheses. If there is a common, well-known English name, then that follows the pharmacological name in parentheses. Because the Chinese often use different names for the same medicinal as well as different species under the same Chinese name, it is extremely important, that the Chinese name of a medicinal be cross-referenced by a pharm-acological name. That way, if one name is ambiguous or unclear, the other name should clarify the medicinal's identity for all concerned.

STANDARD DAILY DOSAGE

This is the standard daily dosage as taught at government sponsored and endorsed Chinese medical colleges in the People's Republic of China and found in such standard English language texts as Bensky and Gamble's *Chinese Herbal Medicine: Materia Medica* and Hong-yen Hsu's *Oriental Materia Medica: A Concise Guide.* These daily doses are the standards for the prescription and administration of bulk-dispensed Chinese medicinals made into water decoctions for oral administration. When this is not the case, any other method of administration is specified, such as "in pills and powders."

That being said, most Westerners availing themselves of the benefits of Chinese medicinals are taking their medications in the form of ready-made pills, powdered extracts, or tinctures. Therefore, it is necessary to say something about the conversion of these standards when looking at the use of some sort of ready-made extract. The easiest way to determine the relative strengths of extracts is to know their extract ratio. For instance, if it takes five pounds (or kilos) of a medicinal or medicinal formula to make one pound (or kilo) of finished product, that is a 5:1 extract ratio. If it takes eight pounds (or kilos) to make one pound (or kilo) of finished product, then this is an 8:1 extract ratio. Similarly, a 10:1 extract ratio means that 10 pounds of herbs were used to make one pound of finished product. The higher the first number, the more highly concentrated is the extract and, therefore, the more potent it is.

If one knows the extract ratio of a Chinese medicinal formula, then one can figure out roughly how much of that ready-made medicine equals how much of bulk-dispensed herbs. For example, three grams of a 5:1 extract powder equal 15 grams of bulk-dispensed herbs, while three grams of a 10:1 extract powder equal 30 grams of bulk-dispensed herbs. If one then wants to know the approximate daily dose of a single ingredient in a ready-made extract formula, one can figure the proportion of that ingredient in the standard form of that prescription and then divide accordingly. For instance, in *Si Jun Zi Tang* (Four Gentlemen Decoction a.k.a. Four Major Herb Combination), the proportions given by Hong-yen Hsu for the individual ingredients are as follows:

> *Ren Shen* (Radix Panacis Ginseng), 4 parts
> *Bai Zhu* (Rhizoma Atractylodis Macrocephalae), 4 parts
> *Fu Ling* (Sclerotium Poriae Cocos), 4 parts
> *Gan Cao* (Radix Glycyrrhizae Uralensis), 1 part

This means that there are a total of 13 parts to this formula (4 + 4 + 4 + 1 = 13). If one wants to know how much *Ren Shen* is in three grams of this formula in a 5:1 extract form, one then multiples 4/13 times 15. In other words, one first multiplies three grams times five (3g x 5 [the extract ratio multiplier] = 15). Then one multiplies 4/13 times 15 (4/13 x 15 = 4.615 grams). Therefore, the answer is 4.615 grams. This means that, if the *Ren Shen* had been taken as part of a bulk-dispensed, water-based decoction in the same proportions as the above formula, the patient would have received 4.615 grams of *Ren Shen*. Since the standard daily dosage range for *Ren Shen* runs from 1-30 grams, this is well within and towards the low end of *Ren Shen*'s standard dosage range.

ADVISORIES

The advisories for each medicinal come from six potential sources. Each source is coded, and a key is listed at the bottom of each page for your convenience. For example, "AH" stands for the American Herbal Products Association (AHPA)'s *Botanical Safety Handbook*.[10] In some cases, such as *Ma Huang* (Herba Ephedrae), where there is general agreement among all sources about its potential toxicity, we have included a summary statement with the most important warnings about the medicinal.

It should be strongly noted that most of these advisories are couched in terms of theoretical possibility. A certain medicinal *could* do such and such or *may* result in such and such based on its chemical constituents or pharmacodynamic actions. However, these advisories are, in no way, definitive and categorically complete. The truth of the matter is that, when it comes to a Chinese medicinal's interactions with every single Western medical drug, we simply do not yet have enough experience and information to make simple, categorically complete, and definitive statements. At this point in time, these advisories are based on theoretical speculation, *in vitro* experiments, animal studies, and anecdotal evidence in humans based on a very few incidents.

In addition, these advisories all deal with the use of individual medicinals used as "singles." However, standard professional Oriental medicine does not use singles (with a few notable exceptions). It uses formulas made up of multiple ingredients according to well-established, time-tested principles and rules. In part, these principles and rules are meant to avoid the creation of adverse interactions and to minimize the potential for toxicity. Therefore, many of these advisories are not very meaningful when read and judged by trained and experienced Oriental medical practitioners. In some cases, the role that a medicinal plays in a particular formula may call for such a low dose as to render it innocuous. In other cases, potential adverse reactions are forestalled or mitigated by other ingredients in a formula. Therefore, practitioners of Western medicine are especially advised not to read too much into these individual advisories in terms of catastrophic potential.

COMMENTS

Comments are our concluding comments about the formula, either expanding on its use or other useful information for practitioners, such as common substitutions.

WHAT ABOUT CONFLICTING INFORMATION?

In many cases, medicinal advisories from different sources may conflict. This may seem confusing at first, but, actually, it is to be expected and may, in the end, be quite useful. For example, many medicinals are considered by AHPA to be "safe when used appropriately." This means that, if the diagnosis, preparation, and dosage are correct, the medicinal will generally have no potential toxicity. However, in the case of common field mint (*Bo He*, Herba Menthae Haplocalycis), Bensky and Gamble offer the caution, "Not recommended for nursing mothers as it may inhibit lactation." This simply means that these authors discovered a source or found a study that indicated some potential for this medicinal's inhibiting lactation. Having this additional information allows the practitioner to make a determination as to whether this medicinal is appropriate for the patient. If the patient is nursing, has had a history of scanty or difficult lactation and *Bo He* is a primary ingredient in the formula under consideration, it may be wiser to either leave it out of the formula or find a substitute formula for treating the problem. In other words, this additional information helps one make an *informed* choice about a particular medicinal and, in the larger context, a particular formula.

LOOKING UP FORMULAS & INDIVIDUAL MEDICINALS

This book has several comprehensive indexes to make finding information within quick and relatively easy. There is a general index which mainly consists of diseases, signs and symptoms, and Western medical terms and medications. This is followed by a formula index in Pinyin as well as a formula index in English. Next, there is a Chinese medicinal index in Pinyin romanization as well as in Latin pharmacological nomenclature. And finally, this book is accompanied by a CD-ROM which is searchable by any term in any of these indexes.

DISCLAIMER

This book is not intended to be a substitute for good medical training and practice, either Western or Oriental. If you have not been trained sufficiently in either, you should not be using this book as a prescription tool for treating patients. Neither the authors of this book or the source books utilized to research and generate this work should be held liable for injuries to patients due to the information contained herein.

ENDNOTES

[1] Bensky, D. & Gamble, A., *Chinese Herbal Medicine: Materia Medica*, Eastland Press, Seattle, 1993

[2] Bensky, D. & Barolet, R., *Chinese Herbal Medicine: Formulas and Strategies,* Eastland Press, Seattle, 1990

[3] Flaws, B., *260 Essential Chinese Medicinals,* 1999; *70 Essential Chinese Herbal Formulas,* Blue Poppy Press, Boulder, CO, 2001

[4] Tyler Varro E., *Physicians' Desk Reference for Herbal Medicines,* Thomson Medical Economics, Montvale, NJ, 2003

[5] Huang, K.C., *The Pharmacology of Chinese Herbs,* 2nd ed., CRC Press, N, 1999

[6] Wiseman, N., ed., *English-Chinese Chinese-English Dictionary of Chinese Medicine,* Hunan Science & Technology Press, Changsha, 1996

[7] Hsu, Hong-yen, *Commonly Used Chinese Herb Formulas with Illustrations,* Oriental Healing Arts Institute, LA, 1980

[8] Flaws, B., *The Secret of Chinese Pulse Diagnosis*, Blue Poppy Press, Boulder, CO, 1995

[9] Hsu, *op. cit.,* p. 264

[10] M. McGuffin, *et. al.,* ed's., American Herbal Products Association's *Botanical Safety Handbook,* CRC Press, NY, 1997.

AN GONG NIU HUANG WAN
(Quiet the Palace Bezoar Pills, a.k.a. Bos & Curcuma Formula)

Category: Orifice-opening
Functions: Clears heat and opens the orifices, sweeps away phlegm and resolves toxins
Chinese medical indications: Heat evils falling into the pericardium with high fever, easy anger, restlessness, deranged speech, spirit clouding, a crimson red tongue, and a rapid pulse
Contraindications: Pregnancy
Western medical indications: Total or partial loss of consciousness due to cerebral vascular accident, infantile convulsions, acute encephalitis, acute meningitis, acute hepatitis, pneumonia, dysentery, uremia, hepatic coma, and schizophrenia
Potential formula toxicities & interactions:
FL/B&B: Do not use in high doses or long-term due to the possibility of mercury toxicity from *Zhu Sha* (Cinnabaris). For best results, formula should not be heated.

POTENTIAL MEDICINAL TOXICITIES & INTERACTIONS:

Niu Huang
(Calculus Bovis, cattle gallstone, bezoar)

Standard daily dosage: 0.15-1g used only in pills and powders
B&G: Contraindicated during pregnancy. Large overdosage in mice led

to diarrhea, coma, and death. According to some traditional sources, antagonizes *Long Gu (Os Draconis), Sheng Di* (uncooked Radix Rehmanniae Glutinosae), and *Long Dan Cao* (Radix Gentianae Longdancao) and counteracts *Niu Xi* (Radix Achyranthis Bidentatae).

Xi Jiao
(Cornu Rhinocerotis, rhinoceros horn)

Standard daily dosage: 1-2g as a powder
B&G: Use with great caution during pregnancy and only in the presence of high fever. According to traditional sources, may antagonize *Chuan Wu* (Radix Aconiti Carmichaeli), *Cao Wu* (Radix Aconiti Kusnezoffii), and *Lei Wan* (Sclerotium Omphaliae Lapidescentis).

Because *Xi Jiao* is from an endangered species, it is now commonly substituted by *Shui Niu Jiao* (Cornu Bubali, water buffalo horn). Standard daily dosage of this ingredient in decoction is 4.5-9g.

She Xiang
(Secretio Moschi Moschiferi, musk)

Standard daily dosage: 0.016-0.15g in pills and powders
B&G: Contraindicated during pregnancy. Use with caution in cases of hypertension.

Huang Lian
(Rhizoma Coptidis Chinensis)

Standard daily dosage: 1.5-9g. The U.S. FDA has banned the inclusion of this medicinal in all dietary supplements.
AH: Do not use during pregnancy. (This medicinal is commonly used during pregnancy in China when indicated by disease and pattern discrimination.)
B&G: Contains berberine. Long-term use may damage the digestive system. According to some traditional sources, antagonizes *Ju Hua* (Flos Chrysanthemi Morifolii), *Xuan Shen* (Radix Scrophulariae Ningpoensis), *Bai Xian Pi* (Cortex Radicis Dictamni Dasycarpi), *Jiang Can* (Bombyx Batryticatus). According to some traditional sources counteracts *Kuan Dong Hua* (Flos Tussilaginis Farfarae) and *Niu Xi* (Radix Achyranthis Bidentatae). Some traditional sources say it should not be taken with pork.
C&C: Contains alkaloids, quercetin, and potassium. Could possibly cause hyperkalemia when used with potassium-sparing diuretics. Could possibly reduce the absorption and therapeutic effect of potassium and sodium iodides, sodium bicarbonate, calcium gluconate, carbonate, and

lactate, aluminum hydroxide, magnesium and ferrous sulfates, and bismuth subcarbonate.

Huang Qin, Tiao Qin
(Radix Scutellariae Baicalensis)

Standard daily dosage: 6-15g
AH: Safe when used appropriately
B&G: According to some traditional sources, counteracts *Dan Pi* (Cortex Radicis Moutan) and *Li Lu* (Rhizoma Et Radix Veratri).
C&C: Contains potassium and glycosides, Could possibly cause hyperkalemia when used with potassium-sparing diuretics. Vitamin C, nicotinic acid, glutamic acid, hydrochloric acid, and other highly acidic substances could possibly reduce the therapeutic effect of this medicinal.

Zhi Zi, Shan Zhi, Shan Zhi Zi
(Fructus Gardeniae Jasminoidis, dried gardenia fruit pod)

Standard daily dosage: 3-12g
AH: Safe when used appropriately
B&G: Contains geniposide which caused diarrhea in mice.
C&C: Contains potassium and glycosides. Could possibly cause hyperkalemia when used with potassium-sparing diuretics. Vitamin C, nicotinic acid, glutamic acid, hydrochloric acid, and other highly acidic substances could possibly reduce the therapeutic effect of this medicinal.

Xiong Huang
(Realgar, arsenic sulfide)

Standard daily dosage: 0.15-0.6 in pills and powders
B&G: Contraindicated during pregnancy

Bing Pian
(Borneol)

Standard daily dosage: 0.3-0.9g in pills and powders
B&G: Use with caution during pregnancy. Do not expose to heat.

Yu Jin
(Tuber Curcumae)

Standard daily dosage: 4.5-9g

B&G: Use with caution during pregnancy. Some traditional sources discourage use with *Ding Xiang* (Flos Caryophylli).
C&C: Contains potassium. Could possibly cause hyperkalemia when used with potassium-sparing diuretics.
PDR: This medicinal should not be used by people with obstructed biliary ducts. Those with gallstones should take it only under the supervision of a physician. Stomach complaints can occur following extended use or in the case of overdose.

Zhu Sha
(Cinnabaris, cinnabar)

Standard daily dosage: 0.2-2.7g in pills and powders
B&G: Contains mercuric sulfide which is highly toxic. Should not be used in large amounts or long-term. To prevent mercury poisoning, do not heat.
GLW: Symptoms of adverse reaction include burning pain in the oral cavity and throat, swelling and distention of the mucosa, bleeding, ulceration, and a metallic taste in the mouth, nausea, vomiting, abdominal pain, diarrhea, mucus in the stools or hemafecia. If severe, there is hemorrhagic enteritis, clenched teeth, fright reversal, and trembling. If the kidneys are poisoned, there is edema, scanty urination, albuminuria, and acute kidney failure, syncope, convulsions, low blood pressure, shock, and eventual respiratory failure.

Zhen Zhu
(Margarita, pearl)

Standard daily dosage: 0.3-0.9g in pills and powders
C&C: Contains calcium. Could possibly reduce the effect of most antibiotics and levadopa, cause digitalis intoxication and heart arrhythmias, hinder the absorption of isoniazid.

COMMENTS

This powerful formula is designed to treat strokes, epilepsy, and other neurological symptoms. It has several toxic substances in it and should only be prescribed by a skilled practitioner. It is typically administered as a ready-made medicine.

BA ZHENG SAN
(Eight Correcting [Ingredients] Powder, a.k.a. Dianthus Formula)

Category: Dampness-dispelling
Functions: Clears heat and drains fire, disinhibits water and frees the flow of strangury
Chinese medical indications: Heat and/or bloody strangury due to damp heat in the lower burner with dark, turbid, scanty, difficult, and painful urination, a dry mouth and parched throat, slimy, yellow tongue fur, and a slippery, rapid pulse
Contraindications: Cold
Western medical indications: Acute urinary tract infection, urinary calculi, cystitis, urethritis, acute prostatitis, acute nephritis, acute pyelonephritis, glomerulonephritis, and acute gonorrhea
Potential formula toxicities & interactions:
FL/B&B: Long-term use may cause weakness, light-headedness, heart palpitations, and diminished appetite. Use with care during pregnancy.

POTENTIAL MEDICINAL TOXICITIES & INTERACTIONS:

Mu Tong
(Caulis Akebiae)

Standard daily dosage: 3-9g
B&G: Contraindicated during pregnancy. Could possibly cause dehydration and renal failure in large doses.
C&C: Contains potassium. Could possibly cause hyperkalemia when used with potassium-sparing diuretics.
PDR: Do not administer during pregnancy. Large doses of the medicinal may lead to gastroenteritis, intestinal colic, and diarrhea due to saponin content.
GLW: Symptoms of adverse reaction include early stage symptoms of poisoning, such as upper abdominal discomfort, vomiting, chest oppression, abdominal pain, and diarrhea. Secondarily, there is frequent urination, urgent urination, facial edema which gradually spreads to the entire body, inability to lie down, unclear consciousness, scanty urination or blocked urination, and increased blood pressure. Some patients present oily stools. In those with acute kidney failure, uremia leads to death.

This medicinal is often substituted with Caulis Aristolochiae

Manchuriensis which contains aristolochic acid. Therefore, it is important that this medicinal only be prescribed in the form of Caulis Akebiae Trifoliatae or Akebiae Quinatae.

Hua Shi
(Talcum)

Standard daily dosage: 9-18g
AH: Safe when used appropriately
B&G: Use with caution during pregnancy. Can stimulate the growth of granulomas in the colon and vagina.
C&C: Contains calcium and magnesium. Could possibly reduce the effect of most antibiotics, levadopa, and prednisolone, cause digitalis intoxication and heart arrhythmias, and hinder the absorption of isoniazid.

Che Qian Zi, Che Qian Ren
(Semen Plantaginis, plantain seeds)

Standard daily dosage: 4.5-9g
B&G: Contraindicated during pregnancy
C&C: Contains glycosides. Highly acidic. Could possibly cause crystalluria and hematuria, reduce the therapeutic effect of sodium bicarbonate, aluminum hydroxide, many antibiotics (especially aminoglycosides and sulfas), reserpine, caffeine, opiates, scopolamine, and berbamin. Vitamin C, nicotinic acid, glutamic acid, hydrochloric acid, and other highly acidic substances could possibly reduce the therapeutic effect of this medicinal.

Qu Mai
(Herba Dianthi, dianthus)

Standard daily dosage: 6-24g
B&G: According to traditional sources, may antagonize *Sang Piao Xiao* (Ootheca Mantidis).
C&C: Contains glycosides. Vitamin C, nicotinic acid, glutamic acid, hydrochloric acid, and other highly acidic substances could possibly reduce the therapeutic effect of this medicinal.

Bian Xu, Bian Xu Cao
(Herba Polygoni Avicularis)

Standard daily dosage: 9-15g
B&G: Could possibly cause dermatitis or gastrointestinal disturbance in horses or sheep.

C&C: Contains potassium. Could possibly cause hyperkalemia when used in large doses with potassium-sparing diuretics.
PDR: No health risks or side effects are known in conjunction with the proper administration of designated therapeutic dosages.

Zhi Zi, Shan Zhi, Shan Zhi Zi
(Fructus Gardeniae Jasminoidis, dried gardenia fruit pod)

Standard daily dosage: 3-12g
AH: Safe when used appropriately
B&G: Contains geniposide which caused diarrhea in mice.
C&C: Contains potassium and glycosides. Could possibly cause hyperkalemia when used with potassium-sparing diuretics. Vitamin C, nicotinic acid, glutamic acid, hydrochloric acid, and other highly acidic substances could possibly reduce the therapeutic effect of this medicinal.

Da Huang, Dai Huang, Chuan Jun, Jun
(Radix Et Rhizoma Rhei, rhubard root)

Standard daily dosage: 3-12g
AH: Not to be used during pregnancy. Not to be used while nursing. Contraindicated in intestinal obstruction, abdominal pain of unknown origin, or any inflammatory condition of the intestines.
BR: Reduces absorption of oral drugs. Overuse may cause hypokalemia and increased toxicity of cardiac glycosides. May aggravate potassium loss from diuretics.
B&G: Use with extreme caution during pregnancy, menstruation, or postpartum. Contraindicated for nursing mothers since active ingredients enter the milk.
C&C: Contains alkaloids, tannic acid, potassium, and glycosides. Could possibly cause hyperkalemia when used with potassium-sparing diuretics. Vitamin C, nicotinic acid, glutamic acid, hydrochloric acid, and other highly acidic substances could possibly reduce the therapeutic effect of this medicinal.
PDR: Consult a physician before using this medicinal during pregnancy or while nursing. Contraindicated in cases of intestinal obstruction, acute inflammatory intestinal disease, appendicitis, and abdominal pain of unknown origin.

Deng Xin Cao, Deng Xin, Deng Cao
(Medulla Junci Effusi, juncus)

Standard daily dosage: 1.5-4.5g
No toxicity or interaction information listed in the sources

Gan Cao
(Radix Glycyrrhizae Uralensis, licorice root)

AH: Not to be used during pregnancy. As a single herb in high doses, it is contraindicated in diabetes, hypertension, and liver disorders. Not for long-term use.

BR: May increase toxicity of cardiac glycosides. May increase potassium loss due to diuretics and laxatives. Possible additive effect to corticosteroids. May be synergistic with insulin in causing hypokalemia and sodium retention.

B&G: According to some traditional sources, incompatible with *Gan Sui* (Radix Euphorbiae Kansui), *Yuan Hua* (Flos Daphnes Genkwae), and *Yuan Zhi* (Radix Polygalae Tenuifoliae). If taken long-term, it may cause hypertension and/or edema. Contains glycyrrhetinic acid which could possibly cause a reduction in thyroid activity and basal metabolic rate.

The research on *Gan Cao* concurs that this medicinal is generally safe when used in small amounts as a harmonizing agent. It should not be taken long-term or as a single herb during pregnancy. When used as a single medicinal or in patients taking other potent Western pharmaceuticals, caution should be exercised to guard against potential toxicity and drug interaction.

COMMENTS

If there is no accompanying constipation, *Da Huang* can commonly be deleted from this formula. When damp heat is a result of a liver-spleen disharmony, as it commonly is in Western patients, this formula needs to be modified or a selection of its ingredients added to some other harmonizing formula.

BAI DU SAN

(Vanquishing Toxins Powder, a.k.a. *Ren Shen Bai Du San*, Ginseng
Vanquishing Toxins Powder, *Bai Du Jia Ren Shen San*, Vanquishing
Toxins Plus Ginseng Powder, Ginseng & Gypsum Combination)

Category: Exterior-resolving
Functions: Effuses sweat and resolves the exterior, scatters wind
and eliminates dampness while simultaneously boosting the qi
Chinese medical indications: External contraction of wind, cold,
and dampness with concomitant righteous qi vacuity, high fever,
severe chills, no sweating, pain and stiffness of the head and nape
of the neck, soreness and pain of the extremities, chest and ductal
glomus and fullness, nasal congestion, cough with profuse
phlegm, slimy, white tongue fur, and a floating, soggy pulse
Contraindications: Heat
Western medical indications: Common cold, upper respiratory
tract infections, flu, emphysema, malaria, early stage dysentery,
early stage measles, acute cellulitis, sores
Potential formula toxicities & interactions: None listed

POTENTIAL MEDICINAL TOXICITIES & INTERACTIONS:

Chai Hu
(Radix Bupleuri)

Standard daily dosage: 3-12g
AH: Safe when used appropriately
B&G: May occasionally cause nausea and vomiting. In that case, the
dose should be reduced significantly.
C&C: Vitamin C, nicotinic acid, glutamic acid, hydrochloric acid, and
other highly acidic substances could possibly reduce the therapeutic
effect of this medicinal.
PDR: Not to be administered during pregnancy. (This medicinal is routinely
used in Chinese medical gynecology during pregnancy as part of formulas
appropriately prescribed on the basis of pattern discrimination.) Overdose may
lead to gastroenteritis, intestinal colic, and diarrhea due to saponin content.

Qian Hu
(Radix Peucedani)

Standard daily dosage: 4.5-9g
B&G: According to traditional sources, may counteract *Li Lu* (Rhizoma
Et Radix Veratri).

C&C: Contains tannic acid. Could possibly reduce the absorption and biologic effect of most antibiotics, isoniazid, chlorpromazine, calcium carbonate and gluconate, atropine, ephedrine, quinine, reserpine, digitalis, vitamin B_1, trypsine, amylase, and pepsin.

Chuan Xiong
(Radix Ligustici Wallichii)

Standard daily dosage: 3-9g (In China today, it is not uncommon for this medicinal to be prescribed up to 15 grams per day in decoction.)

AH: Do not use during pregnancy. (This medicinal is routinely used in Chinese medical gynecology during pregnancy as part of formulas appropriately prescribed on the basis of pattern discrimination.)

B&G: Not for patients with migraine headache or excessive menstrual bleeding. Overdosage causes vomiting and dizziness. According to some traditional texts, antagonizes *Shan Zhu Yu* (Fructus Corni Officinalis) and *Huang Qi* (Radix Astragali Membranacei), counteracts *Hua Shi* (Talcum) and *Huang Lian* (Rhizoma Coptidis Chinensis), and is incompatible with *Li Lu* (Rhizoma Et Radix Veratri).

C&C: Contains alkaloids and potassium. Could possibly cause hyperkalemia when used with potassium-sparing diuretics. Could possibly reduce the absorption and therapeutic effect of potassium and sodium iodides, sodium bicarbonate, aluminum hydroxide, and magnesium sulfate.

Zhi Ke, Zhi Qiao
(Fructus Citri Aurantii)

Standard daily dose: 3-9g

AH: Safe when used appropriately

B&G: Use with caution during pregnancy.

C&C: Contains tannic acid. Highly acidic. Could possibly cause crystalluria and hematuria. Could possibly reduce the absorption and biologic effect of most antibiotics, isoniazid, chlorpromazine, calcium carbonate and gluconate, atropine, ephedrine, quinine, reserpine, digitalis, vitamin B_1, trypsine, amylase, and pepsin, sodium bicarbonate, aluminum hydroxide, caffeine, opiates, scopolamine, and berbamin.

PDR: May cause UV-sensitivity in light-skinned individuals. Otherwise, no health hazards are known in conjunction with the proper administration of designated therapeutic dosages.

Qiang Huo
(Radix Et Rhizoma Notopterygii)

Standard daily dosage: 6-15g

AH: Safe when used appropriately

Du Huo
(Radix Angelicae Pubescentis)

Standard daily dosage: 3-9g
AH: Patients should avoid prolonged exposure to sunlight.

Fu Ling, Bai Fu Ling, Yun Ling
(Sclerotium Poriae Cocos)

Standard daily dosage: 9-15g
B&G: Large doses or long-term use is discouraged. Contraindicated in patients with frequent, copious urination. According to traditional sources, may counteract *Di Yu* (Radix Sanguisorbae Officinalis), *Qin Jiao* (Radix Gentianae Qinjiao), and *Bie Jia* (Carapax Amydae Sinensis).
C&C: Contains potassium. Could possibly cause hyperkalemia when used with potassium-sparing diuretics.

Jie Geng
(Radix Platycodi Grandiflori, bellflower root)

Standard daily dosage: 3-9g
AH: Contraindicated in hemoptysis, especially in cases of tuberculosis. Use with caution in bleeding peptic ulcer.
B&G: Contraindicated in patients with hemoptysis. According to some traditional sources, counteracts *Long Dan Cao* (Radix Gentianae Longdancao) and *Long Yan Rou* (Arillus Euphoriae Longanae).
C&C: Contains calcium and glycosides. Could possibly reduce the effect of most antibiotics, cause digitalis intoxication and heart arrhythmias, hinder the absorption of isoniazid, and reduce the biological effect of levadopa. Vitamin C, nicotinic acid, glutamic acid, hydrochloric acid, and other highly acidic substances could possibly reduce the therapeutic effect of this medicinal.

Ren Shen
(Radix Panacis Ginseng, ginseng)

Standard daily dosage: 1-30g
AH: Contraindicated in hypertension
BR: May cause manic episodes in patients on MAO-inhibitors. May cause hypertension if consumed with caffeine. Possible additive effects to insulin. May reduce the anticoagulative effect of warfarin (Coumadin).

B&G: Contraindicated for hypertensive patients. Overdose can lead to headache, insomnia, heart palpitations, and a rise in blood pressure. A traditional antidote is mung bean soup.

C&C: Vitamin C, nicotinic acid, glutamic acid, hydrochloric acid, and other highly acidic substances could possibly reduce the therapeutic effect of this medicinal.

PDR: Contraindicated in patients with hypertension. Not recommended in large doses during pregnancy or lactation due to potential neonatal androgenization. Enhances the effect of insulin and other antidiabetic agents. Use with MAO-inhibitors may cause headaches, tremors, and manias.

Gan Cao
(Radix Glycyrrhizae Uralensis, licorice root)

Standard daily dosage: 2-12g

AH: Do not use during pregnancy. (This medicinal is routinely used in China during pregnancy when its use is indicated by pattern discrimination.) As a single herb in high doses, it is contraindicated in diabetes, hypertension, and liver disorders. Not for long-term use.

BR: May increase toxicity of cardiac glycosides. May increase potassium loss due to diuretics and laxatives. Possible additive effect to corticosteroids. May be synergistic with insulin in causing hypokalemia and sodium retention.

B&G: According to some traditional sources, is incompatible with *Gan Sui* (Radix Euphorbiae Kansui), *Yuan Hua* (Flos Daphnes Genkwae), and *Yuan Zhi* (Radix Polygalae Tenuifoliae). If taken long-term, it may cause hypertension and/or edema. Contains glycyrrhetinic acid which could possibly cause a reduction in thyroid activity and basal metabolic rate.

The research on *Gan Cao* concurs that this medicinal is generally safe when used in small amounts as an envoy. It should not be taken long-term or as a single herb during pregnancy. When used as a single medicinal or in patients taking other potent Western pharmaceuticals, caution should be exercised to guard against potential toxicity and drug interaction.

Bo He
(Herba Menthae Haplocalycis, field mint)

Standard daily dose: 1.5-6g

AH: Safe when used appropriately

B&G: Not recommended for nursing mothers as it may inhibit lactation.

Sheng Jiang
(uncooked Rhizoma Zingiberis Officinalis, fresh ginger)

Standard daily dose: 3-9g
AH: Safe when used appropriately
BR: Reduces vomiting caused by chemotherapeutic drugs. Increases the absorption of oral drugs.
PDR: Recommended safe dosage limit is six grams (6g). Avoid larger doses if being used to treat morning sickness or if used in patients taking anticoagulants.

COMMENTS

Dang Shen (Radix Codonopsitis Pilosulae) is commonly substituted for *Ren Shen* in this formula. This formula deserves to be more commonly prescribed than it is in the West where *Ma Huang Tang* (Ephedra Decoction) or *Ge Gen Tang* (Pueraria Decoction) are often erroneously prescribed in its stead based on the main symptoms of fever with upper back and nape of the neck stiffness. Such patients commonly suffer from a root vacuity and only a tip or branch repletion and, therefore, need a formula which supplements and drains, supports and attacks at the same time in a balanced manner.

BAI HE GU JIN TANG
(Lily Secure the Lungs Decoction, a.k.a. Lily Combination)

Category: Dryness-treating
Functions: Nourishes yin and moistens the lungs, transforms phlegm, and stops cough
Chinese medical indications: Coughing and panting due to a lung-kidney yin vacuity with blood-streaked phlegm, wheezing, a dry, sore throat, heat in the centers of the palms and soles, night sweats, a red tongue with scanty fur, and a fine, rapid pulse
Contraindications: Spleen vacuity and/or food stagnation
Western medical indications: Chronic bronchitis, bronchiectasis, hemoptysis, chronic pharyngitis, laryngitis, polyps on the vocal cords, carcinoma of the larynx, spontaneous pneumothorax, cor pulmonale, silicosis, and pulmonary tuberculosis
Potential formula toxicities & interactions: None listed

POTENTIAL MEDICINAL TOXICITIES & INTERACTIONS:

Bai He
(Bulbus Lilii, lily bulb)

Standard daily dosage: 9-30g
AH: Safe when used appropriately
C&C: Contains alkaloids. Could possibly reduce the absorption and therapeutic effect of potassium and sodium iodides, sodium bicarbonate, aluminum hydroxide, and magnesium sulfate.

Sheng Di, Sheng Di Huang
(uncooked Radix Rehmanniae Glutinosae)

Standard daily dosage: 9-30g
AH: Contraindicated in patients with diarrhea or lack of appetite
B&G: Contraindicated in pregnant women with anemias or digestive weakness
C&C: Contains potassium. Could possibly cause hyperkalemia when used with potassium-sparing diuretics.
PDR: No health risks or side effects are known in conjunction with the proper administration of designated therapeutic dosages.

Shu Di, Shu Di Huang
(cooked Radix Rehmanniae Glutinosae)

Standard daily dosage: 9-30g
AH: Contraindicated in patients with diarrhea or indigestion
B&G: Overuse can lead to abdominal distention and loose stools. Side effects include diarrhea, abdominal pain, dizziness, lethargy, and heart palpitations which often disappear upon continued administration of the medicinal.
PDR: No health risks or side effects are known in conjunction with the proper administration of designated therapeutic dosages.

Mai Men Dong, Mai Dong
(Tuber Ophiopogoni Japonici)

Standard daily dosage: 6-15g

AH: Safe when used appropriately
B&G: According to some traditional sources, antagonizes *Kuan Dong Hua* (Flos Tussilaginis Farfarae) and counteracts *Ku Shen* (Radix Sophorae Flavescentis) and *Bai Mu Er* (Fructificatio Tremellae Fuciformis).
C&C: Contains glycosides. Vitamin C, nicotinic acid, glutamic acid, hydrochloric acid, and other highly acidic substances could possibly reduce the therapeutic effect of this medicinal.

Xuan Shen, Yuan Shen
(Radix Scrophulariae Ningpoensis)

Standard daily dosage: 9-30g
C&C: Contains alkaloids, potassium, and glycosides. Could possibly cause hyperkalemia when used with potassium-sparing diuretics. Could possibly reduce the absorption and therapeutic effect of potassium and sodium iodides, sodium bicarbonate, aluminum hydroxide, and magnesium sulfate. Vitamin C, nicotinic acid, glutamic acid, hydrochloric acid, and other highly acidic substances could possibly reduce the therapeutic effect of this medicinal.

Chuan Bei Mu
(Bulbus Fritillariae Cirrhosae)

Standard daily dosage: 3-12g
AH: Not to be used during pregnancy. (This medicinal is commonly used in China during pregnancy to treat coughing and panting when indicated by pattern discrimination.)
B&G: According to traditional sources, incompatible with *Wu Tou*

(Radix Aconiti) and counteracts *Qin Jiao* (Radix Gentianae Qinjiao).
C&C: Contains alkaloids. Could possibly reduce the absorption and
therapeutic effect of potassium and sodium iodides, sodium bicarbonate,
aluminum hydroxide, and magnesium sulfate.

Jie Geng
(Radix Platycodi Grandiflori, bellflower root)

Standard daily dosage: 3-9g
AH: Contraindicated in hemoptysis, especially in cases of tuberculosis.
Use with caution in bleeding peptic ulcer.
B&G: Contraindicated in patients with hemoptysis. According to some
traditional sources, counteracts *Long Dan Cao* (Radix Gentianae
Longdancao) and *Long Yan Rou* (Arillus Euphoriae Longanae).
C&C: Contains calcium and glycosides. Could possibly reduce the effect of
most antibiotics, cause digitalis intoxication and heart arrhythmias, hinder the
absorption of isoniazid, and reduce the biological effect of levadopa. Vitamin
C, nicotinic acid, glutamic acid, hydrochloric acid, and other highly acidic
substances could possibly reduce the therapeutic effect of this medicinal.

Dang Gui
(Radix Angelicae Sinensis)

Standard daily dosage: 3-15g
AH: Do not use during pregnancy. (This medicinal is routinely used in
Chinese medical gynecology during pregnancy as part of formulas
appropriately prescribed on the basis of pattern discrimination.)
B&G: Use with caution in patients with diarrhea or abdominal distention.
C&C: Contains potassium. Could possibly cause hyperkalemia when
used with potassium-sparing diuretics. May exaggerate the anticoagula-
tive effect of warfarin (Coumadin).

Bai Shao, Shao Yao
(Radix Albus Paeoniae Lactiflorae, white peony root)

Standard daily dosage: 6-30g
AH: Safe when used appropriately
B&G: Use with caution in debilitated patients with diarrhea. According
to some traditional sources, antagonizes *Shi Hu* (Herba Dendrobii) and
Mang Xiao (Mirabilitum), counteracts *Bie Jia* (Carapax Amydae Sinensis)
and *Xiao Ji* (Herba Cephalanoploris Segeti), and is incompatible with *Li
Lu* (Rhizoma Et Radix Veratri).
C&C: Contains calcium, tannic acid, potassium, and glycosides. Could
possibly cause hyperkalemia when used with potassium-sparing diuret-

ics. Could possibly reduce the effect of most antibiotics, cause digitalis intoxication and heart arrhythmias, could possibly reduce the absorption and therapeutic effect of levadopa, isoniazid, chlorpromazine, calcium carbonate and gluconate, atropine, ephedrine, quinine, reserpine, vitamin B$_1$, trypsine, amylase, and pepsin. Vitamin C, nicotinic acid, glutamic acid, hydrochloric acid, and other highly acidic substances could possibly reduce the therapeutic effect of this medicinal.

Gan Cao
(Radix Glycyrrhizae Uralensis, licorice)

Standard daily dosage: 2-12g

AH: Do not use during pregnancy. (This medicinal is routinely used in Chinese medical gynecology during pregnancy as part of formulas appropriately prescribed on the basis of pattern discrimination.) As a single herb in high doses, it is contraindicated in diabetes, hypertension, and liver disorders. Not for long-term use.

BR: May increase toxicity of cardiac glycosides. May increase potassium loss due to diuretics and laxatives. Possible additive effect to corticosteroids. May be synergistic with insulin in causing hypokalemia and sodium retention.

B&G: According to some traditional sources, is incompatible with *Gan Sui* (Radix Euphorbiae Kansui), *Yuan Hua* (Flos Daphnes Genkwae), and *Yuan Zhi* (Radix Polygalae Tenuifoliae). If taken long-term, it may cause hypertension and/or edema. Contains glycyrrhetinic acid which could possibly cause a reduction in thyroid activity and basal metabolic rate.

The research on *Gan Cao* concurs that this medicinal is generally safe when used in small amounts as an envoy. It should not be taken long-term or as a single herb during pregnancy. When used as a single medicinal or in patients taking other potent Western pharmaceuticals, caution should be exercised to guard against potential toxicity and drug interaction.

BAI HU TANG
(White Tiger Decoction, a.k.a. Gypsum Combination)

Category: Qi aspect heat-clearing
Functions: Clears heat and engenders fluids
Chinese medical indications: *Yang ming* blazing heat (*i.e.*, heat evils entering the qi aspect) with high fever, profuse sweating, aversion to heat, a red facial complexion, severe thirst, easy anger, and a flooding, rapid pulse
Contraindications: Spleen qi vacuity fever or true cold and false heat
Western medical indications: High fever due to infectious illnesses such as gingivitis, encephalitis B, epidemic meningitis, lobar pneumonia, erysipelas, scarlatina, measles, common cold, flus. Also useful in treating diabetes mellitus, eczema, pruritus, and some anxiety and emotional disorders.
Potential formula toxicities & interactions: None listed

POTENTIAL MEDICINAL TOXICITIES & INTERACTIONS:

Shi Gao
(Gypsum Fibrosum)

Standard daily dosage: 9-30g
B&G: Could possibly cause gastric upset in some patients.
C&C: Contains calcium. Could possibly reduce the effect of most antibiotics and levadopa, cause digitalis intoxication and heart arrhythmias, and hinder the absorption of isoniazid.

Zhi Mu
(Rhizoma Anemarrhenae Aspheloidis)

Standard daily dosage: 6-12g
AH: Safe when used appropriately
B&G: May cause diarrhea in some patients.
C&C: Contains potassium and glycosides. Could possibly cause hyperkalemia when used with potassium-sparing diuretics. Vitamin C, nicotinic acid, glutamic acid, hydrochloric acid, and other highly acidic substances could possibly reduce the therapeutic effect of this medicinal.
PDR: No health hazards are known in conjunction with the proper administration of designated therapeutic dosages.

Gan Cao
(Radix Glycyrrhizae Uralensis, licorice)

Standard daily dosage: 2-12g
AH: Do not use during pregnancy. (This medicinal is routinely used in Chinese medical gynecology during pregnancy as part of formulas appropriately prescribed on the basis of pattern discrimination.) As a single herb in high doses, it is contraindicated in diabetes, hypertension, and liver disorders. Not for long-term use.
BR: May increase toxicity of cardiac glycosides. May increase potassium loss due to diuretics and laxatives. Possible additive effect to corticosteroids. May be synergistic with insulin in causing hypokalemia and sodium retention.
B&G: According to some traditional sources, is incompatible with *Gan Sui* (Radix Euphorbiae Kansui), *Yuan Hua* (Flos Daphnes Genkwae), and *Yuan Zhi* (Radix Polygalae Tenuifoliae). If taken long-term, it may cause hypertension and/or edema. Contains glycyrrhetinic acid which could possibly cause a reduction in thyroid activity and basal metabolic rate.

The research on *Gan Cao* concurs that this medicinal is generally safe when used in small amounts as an envoy. It should not be taken long-term or as a single herb during pregnancy. When used as a single medicinal or in patients taking other potent Western pharmaceuticals, caution should be exercised to guard against potential toxicity and drug interaction.

Geng Mi
(Semen Oryzae Sativae, polished rice)

Standard daily dosage: 15-30g

No toxicity or interaction information listed in the sources

BAI TOU WENG TANG
(Pulsatilla Decoction, a.k.a. Anemone Combination)

Category: Heat-clearing
Functions: Clears heat and resolves toxins, cools the blood and stops dysentery
Chinese medical indications: Heat toxins burning and damaging the stomach and intestines with abdominal pain, tenesmus, perianal burning, diarrhea with pus and blood (but more blood than pus), thirst, a red tongue with yellow fur, and a slippery, bowstring, rapid pulse
Contraindications: Spleen qi vacuity weakness
Western medical indications: Acute enteritis, postpartum enteritis, acute bacillary dysentery, amoebic dysentery, ulcerative colitis, abnormal vaginal discharge, urinary tract infections, acute conjunctivitis
Potential formula toxicities & interactions:
FL/B&B: Not to be used for long periods of time in patients with digestive weakness.

POTENTIAL MEDICINAL TOXICITIES & INTERACTIONS:

Bai Tou Weng
(Radix Pulsatillae Chinensis)

Standard daily dosage: 6-15g
B&G: Contraindicated in patients with chronic dysenteric disorders with damaged or weak digestive systems.
C&C: Contains glycosides. Vitamin C, nicotinic acid, glutamic acid, hydrochloric acid, and other highly acidic substances could possibly reduce the therapeutic effect of this medicinal.
GLW: The first symptom of internal poisoning by this medicinal is a burning sensation in the mouth along with swelling of the oral cavity. This is followed by severe abdominal pain, diarrhea with the expulsion of black, putrid stools which may contain threads of blood, heart arrhythmia and weakness, low blood pressure, circulatory failure, difficulty breathing, and dilation of the pupils. Death typically occurs within 10 hours of ingestion in severe cases.

Huang Lian
(Rhizoma Coptidis Chinensis)

Standard daily dosage: 1.5-9g
AH: Not to be used during pregnancy (This medicinal is commonly used during pregnancy in China when indicated by disease and pattern discrimination.)

B&G: Contains berberine. Long-term use may damage the digestive system. According to some traditional sources, antagonizes *Ju Hua* (Flos Chrysanthemi Morifolii), *Xuan Shen* (Radix Scrophulariae Ningpoensis), *Bai Xian Pi* (Cortex Radicis Dictamni Dasycarpi), and *Jiang Can* (Bombyx Batryticatus). According to some traditional sources counteracts *Kuan Dong Hua* (Flos Tussilaginis Farfarae) and *Niu Xi* (Radix Achyranthis Bidentatae). Some traditional sources say it should not be taken with pork.

C&C: Contains alkaloids, quercetin, and potassium. Could possibly cause hyperkalemia when used with potassium-sparing diuretics. Could possibly reduce the absorption and therapeutic effect of potassium and sodium iodides, sodium bicarbonate, calcium gluconate, carbonate, and lactate, aluminum hydroxide, magnesium and ferrous sulfates, and bismuth subcarbonate.

Huang Bai, Huang Bo
(Cortex Phellodendri)

Standard daily dosage: 3-12g

AH: Not to be used during pregnancy (This medicinal is commonly used during pregnancy in China.)

B&G: Chinese literature reports one case of a patient who developed a skin rash after ingestion.

C&C: Contains alkaloids and quercetin. Could possibly reduce the absorption and therapeutic effect of potassium and sodium iodides, sodium bicarbonate, calcium gluconate, carbonate, and lactate, aluminum hydroxide, magnesium and ferrous sulfates, and bismuth subcarbonate.

Qin Pi
(Cortex Fraxini)

Standard daily dosage: 4.5-15g

B&G: According to some traditional sources, antagonizes *Wu Zhu Yu* (Fructus Evodiae Rutecarpae).

C&C: Contains glycosides. Vitamin C, nicotinic acid, glutamic acid, hydrochloric acid, and other highly acidic substances could possibly reduce the therapeutic effect of this medicinal.

COMMENTS

While this formula is a very famous one for the treatment of damp heat diarrhea and dysentery, it is rarely prescribed in this simple, discrete form. For instance, it is commonly modified for either predominant heat or predominant dampness, accompanying qi stagnation and/or blood stasis, and for accompanying qi and/or yin vacuity.

BAN XIA HOU PO TANG
(Pinellia & Magnolia Decoction)

Category: Qi-rectifying
Functions: Moves the qi and downbears counterflow, transforms phlegm and dissipates binding
Chinese medical indications: Phlegm dampness with upward counterflow of the lung and/or stomach qi manifesting as plum pit qi, chest and abdominal oppression and fullness, possible nausea and vomiting, possible cough with profuse phlegm, slimy, white tongue fur, and a bowstring, slippery pulse
Contraindications: Depressive or vacuity heat
Western medical indications: Neurotic esophageal stenosis, gastrointestinal neurosis, chronic laryngitis, tracheitis, neurasthenia, morning sickness, bronchitis, hysteria, neurosis, recurrent palpitations, asthma, pertussis, toxemia during pregnancy, and edema
Potential formula toxicities & interactions: None listed

POTENTIAL MEDICINAL TOXICITIES & INTERACTIONS:

Ban Xia
(Rhizoma Pinelliae Ternatae)

Standard daily dosage: 4.5-12g
AH: Do not use during pregnancy. (This medicinal is routinely used during pregnancy in China when indicated by disease and pattern discrimination.) Contraindicated in all hemorrhagic disorders.
B&G: Safe as long as it is properly prepared. Must be decocted with other herbs and not taken alone or uncooked. Toxic effects due to improper preparation or dosage include burning and numbness in throat and lips, nausea, and a feeling of pressure in the chest. Antidote is oral administration of raw ginger. Use with caution in patients with fever. According to some traditional sources, incompatible with *Wu Tou* (Radix Aconiti).
C&C: Contains alkaloids and glycosides. Could possibly reduce the absorption and therapeutic effect of potassium and sodium iodides, sodium bicarbonate, aluminum hydroxide, and magnesium sulfate. Vitamin C, nicotinic acid, glutamic acid, hydrochloric acid, and other highly acidic substances could possibly reduce the therapeutic effect of this medicinal.
GLW: Poisoning occurs within 15 minutes to three hours after ingestion

of a suitable amount. Initially, there is burning pain in the mouth, tongue, and throat, and enlargement of the tongue. This is then followed by drooling, ulceration of the oral mucosa, unclear speech, difficulty swallowing, dizziness, low-grade fever, heart palpitations, numbness of the extremities, a somber white facial complexion, and a weak, forceless pulse. If severe, there may be convulsions and respiratory failure leading to death.

Hou Po, Chuan Po
(Cortex Magnoliae Officinalis)

Standard daily dosage: 3-9g
AH: Do not use during pregnancy. (This medicinal is commonly used in China during pregnancy, especially for the treatment of nausea and vomiting.)
B&G: Use with caution during pregnancy. According to some traditional sources, antagonizes *Ze Xie* (Rhizoma Alismatis Orientalis) and *Han Shui Shi* (Calcitum).
C&C: Contains tannic acid and potassium. Could possibly cause hyperkalemia when used with potassium-sparing diuretics. Could possibly reduce the absorption and biologic effect of most antibiotics, isoniazid, chlorpromazine, calcium carbonate and gluconate, atropine, ephedrine, quinine, reserpine, digitalis, vitamin B_1, trypsine, amylase, and pepsin.
PDR: No health risks or side effects are known in conjunction with the proper administration of designated therapeutic dosages.

Fu Ling, Bai Fu Ling, Yun Ling
(Sclerotium Poriae Cocos)

Standard daily dosage: 9-15g
B&G: Large doses or long-term use is discouraged. Contraindicated in patients with frequent, copious urination. According to traditional sources, may counteract *Di Yu* (Radix Sanguisorbae Officinalis), *Qin Jiao* (Radix Gentianae Qinjiao), and *Bie Jia* (Carapax Amydae Sinensis).
C&C: Contains potassium. Could possibly cause hyperkalemia when used with potassium-sparing diuretics.

Sheng Jiang
(uncooked Rhizoma Zingiberis Officinalis, fresh ginger)

Standard daily dose: 3-9g
BR: Reduces vomiting caused by chemotherapeutic drugs. Increases absorption of oral drugs.

PDR: Recommended safe dosage limit is six grams (6g). Avoid larger doses if being used to treat morning sickness or if used in patients taking anticoagulants.

Zi Su Ye, Su Ye, Zi Su
(Folium Perillae Frutescentis, beefsteak leaves)

Standard daily dosage: 3-9g
PDR: Use during pregnancy is contraindicated because perillaldehyde has been demonstrated to have a mutagenic effect in some in vitro studies. Studies showed that large doses can trigger pulmonary edema.

BAN XIA XIE XIN TANG
(Pinellia Drain the Heart Decoction, a.k.a. Pinellia Combination)

Category: Harmonizing
Functions: Harmonizes the stomach and downbears counterflow, fortifies the spleen and eliminates glomus
Chinese medical indications: Spleen vacuity and stomach and intestinal damp heat with stomach duct glomus and distention, nausea and vomiting, borborygmus, diarrhea, torpid intake, thin, yellow, slimy tongue fur, and a bowstring, slippery, rapid pulse
Contraindications: None listed
Western medical indications: Acute and chronic gastritis, enteritis, indigestion, pediatric vomiting and diarrhea, chronic hepatitis, early stage cirrhosis, and gastric ulcers
Potential formula toxicities & interactions: None listed

POTENTIAL MEDICINAL TOXICITIES & INTERACTIONS:

Ban Xia
(Rhizoma Pinelliae Ternatae)

Standard daily dosage: 4.5-12g
AH: Do not use during pregnancy. (This medicinal is routinely used during pregnancy in China when indicated by disease and pattern discrimination.) Contraindicated in all hemorrhagic disorders.
B&G: Safe as long as it is properly prepared. Must be decocted with other herbs and not taken alone or uncooked. Toxic effects due to improper preparation or dosage include burning and numbness in throat and lips, nausea, and a feeling of pressure in the chest. Antidote is oral administration of raw ginger. Use with caution in patients with fever. According to some traditional sources, incompatible with *Wu Tou* (Radix Aconiti).
C&C: Contains alkaloids and glycosides. Could possibly reduce the absorption and therapeutic effect of potassium and sodium iodides, sodium bicarbonate, aluminum hydroxide, magnesium sulfate. Vitamin C, nicotinic acid, glutamic acid, hydrochloric acid, and other highly acidic substances could possibly reduce the therapeutic effect of this medicinal.
GLW: Poisoning occurs within 15 minutes to three hours after ingestion of a suitable amount. Initially, there is burning pain in the mouth, tongue, and throat, and enlargement of the tongue. This is then followed by drooling, ulceration of the oral mucosa, unclear speech, difficulty swallowing, dizziness, low-grade fever, heart palpitations, numbness of

the extremities, a somber white facial complexion, and a weak, forceless pulse. If severe, there may be convulsions and respiratory failure leading to death.

Huang Qin, Tiao Qin
(Radix Scutellariae Baicalensis)

Standard daily dosage: 6-15g
AH: Safe when used appropriately
B&G: According to some traditional sources, counteracts *Dan Pi* (Cortex Radicis Moutan) and *Li Lu* (Rhizoma Et Radix Veratri).
C&C: Contains potassium and glycosides. Could possibly cause hyperkalemia when used with potassium-sparing diuretics. Vitamin C, nicotinic acid, glutamic acid, hydrochloric acid, and other highly acidic substances could possibly reduce the therapeutic effect of this medicinal.

Gan Jiang
(dry Rhizoma Zingiberis Officinalis, dry ginger)

Standard daily dosage: 3-12g
AH: Do not use during pregnancy. Patients with gallstones should consult a practitioner prior to use.
B&G: Use with caution during pregnancy.

Ren Shen
(Radix Panacis Ginseng, ginseng)

Standard daily dosage: 1-30g
BR: May cause manic episodes in patients on MAO-inhibitors. May cause hypertension if consumed with caffeine. Possible additive effects to insulin. May reduce the anticoagulative effect of warfarin (Coumadin).
B&G: Contraindicated for hypertensive patients. Overdose can lead to headache, insomnia, heart palpitations, and a rise in blood pressure. A traditional antidote is mung bean soup.
C&C: Vitamin C, nicotinic acid, glutamic acid, hydrochloric acid, and other highly acidic substances could possibly reduce the therapeutic effect of this medicinal.
PDR: Contraindicated in patients with hypertension. Not recommended in large doses during pregnancy or lactation due to potential neonatal androgenization. Enhances the effect of insulin and other antidiabetic agents. Use with MAO-inhibitors may cause headaches, tremors, and manias.

Gan Cao
(Radix Glycyrrhizae Uralensis, licorice)

Standard daily dosage: 2-12g
AH: Do not use during pregnancy. (This medicinal is routinely used in Chinese medical gynecology during pregnancy as part of formulas appropriately prescribed on the basis of pattern discrimination.) As a single herb in high doses, it is contraindicated in diabetes, hypertension, and liver disorders. Not for long-term use.
BR: May increase toxicity of cardiac glycosides. May increase potassium loss due to diuretics and laxatives. Possible additive effect to corticosteroids. May be synergistic with insulin in causing hypokalemia and sodium retention.
B&G: According to some traditional sources, is incompatible with *Gan Sui* (Radix Euphorbiae Kansui), *Yuan Hua* (Flos Daphnes Genkwae), and *Yuan Zhi* (Radix Polygalae Tenuifoliae). If taken long-term, it may cause hypertension and/or edema. Contains glycyrrhetinic acid which could possibly cause a reduction in thyroid activity and basal metabolic rate.

The research on *Gan Cao* concurs that this medicinal is generally safe when used in small amounts as an envoy. It should not be taken long-term or as a single herb during pregnancy. When used as a single medicinal or in patients taking other potent Western pharmaceuticals, caution should be exercised to guard against potential toxicity and drug interaction.

Huang Lian
(Rhizoma Coptidis Chinensis)

Standard daily dosage: 1.5-9g
AH: Not to be used during pregnancy. (This medicinal is commonly used during pregnancy in China when indicated by disease and pattern discrimination.)
B&G: Contains berberine. Long-term use may damage the digestive system. According to some traditional sources, antagonizes *Ju Hua* (Flos Chrysanthemi Morifolii), *Xuan Shen* (Radix Scrophulariae Ningpoensis), *Bai Xian Pi* (Cortex Radicis Dictamni Dasycarpi), and *Jiang Can* (Bombyx Batryticatus). According to some traditional sources counteracts *Kuan Dong Hua* (Flos Tussilaginis Farfarae) and *Niu Xi* (Radix Achyranthis Bidentatae). Some traditional sources say it should not be taken with pork.
C&C: Contains alkaloids, quercetin, and potassium. Could possibly cause hyperkalemia when used with potassium-sparing diuretics. Could possibly reduce the absorption and therapeutic effect of potassium and sodium iodides, sodium bicarbonate, calcium gluconate, carbonate, and lactate, aluminum hydroxide, magnesium and ferrous sulfates, and bismuth subcarbonate.

Da Zao, Hong Zao
(Fructus Zizyphi Jujubae, red dates)

Standard daily dosage: 10-30g (3-12 pieces)
AH: Safe when used appropriately
PDR: No health risks or side effects are known in conjunction with the proper administration of designated therapeutic dosages.

COMMENTS

Dang Shen (Radix Codonopsitis Pilosulae) is commonly substituted for *Ren Shen* in this formula. *Gan Cao* may be either uncooked or mix-fried depending on whether it is being primarily used for clearing heat or fortifying the spleen. Two variations of this formula are *Gan Cao Xie Xin Tang* (Licorice Drain the Heart Decoction) and *Sheng Jiang Xie Xin Tang* (Uncooked Ginger Drain the Heart Decoction). The former is used for a spleen-stomach-intestinal disharmony in which spleen vacuity has resulted in heart qi vacuity. The latter is used when there is a spleen-stomach-intestinal disharmony with less vacuity cold and more pronounced dampness.

BAO HE WAN
(Protecting Harmony Pills, a.k.a. Citrus & Crataegus Formula)

Category: Food-dispersing, stagnation-abducting
Functions: Disperses food and harmonizes the stomach
Chinese medical indications: Food stagnation with chest and abdominal glomus and fullness, putrid-smelling belching and burping, acid regurgitation, nausea and vomiting, aversion to food, yellow, slimy tongue fur, and a slippery pulse
Contraindications: Spleen vacuity
Western medical indications: Indigestion, diarrhea, abdominal pain, gastrointestinal flu, belching, acute exacerbation of chronic gastritis, hepatitis, acute pancreatitis, and acute and chronic cholecystitis
Potential formula toxicities & interactions: None listed

POTENTIAL MEDICINAL TOXICITIES AND INTERACTIONS:

Shan Zha
(Fructus Crataegi, hawthorne berries)

Standard daily dosage: 9-15g
AH: Safe when used appropriately
BR: Possible additive effect to digitalis, digoxin, and cardiac glycosides
C&C: Contains glycosides. Could possibly cause digitalis intoxication and heart arrhythmias. Vitamin C, nicotinic acid, glutamic acid, hydrochloric acid, and other highly acidic substances could possibly reduce the therapeutic effect of this medicinal.
PDR: Contraindicated in the first trimester of pregnancy and for children under 12 years of age. High doses can produce hypotension, cardiac arrhythmia, and sedation in susceptible patients. In patients with a history of cardiac problems, heart rate and blood pressure should be monitored on a regular basis.

Shen Qu
(Massa Medica Fermentata)

Standard daily dosage: 6-15g
B&G: Use with caution during pregnancy.
C&C: Contains amylase. Tetracyclines, sulphanomides, and aspirin could possibly reduce the therapeutic effect of this medicinal.

Lai Fu Zi
(Semen Raphani Sativi, radish seeds)

Standard daily dosage: 6-15g
PDR: No health risks or side effects are known in conjunction with the proper administration of designated therapeutic dosages.

Chen Pi, Ju Pi, Ju Hong
(Pericarpium Citri Reticulatae, tangerine peel)

Standard daily dosage: 3-9g
C&C: Contains potassium. Could possibly cause hyperkalemia when used with potassium-sparing diuretics.

Ban Xia
(Rhizoma Pinelliae Ternatae)

Standard daily dosage: 4.5-12g
AH: Do not use during pregnancy. (This medicinal is routinely used during pregnancy in China when indicated by disease and pattern discrimination.) Contraindicated in all hemorrhagic disorders.
B&G: Safe as long as it is properly prepared. Must be decocted with other herbs and not taken alone or uncooked. Toxic effects due to improper preparation or dosage include burning and numbness in throat and lips, nausea, and a feeling of pressure in the chest. Antidote is oral administration of raw ginger. Use with caution in patients with fever. According to some traditional sources, incompatible with *Wu Tou* (Radix Aconiti).
C&C: Contains alkaloids and glycosides. Could possibly reduce the absorption and therapeutic effect of potassium and sodium iodides, sodium bicarbonate, aluminum hydroxide, magnesium sulfate. Vitamin C, nicotinic acid, glutamic acid, hydrochloric acid, and other highly acidic substances could possibly reduce the therapeutic effect of this medicinal.
GLW: Poisoning occurs within 15 minutes to three hours after ingestion of a suitable amount. Initially, there is burning pain in the mouth, tongue, and throat, and enlargement of the tongue. This is then followed by drooling, ulceration of the oral mucosa, unclear speech, difficulty swallowing, dizziness, low-grade fever, heart palpitations, numbness of the extremities, a somber white facial complexion, and a weak, forceless pulse. If severe, there may be convulsions and respiratory failure leading to death.

Fu Ling, Bai Fu Ling, Yun Ling
(Sclerotium Poriae Cocos)

Standard daily dosage: 9-15g
B&G: Large doses or long-term use is discouraged. Contraindicated in patients with frequent, copious urination. According to traditional sources, may counteract *Di Yu* (Radix Sanguisorbae Officinalis), *Qin Jiao* (Radix Gentianae Qinjiao), and *Bie Jia* (Carapax Amydae Sinensis).
C&C: Contains potassium. Could possibly cause hyperkalemia when used with potassium-sparing diuretics.

Lian Qiao
(Fructus Forsythiae Suspensae, dried forsythia fruit pods)

Standard daily dosage: 6-15g
AH: Not to be used during pregnancy. (This medicinal is commonly used in China during pregnancy for the treatment of wind heat external contractions and heat toxins.)
B&G: Contraindicated in patients with diarrhea, carbuncles that have already ulcerated, and skin ulcers.
C&C: Contains potassium and glycosides. Could possibly cause hyperkalemia when used with potassium-sparing diuretics. Vitamin C, nicotinic acid, glutamic acid, hydrochloric acid, and other highly acidic substances could possibly reduce the therapeutic effect of this medicinal.

Mai Ya
(Fructus Germinatus Hordei Vulgaris, malted barley)

Standard daily dosage: 12-30g
AH: Not to be used during pregnancy.
B&G: According to one traditional source, long-term use may damage the kidneys.
C&C: Contains amylase. Tetracyclines, sulphanomides, and aspirin could possibly reduce the therapeutic effect of this medicinal.

BEI MU GUA LOU SAN
(Fritillaria & Trichosanthes Powder)

Category: Phlegm-transforming, dryness-moistening
Functions: Moistens the lungs and clears heat, rectifies the qi
and transforms phlegm
Chinese medical indications: Lung dryness cough with difficult-
to-expectorate phlegm, a dry, sore throat, possible wheezing, a
dry, red tongue with scanty fur, and a fine, rapid, forceful pulse
Contraindications: Yin vacuity cough
Western medical indications: Chronic bronchitis, lung abscess,
breast abscess
Potential formula toxicities & interactions: None listed

POTENTIAL MEDICINAL TOXICITIES & INTERACTIONS:

Chuan Bei Mu
(Bulbus Fritillariae Cirrhosae)

Standard daily dosage: 3-12g
AH: Not to be used during pregnancy. (This medicinal is commonly
used in China during pregnancy to treat coughing and panting when
indicated by pattern discrimination.)
B&G: According to traditional sources, incompatible with *Wu Tou*
(Radix Aconiti) and counteracts *Qin Jiao* (Radix Gentianae Qinjiao).
C&C: Contains alkaloids. Could possibly reduce the absorption and
therapeutic effect of potassium and sodium iodides, sodium bicarbonate,
aluminum hydroxide, and magnesium sulfate.

Gua Lou, Quan Gua Lou
(Fructus Trichosanthis Kirlowii)

Standard daily dosage: 9-30g
AH: Safe when used appropriately
B&G: According to traditional sources, incompatible with *Wu Tou*
(Radix Aconiti). Contains peimine, which is fatal in animals at doses of
nine milligram per kilogram of body weight (9mg/kg). Symptoms of
toxicity include reduced breathing, mydriasis, tremors, and coma.
C&C: Contains alkaloids and glycosides. Could possibly reduce the
absorption and therapeutic effect of potassium and sodium iodides, sodium bicarbonate, aluminum hydroxide, and magnesium sulfate. Vitamin C,
nicotinic acid, glutamic acid, hydrochloric acid, and other highly acidic
substances could possibly reduce the therapeutic effect of this medicinal.

Tian Hua Fen, Hua Fen
(Radix Trichosanthis Kirlowii)

Standard daily dosage: 9-15g
AH: Not to be used during pregnancy.
B&G: Contraindicated in pregnant patients and in patients with diarrhea.
C&C: Contains potassium and glycosides. Could possibly cause hyperkalemia when used with potassium-sparing diuretics. Vitamin C, nicotinic acid, glutamic acid, hydrochloric acid, and other highly acidic substances could possibly reduce the therapeutic effect of this medicinal.

Fu Ling, Bai Fu Ling, Yun Ling
(Sclerotium Poriae Cocos)

Standard daily dosage: 9-15g
B&G: Large doses or long-term use is discouraged. Contraindicated in patients with frequent, copious urination. According to traditional sources, may counteract *Di Yu* (Radix Sanguisorbae Officinalis), *Qin Jiao* (Radix Gentianae Qinjiao), and *Bie Jia* (Carapax Amydae Sinensis).
C&C: Contains potassium. Could possibly cause hyperkalemia when used with potassium-sparing diuretics.

Chen Pi, Ju Pi, Ju Hong
(Pericarpium Citri Reticulatae, tangerine peel)

Standard daily dosage: 3-9g
C&C: Contains potassium. Could possibly cause hyperkalemia when used with potassium-sparing diuretics.

Jie Geng
(Radix Platycodi Grandiflori, bellflower root)

Standard daily dosage: 3-9g
AH: Contraindicated in hemoptysis, especially in cases of tuberculosis. Use with caution in bleeding peptic ulcer.
B&G: Contraindicated in patients with hemoptysis. According to some traditional sources, counteracts *Long Dan Cao* (Radix Gentianae Longdancao) and *Long Yan Rou* (Arillus Euphoriae Longanae).

C&C: Contains calcium and glycosides. Could possibly reduce the effect of most antibiotics, cause digitalis intoxication and heart arrhythmias, hinder the absorption of isoniazid, and reduce the biological effect of levadopa. Vitamin C, nicotinic acid, glutamic acid, hydrochloric acid, and other highly acidic substances could possibly reduce the therapeutic effect of this medicinal.

BU ZHONG YI QI TANG
(Supplement the Center & Boost the Qi Decoction,
a.k.a. Ginseng & Astragalus Combination)

Category: Qi-supplementing
Functions: Supplements the center and boosts the qi, upbears yang and lifts the fallen
Chinese medical indications: Spleen qi vacuity or central qi falling downward with fatigue, loss of strength, shortness of breath, disinclination to speak and/or a weak, faint voice, loose stools, torpid intake, possible spontaneous perspiration, possible recurrent or enduring low-grade fever, a somber white facial complexion, an enlarged, fat tongue with teeth-marks on its edges and thin, white fur, and forceless, possibly weak or short pulse
Contraindications: Fever due to yin vacuity
Western medical indications: Debility after prolonged illness, prolapsed uterus or rectum, chronic hemorrhoids, gastroptosis, hernia, chronic diarrhea, functional uterine bleeding, habitual miscarriage, various postpartum problems (including urinary incontinence, lochioschesis, agalactia), myasthenia gravis, chronic bronchitis, chronic hepatitis, tuberculosis, neurasthenia, impotence, corneal ulcers, cerebral arteriosclerosis, pernicious anemia, leukopenia, chronic nephritis
Potential formula toxicities & interactions: None listed

POTENTIAL MEDICINAL TOXICITIES & INTERACTIONS:

Huang Qi, Bei Qi
(Radix Astragali Membranacei, astragalus)

Standard daily dosage: 9-60g
AH: Safe when used appropriately
C&C: Contains alkaloids and potassium. Could possibly cause hyper-kalemia when used with potassium-sparing diuretics. Could possibly reduce the absorption and therapeutic effect of potassium and sodium iodides, sodium bicarbonate, aluminum hydroxide, and magnesium sul-fate.
PDR: Caution should be taken with patients receiving immunosuppres-sive therapy, such as transplant patients or patients with autoimmune dis-

orders. May cause neurological dysfunction in high doses. May potentiate the risk of bleeding when used concomitantly with anticoagulants, antiplatelets, or antithrombotic agents.

Ren Shen
(Radix Panacis Ginseng, ginseng)

Standard daily dosage: 1-30g
AH: Contraindicated in hypertension
BR: May cause manic episodes in patients on MAO-inhibitors. May cause hypertension if consumed with caffeine. Possible additive effects to insulin. May reduce the anticoagulative effect of warfarin (Coumadin).
B&G: Contraindicated for hypertensive patients. Overdose can lead to headache, insomnia, heart palpitations, and a rise in blood pressure. A traditional antidote is mung bean soup.
C&C: Vitamin C, nicotinic acid, glutamic acid, hydrochloric acid, and other highly acidic substances could possibly reduce the therapeutic effect of this medicinal.
PDR: Contraindicated in patients with hypertension. Not recommended in large doses during pregnancy or lactation due to potential neonatal androgenization. Enhances the effect of insulin and other antidiabetic agents. Use with MAO-inhibitors may cause headaches, tremors, and manias.

Bai Zhu
(Rhizoma Atractylodis Macrocephalae)

Standard daily dosage: 4.5-9g
AH: Safe when used appropriately
B&G: When rats were fed 0.5g/kg of this medicinal for two months, they developed a mild lymphopenia and anemia but suffered no damage to the brain, heart, or liver.

Gan Cao
(Radix Glycyrrhizae Uralensis, licorice)

Standard daily dosage: 2-12g
AH: Do not use during pregnancy. (This medicinal is routinely used in Chinese medical gynecology during pregnancy as part of formulas appropriately prescribed on the basis of pattern discrimination.) As a single herb in high doses, it is contraindicated in diabetes, hypertension, and liver disorders. Not for long-term use.
BR: May increase toxicity of cardiac glycosides. May increase potassium loss due to diuretics and laxatives. Possible additive effect to corti-

costeroids. May be synergistic with insulin in causing hypokalemia and sodium retention.

B&G: According to some traditional sources, incompatible with *Gan Sui* (Radix Euphorbiae Kansui), *Yuan Hua* (Flos Daphnes Genkwae), and *Yuan Zhi* (Radix Polygalae Tenuifoliae). If taken long-term, it may cause hypertension and/or edema. Contains glycyrrhetinic acid which could possibly cause a reduction in thyroid activity and basal metabolic rate.

The research on *Gan Cao* concurs that this medicinal is generally safe when used in small amounts as an envoy. It should not be taken long-term or as a single herb during pregnancy. When used as a single medicinal or in patients taking other potent Western pharmaceuticals, caution should be exercised to guard against potential toxicity and drug interaction.

Dang Gui
(Radix Angelicae Sinensis)

Standard daily dosage: 3-15g
AH: Do not use during pregnancy. (This medicinal is routinely used in Chinese medical gynecology during pregnancy as part of formulas appropriately prescribed on the basis of pattern discrimination.)
B&G: Use with caution in patients with diarrhea or abdominal distention.
C&C: Contains potassium. Could possibly cause hyperkalemia when used with potassium-sparing diuretics. May exaggerate the anticoagulative effect of warfarin (Coumadin).

Chen Pi, Ju Pi, Ju Hong
(Pericarpium Citri Reticulatae, tangerine peel)

Standard daily dosage: 3-9g
AH: Safe when used appropriately
C&C: Contains potassium. Could possibly cause hyperkalemia when used with potassium-sparing diuretics.

Sheng Ma
(Rhizoma Cimicifugae, black cohosh)

Standard daily dosage: 1.5-9g
AH: Do not use during pregnancy. (This medicinal is commonly used during pregnancy in China.) Not to be used while nursing.
B&G: Contraindicated in cases of fully erupted measles and in patients with breathing difficulties. Overdose causes headaches, dizziness, vomiting, tremors, gastroenteritis, and pathologic erections.
C&C: Vitamin C, nicotinic acid, glutamic acid, hydrochloric acid, and

other highly acidic substances could possibly reduce the therapeutic effect of this medicinal.

PDR: Not for use during pregnancy due to an increased risk of spontaneous abortion. (However, this medicinal is routinely used as part of this formula in Chinese medical gynecology for the treatment of threatened abortion due to spleen qi vacuity not containing the fetus. Therefore, this contraindication is not absolute.) Contains glycosides which may potentiate the effect of antihypertensive medications and result in hypotension.

Chai Hu
(Radix Bupleuri)

Standard daily dosage: 3-12g

AH: Safe when used appropriately

B&G: May occasionally cause nausea and vomiting, in which case the dose should then be reduced significantly.

C&C: Vitamin C, nicotinic acid, glutamic acid, hydrochloric acid, and other highly acidic substances could possibly reduce the therapeutic effect of this medicinal.

PDR: Not to be administered during pregnancy. (This medicinal is routinely used in Chinese medical gynecology during pregnancy as part of formulas appropriately prescribed on the basis of pattern discrimination.) Overdose may lead to gastroenteritis, intestinal colic, and diarrhea due to saponin content.

COMMENTS

Dang Shen (Radix Codonopsitis Pilosulae) is commonly substituted for *Ren Shen* in this formula. This formula has a wider scope of application than simply downward falling of the central qi. It may also be used for liver-spleen disharmonies where spleen qi vacuity is marked. In that case, the amount of *Chai Hu* may be increased so that it more forcefully courses the liver and rectifies the qi. Because a liver-spleen disharmony is such a commonly seen pattern, this formula is very commonly used when modified with appropriate additions and subtractions to treat a large variety of conditions.

CANG ER ZI SAN
(Xanthium Powder)

Category: Exterior-resolving
Functions: Dispels wind, stops pain, and frees the flow of the nose
Chinese medical indications: Deep source nasal congestion with profuse, purulent, foul-smelling nasal discharge, nasal congestion, dizziness, frontal headache, thin, white or yellow tongue fur, and a floating pulse
Note: While deep source nasal discharge typically involves lung heat, this formula can be used to treat either hot or cold patterns of nasal congestion simply based on the treatment principles of aromatically and penetratingly free the flow of the nose.
Contraindications: None listed
Western medical indications: Acute or chronic sinusitis, acute, chronic, and allergic rhinitis
Potential formula toxicities & interactions: None listed

POTENTIAL MEDICINAL TOXICITIES & INTERACTIONS:

Cang Er Zi
(Fructus Xanthii Sibirici)

Standard daily dosage: 3-9g
B&G: Safe as long as it is properly prepared. Must be decocted properly with other medicinals and should not be taken alone or uncooked. Toxic effects due to improper preparation or dosage include CNS deficits as well as nephro- and hepatoxicity which can lead to coma and death.
C&C: Contains alkaloids and glycosides. Could possibly reduce the absorption and therapeutic effect of potassium and sodium iodides, sodium bicarbonate, aluminum hydroxide, and magnesium sulfate. Vitamin C, nicotinic acid, glutamic acid, hydrochloric acid, and other highly acidic substances could possibly reduce the therapeutic effect of this medicinal.
GLW: There is a latency period of 1-7 days after poisoning. The initial symptoms include dizziness, headache, fatigue, nausea, vomiting, abdominal pain, diarrhea, fever, malar flushing, and conjunctival hyperemia. In more serious cases, there is vexation, agitation, and restlessness or somnolence, liver area pain, liver enlargement, jaundice, and gastrointestinal tract bleeding. This is followed by dimming of conscious-

ness, fright reversal, heart arrhythmia, shock, and urinary block. Either kidney or respiratory failure may lead to death.

Xin Yi Hua
(Flos Magnoliae Liliflorae)

Standard daily dosage: 3-9g
AH: Safe when used appropriately
B&G: Overdose may cause dizziness or redness of the eyes.

Bai Zhi
(Radix Angelicae Dahuricae, angelica root)

Standard daily dosage: 3-9g
AH: Safe when used appropriately

Bo He
(Herba Menthae Haplocalycis, field mint)

Standard daily dose: 1.5-6g
B&G: Not recommended for nursing mothers as it may inhibit lactation.

COMMENTS

This formula only treats the tip or branch symptom of nasal congestion. Therefore, it is rarely used by itself in this simple, discrete form. More commonly, unless used in ready-made form for symptomatic relief only, these ingredients are added to another formula to treat the root of nasal congestion.

CHAI HU JIA LONG GU MU LI TANG
(Bupleurum Plus Dragon Bone & Oyster Shell Decoction,
a.k.a. Bupleurum & Dragon Bone Combination)

Category: Heavy, settling, spirit-quieting
Functions: Frees the flow of the three yang aspects and quiets the spirit
Chinese medical indications: Replete heat harassing the heart spirit with chest oppression, easy anger, restlessness, insomnia, heart palpitations, deranged speech, a red tongue with thick, slimy, yellow fur, and a bowstring, possibly slippery, rapid pulse
Contraindications: None listed
Western medical indications: Neurosis, schizophrenia, hysteria, epilepsy, hypertension, first or second degree A-V block, hyperthyroidism, Meniere's disease, spasm of the sternocleidomastoid muscle, gastritis, menopausal syndrome, and postconcussion syndrome
Potential formula toxicities & interactions:
B&B: The original recipe for this formula called for the inclusion of *Qian Dan* (Minium), a form of lead which is toxic. Modern day formulations substitute either uncooked *Tie Luo* (Frusta Ferri) or *Dai Zhe Shi* (Haemititum) or simply omit this medicinal altogether.

POTENTIAL MEDICINAL TOXICITIES & INTERACTIONS:

Chai Hu
(Radix Bupleuri)

Standard daily dosage: 3-12g
AH: Safe when used appropriately
B&G: May occasionally cause nausea and vomiting, in which case the dose should then be reduced significantly.
C&C: Vitamin C, nicotinic acid, glutamic acid, hydrochloric acid, and other highly acidic substances could possibly reduce the therapeutic effect of this medicinal.
PDR: Not to be administered during pregnancy.[25] Overdose may lead to gastroenteritis, intestinal colic, and diarrhea due to saponin content.

Huang Qin, Tiao Qin
(Radix Scutellariae Baicalensis)

Standard daily dosage: 6-15g
AH: Safe when used appropriately
B&G: According to some traditional sources, counteracts *Dan Pi* (Cortex Radicis Moutan) and *Li Lu* (Rhizoma Et Radix Veratri).
C&C: Contains potassium and glycosides. Could possibly cause hyperkalemia when used with potassium-sparing diuretics. Vitamin C, nicotinic acid, glutamic acid, hydrochloric acid, and other highly acidic substances could possibly reduce the therapeutic effect of this medicinal.

Ban Xia
(Rhizoma Pinelliae Ternatae)

Standard daily dosage: 4.5-12g
AH: Do not use during pregnancy. (This medicinal is routinely used during pregnancy in China when indicated by disease and pattern discrimination.) Contraindicated in all hemorrhagic disorders.
B&G: Safe as long as it is properly prepared. Must be decocted with other herbs and not taken alone or uncooked. Toxic effects due to improper preparation or dosage include burning and numbness in throat and lips, nausea, and a feeling of pressure in the chest. Antidote is oral administration of raw ginger. Use with caution in patients with fever. According to some traditional sources, incompatible with *Wu Tou* (Radix Aconiti).
C&C: Contains alkaloids and glycosides. Could possibly reduce the absorption and therapeutic effect of potassium and sodium iodides, sodium bicarbonate, aluminum hydroxide, and magnesium sulfate. Vitamin C, nicotinic acid, glutamic acid, hydrochloric acid, and other highly acidic substances could possibly reduce the therapeutic effect of this medicinal.
GLW: Poisoning occurs within 15 minutes to three hours after ingestion of a suitable amount. Initially, there is burning pain in the mouth, tongue, and throat, and enlargement of the tongue. This is then followed by drooling, ulceration of the oral mucosa, unclear speech, difficulty swallowing, dizziness, low-grade fever, heart palpitations, numbness of the extremities, a somber white facial complexion, and a weak, forceless pulse. If severe, there may be convulsions and respiratory failure leading to death.

Ren Shen
(Radix Panacis Ginseng, ginseng)

Standard daily dosage: 1-30g
AH: Safe when used appropriately
BR: May cause manic episodes in patients on MAO-inhibitors. May cause hypertension if consumed with caffeine. Possible additive effects to insulin. May reduce the anticoagulative effect of warfarin (Coumadin).
B&G: Contraindicated for hypertensive patients. Overdose can lead to headache, insomnia, heart palpitations, and a rise in blood pressure. A traditional antidote is mung bean soup.
C&C: Vitamin C, nicotinic acid, glutamic acid, hydrochloric acid, and other highly acidic substances could possibly reduce the therapeutic effect of this medicinal.
PDR: Contraindicated in patients with hypertension. Not recommended in large doses during pregnancy or lactation due to potential neonatal androgenization. Enhances the effect of insulin and other antidiabetic agents. Use with MAO-inhibitors may cause headaches, tremors, and manias.

Sheng Jiang
(uncooked Rhizoma Zingiberis Officinalis, fresh ginger)

Standard daily dose: 3-9g
AH: Safe when used appropriately
BR: Reduces vomiting caused by chemotherapeutic drugs. Increases absorption of oral drugs.
PDR: Recommended safe dosage limit is six grams (6g). Avoid larger doses if being used to treat morning sickness or if used in patients taking anticoagulants.

Gui Zhi
(Ramulus Cinnamomi Cassiae, cinnamon twigs)

Standard daily dosage: 3-15g
AH: Safe when used appropriately
B&G: Use with caution in the presence of fever, during pregnancy, or during excessive menstruation.
PDR: Contraindicated during pregnancy.

Fu Ling, Bai Fu Ling, Yun Ling
(Sclerotium Poriae Cocos)

Standard daily dosage: 9-15g
B&G: Large doses or long-term use is discouraged. Contraindicated in patients with frequent, copious urination. According to traditional sources, may counteract *Di Yu* (Radix Sanguisorbae Officinalis), *Qin Jiao* (Radix Gentianae Qinjiao), and *Bie Jia* (Carapax Amydae Sinensis).
C&C: Contains potassium. Could possibly cause hyperkalemia when used with potassium-sparing diuretics.

Long Gu
(Os Draconis, fossilized bone)

Standard daily dosage: 15-30g
B&G: According to some traditional sources, counteracts *Shi Gao* (Gypsum Fibrosum) and should not be mixed with fish.
C&C: Contains calcium, iron, magnesium, aluminum, and potassium. Could possibly cause hyperkalemia when used with potassium-sparing diuretics. Could possibly reduce the effect of most antibiotics, levadopa, and prednisolone, cause digitalis intoxication and heart arrhythmias, and hinder the absorption of isoniazid.

Mu Li
(Concha Ostreae, oyster shell)

Standard daily dosage: 15-30g
B&G: Contraindicated when the patient has high fever without sweating. Overdose may lead to indigestion or constipation. According to some traditional sources, works synergistically with *Bei Mu* (Bulbus Fritillariae), *Gan Cao* (Radix Glycyrrizae Uralensis), *Niu Xi* (Radix Achyranthis Bidentatae), and *Yuan Zhi* (Radix Polygalae Tenuifoliae) and has adverse effects when combined with *Ma Huang* (Herba Ephedrae), *Wu Zhu Yu* (Fructus Evodiae Rutecarpae), and *Xi Xin* (Herba Asari Cum Radice).
C&C: Contains calcium, iron, magnesium, and aluminum. Could possibly reduce the effects of most antibiotics, levadopa, and prednisolone, cause digitalis intoxication and heart arrhythmias, and hinder the absorption of isoniazid.

The U.S. FDA has banned the inclusion of this medicinal in all dietary supplements.

Da Huang, Dai Huang, Chuan Jun, Jun
(Radix Et Rhizoma Rhei, rhubarb root)

Standard daily dosage: 3-12g
AH: Do not use during pregnancy. Not to be used while nursing. Contraindicated in intestinal obstruction, abdominal pain of unknown origin, or any inflammatory condition of the intestines.
BR: Reduces absorption of oral drugs. Overuse may cause hypokalemia and increased toxicity of cardiac glycosides. May aggravate potassium loss from diuretics.
B&G: Use with extreme caution during pregnancy, menstruation, or postpartum. Contraindicated for nursing mothers since active ingredients enter the milk.
C&C: Contains alkaloids, tannic acid, potassium, and glycosides. Could possibly cause hyperkalemia when used with potassium-sparing diuretics. Vitamin C, nicotinic acid, glutamic acid, hydrochloric acid, and other highly acidic substances could possibly reduce the therapeutic effect of this medicinal.
PDR: Consult a physician before using this medicinal during pregnancy or while nursing. Contraindicated in cases of intestinal obstruction, acute inflammatory intestinal disease, appendicitis and abdominal pain of unknown origin.

Da Zao, Hong Zao
(Fructus Zizyphi Jujubae, red dates)

Standard daily dosage: 10-30g (3-12 pieces)
AH: Safe when used appropriately
PDR: No health risks or side effects are known in conjunction with the proper administration of designated therapeutic dosages.

Dai Zhe Shi
(Haemititum, hematite)

Standard daily dosage: 9-30g
B&G: Use with caution during pregnancy. Signs of toxicity include weakness, slowness of movement, and paroxysmal spasms leading to paralysis and death. Two grams daily for seven days caused death in mice. Researchers have found small amounts of arsenic salts in some samples accounting for its toxicity. According to some traditional sources, counteracts *Fu Zi* (Radix Lateralis Praeparatus Aconiti Carmichaeli).
C&C: Contains iron. Could possibly reduce the effect of most antibi-

otics, levadopa, and prednisolone and hinder the absorption of isoniazid.

COMMENTS

Dang Shen (Radix Codonopsitis Pilosulae) is commonly substituted for *Ren Shen* in this formula. *Da Huang* is typically omitted if there is no concomitant constipation. Originally, this formula contained *Huang Dan* (Minium, a form of lead). Nowadays, *Dai Zhe Shi* is usually substituted or the ingredient is left out altogether. Like many other famous formulas, this one treats a liver-spleen disharmony with depressive heat. In this case, the spleen disharmony has resulted in lack of construction and nourishment of the heart spirit, while depressive heat has counterflowed upward to also harass the spirit.

CHUAN XIONG CHA TIAO SAN
(Ligusticum Mixed with Tea Powder,
a.k.a. Cnidium & Tea Formula)

Category: Exterior-resolving
Functions: Courses wind and stops pain
Chinese medical indications: External contraction wind evil
headache accompanied by fever, aversion to wind, dizziness,
nasal congestion, thin, white tongue fur, and a floating pulse
Contraindications: Ascendant liver yang hyperactivity with liver
blood-kidney yin vacuity or qi and blood dual vacuity headache
Western medical indications: Headache from common cold or
flu, migraine, tension headache, neurogenic headache, acute and
chronic rhinitis and sinusitis, and vertigo
Potential formula toxicities & interactions: None listed

POTENTIAL MEDICINAL TOXICITIES & INTERACTIONS:

Bo He
(Herba Menthae Haplocalycis, field mint)

Standard daily dose: 1.5-6g
AH: Safe when used appropriately
B&G: Not recommended for nursing mothers as it may inhibit lactation.

Chuan Xiong
(Radix Ligustici Wallichii)

Standard daily dosage: 3-9g (In China today, it is not uncommon for
this medicinal to be prescribed up to 15 grams per day in decoction.)
AH: Do not use during pregnancy. (This medicinal is routinely used in
Chinese medical gynecology during pregnancy as part of formulas
appropriately prescribed on the basis of pattern discrimination.)
B&G: Not for patients with migraine headache or excessive menstrual
bleeding. Overdosage causes vomiting and dizziness. According to some
traditional texts, antagonizes *Shan Zhu Yu* (Fructus Corni Officinalis)
and *Huang Qi* (Radix Astragali Membranacei), counteracts *Hua Shi*
(Talcum) and *Huang Lian* (Rhizoma Coptidis Chinensis), and is incompatible with *Li Lu* (Rhizoma Et Radix Veratri).
C&C: Contains alkaloids and potassium. Could possibly cause hyperkalemia when used with potassium-sparing diuretics. Could possibly
reduce the absorption and therapeutic effect of potassium and sodium

iodides, sodium bicarbonate, aluminum hydroxide, and magnesium sulfate.

Bai Zhi
(Radix Angelicae Dahuricae, angelica root)

Standard daily dosage: 3-9g
AH: Safe when used appropriately

Qiang Huo
(Radix Et Rhizoma Notopterygii)

Standard daily dosage: 6-15g

No toxicity or interaction information listed in the sources

Xi Xin
(Herba Asari Cum Radice)

Standard daily dosage: 1-3g
AH: Do not use during pregnancy. Contains aristolochic acid (AA). Do not exceed recommended dose.
B&G: Nephrotoxic. Use with caution in patients with renal problems. According to some traditional sources, may antagonize *Shan Zhu Yu* (Fructus Corni Officinalis) and *Huang Qi* (Radix Astragali Membranacei).
PDR: Not to be used during pregnancy.
GLW: Symptoms of adverse reaction include headache, vomiting, vexation and agitation, sweating, stiffness of the neck, oral thirst, a rapid pulse, increased body temperature and blood pressure, slightly dilated pupils, a red flushed face, twitching muscles, generalized tension which may become convulsions, clenched teeth, arched-back rigidity, unclear thinking, cramping of the four limbs, dimming of consciousness, urinary block, and, eventually, death due to respiratory paralysis.

Xi Xin is on the FDA's "B List" of herbs which may potentially contain aristolochic acid (AA). *Xi Xin* is harvested in China mostly from *Asarum sieboldi* and *Asarum heteropoides*, neither of which have conclusively been shown to contain AA. However, other species of *Asarum* are sometimes substituted, and these may contain AA. As of this writing, the FDA has set no acceptable limit to AA consumption by humans.

Jing Jie Sui, Jing Jie
(Herba Seu Flos Schizonepetae Tenuifoliae)

Standard daily dosage: 3-9g

No toxicity or interaction information listed in the sources

Fang Feng
(Radix Ledebouriellae Divaricatae)

Standard daily dosage: 3-9g
AH: Safe when used appropriately
B&G: According to some traditional sources, may antagonize *Gan Jiang* (dry Rhizoma Zingiberis Officinalis), *Li Lu* (Rhizoma Et Radix Veratri) and counteracts *Bei Xie* (Rhizoma Dioscoreae Hypoglaucae).
C&C: Contains glycosides. Vitamin C, nicotinic acid, glutamic acid, hydrochloric acid, and other highly acidic substances could possibly reduce the therapeutic effect of this medicinal.

Gan Cao
(Radix Glycyrrhizae Uralensis, licorice)

Standard daily dosage: 2-12g
AH: Do not use during pregnancy. (This medicinal is routinely used in Chinese medical gynecology during pregnancy as part of formulas appropriately prescribed on the basis of pattern discrimination.) As a single herb in high doses, it is contraindicated in diabetes, hypertension, and liver disorders. Not for long-term use.
BR: May increase toxicity of cardiac glycosides. May increase potassium loss due to diuretics and laxatives. Possible additive effect to corticosteroids. May be synergistic with insulin in causing hypokalemia and sodium retention.
B&G: According to some traditional sources, incompatible with *Gan Sui* (Radix Euphorbiae Kansui), *Yuan Hua* (Flos Daphnes Genkwae), and *Yuan Zhi* (Radix Polygalae Tenuifoliae). If taken long-term, it may cause hypertension and/or edema. Contains glycyrrhetinic acid which could possibly cause a reduction in thyroid activity and basal metabolic rate.

The research on *Gan Cao* concurs that this medicinal is generally safe when used in small amounts as an envoy. It should not be taken long-term or as a single herb during pregnancy. When used as a single medicinal or in patients taking other potent Western pharmaceuticals, caution should be exercised to guard against potential toxicity and drug interaction.

COMMENTS

This formula is commonly used for the firstaid relief of various types of repletion pattern headaches. Its ingredients free the flow of the qi and blood in all portions of the head, front, back, sides, and top. Unless combined with supplementing formulas, it is inappropriate for treating vacuity pattern headaches.

DA CHENG QI TANG
(Major Order the Qi Decoction,
a.k.a. Major Rhubarb Combination)

Category: Draining & precipitating
Functions: Harshly or sternly precipitates heat binding
Chinese medical indications: Internal heat accumulation with constipation, flatulence, abdominal glomus and fullness, abdominal pain which refuses pressure, a tense, firm abdomen, dry, yellow or dry, black tongue fur with prickles, and a confined, replete pulse
Contraindications: Vacuity weakness
Western medical indications: Acute pneumonia, typhoid, flu, measles, meningitis, hypertension, tetanus, beriberi, habitual constipation, appendicitis, intestinal obstruction, acute abdominal pain, neurosis, food poisoning, obesity, dysentery, hemorrhoids
Potential formula toxicities & interactions:
FL/B&B: Prohibited during pregnancy. If inappropriately prescribed, may cause vomiting and severe diarrhea, especially in debilitated patients.

POTENTIAL MEDICINAL TOXICITIES & INTERACTIONS:

Da Huang, Dai Huang, Chuan Jun, Jun
(Radix Et Rhizoma Rhei, rhubard root)

Standard daily dosage: 3-12g
AH: Do not use during pregnancy. Not to be used while nursing. Contraindicated in intestinal obstruction, abdominal pain of unknown origin, or any inflammatory condition of the intestines.
BR: Reduces absorption of oral drugs. Overuse may cause hypokalemia and increased toxicity of cardiac glycosides. May aggravate potassium loss from diuretics.
B&G: Use with extreme caution during pregnancy, menstruation, or postpartum. Contraindicated for nursing mothers since active ingredients enter the milk.
C&C: Contains alkaloids, tannic acid, potassium, and glycosides. Could possibly cause hyperkalemia when used with potassium-sparing diuretics. Vitamin C, nicotinic acid, glutamic acid, hydrochloric acid, and other highly acidic substances could possibly reduce the therapeutic effect of this medicinal.

PDR: Consult a physician before using this medicinal during pregnancy or while nursing. Contraindicated in cases of intestinal obstruction, acute inflammatory intestinal disease, appendicitis and abdominal pain of unknown origin.

Hou Po, Chuan Po
(Cortex Magnoliae Officinalis)

Standard daily dosage: 3-9g
AH: Not to be used during pregnancy (This medicinal is commonly used in China during pregnancy, especially for the treatment of nausea and vomiting.)
B&G: Use with caution during pregnancy. According to some traditional sources, antagonizes *Ze Xie* (Rhizoma Alismatis Orientalis) and *Han Shui Shi* (Calcitum).
C&C: Contains tannic acid and potassium. Could possibly cause hyperkalemia when used with potassium-sparing diuretics and reduce the absorption and biologic effect of most antibiotics, isoniazid, chlorpromazine, calcium carbonate and gluconate, atropine, ephedrine, quinine, reserpine, digitalis, vitamin B_1, trypsine, amylase, and pepsin.
PDR: No health risks or side effects are known in conjunction with the proper administration of designated therapeutic dosages.

Zhi Shi
(Fructus Immaturus Citri Aurantii, immature bitter orange)

Standard daily dosage: 3-9
B&G: Use with caution during pregnancy or in debilitated patients.
C&C: Contains tannic acid. Highly acidic. Could possibly cause crystalluria and hematuria and reduce the absorption and biologic effect of most antibiotics, isoniazid, chlorpromazine, calcium carbonate and gluconate, atropine, ephedrine, quinine, reserpine, digitalis, vitamin B_1, trypsine, amylase, and pepsin, sodium bicarbonate, aluminum hydroxide, reserpine, caffeine, opiates, scopolamine, and berbamin.

Mang Xiao
(Mirabilitum, Glauber's salt)

Standard daily dosage: 3-9g
B&G: Contraindicated during pregnancy, postpartum, and during menstruation. Use with caution when fever is present and in the elderly.

COMMENTS

Although a famous classical formula, this formula is not commonly indicated in the West where most users of Chinese medicine manifest vacuity and repletion at the same time.

DA HUANG FU ZI TANG

(Rhubarb & Aconite Decoction, a.k.a. Rhubarb & Aconite
Combination)

Category: Attacking & precipitating
Functions: Warms yang and dissipates cold, drains binding and
moves stagnation
Chinese medical indications: Internal cold accumulation with
abdominal pain, constipation, rib-side pain, aversion to cold,
low-grade fever, cold hands and feet, white, slimy tongue fur,
and a confined, tight or bowstring pulse
Contraindications: Heat
Western medical indications: Stomach and intestinal spasms,
pyelonephritis, kidney stones, gallstones, pancreatitis, intestinal
colic, hernia pain, sciatica, intercostal neuralgia, migraines,
chronic colitis, chronic pelvic inflammation
Potential formula toxicities & interactions: None listed

POTENTIAL MEDICINAL TOXICITIES & INTERACTIONS:

Da Huang, Dai Huang, Chuan Jun, Jun
(Radix Et Rhizoma Rhei, rhubarb root)

Standard daily dosage: 3-12g
AH: Do not use during pregnancy. Not to be used while nursing.
Contraindicated in intestinal obstruction, abdominal pain of unknown
origin, or any inflammatory condition of the intestines.
BR: Reduces absorption of oral drugs. Overuse may cause hypokalemia
and increased toxicity of cardiac glycosides. May aggravate potassium
loss from diuretics.
B&G: Use with extreme caution during pregnancy, menstruation, or
postpartum. Contraindicated for nursing mothers since active ingredients
enter the milk.
C&C: Contains alkaloids, tannic acid, potassium, and glycosides. Could
possibly cause hyperkalemia when used with potassium-sparing diuretics. Vitamin C, nicotinic acid, glutamic acid, hydrochloric acid, and
other highly acidic substances could possibly reduce the therapeutic
effect of this medicinal.
PDR: Consult a physician before using this medicinal during pregnancy
or while nursing. Contraindicated in cases of intestinal obstruction,
acute inflammatory intestinal disease, appendicitis and abdominal pain
of unknown origin.

Fu Zi, Shu Fu Zi, Fu Pian
(Radix Lateralis Praeparatus Aconiti Carmichaeli,
wolfsbane, monkshood)

Standard daily dosage: 1.5-15g

AH: To be used only under the supervision of an expert qualified in the appropriate use of this substance

B&G: Contraindicated during pregnancy. A very toxic medicinal which can be fatal if ingested in its uncooked form or in an inappropriate dose. It is generally combined with *Gan Cao* (Radix Glycyrhizae Uralensis) and *Gan Jiang* (dry Rhizoma Zingiberis Officinalis) in decoctions to reduce its toxicity. Symptoms of toxicity include drooling, gastric upset, light-headedness, blurred vision, and numbness and tingling of the extremities. More severe symptoms include premature atrial contractions, dyspnea, and reduced temperature and blood pressure. Emergency measures include the administration of atropine.

C&C: Contains alkaloids. Could possibly reduce the absorption and therapeutic effect of potassium and sodium iodides, sodium bicarbonate, aluminum hydroxide, and magnesium sulfate.

PDR: Contains nor-diterpene alkaloids, including aconitine. Highly toxic; small doses can be fatal.

GLW: If mild poisoning, there is a burning hot sensation in the mouth and on the tongue, numbness, and pain which gradually spreads to the four limbs and then to the whole body, nausea, vomiting, dizziness, heart palpitations, rapid breathing, vexation, agitation, restlessness, drooling. If more severe poisoning, there may be generalized sweating, paralysis, convulsions, urinary incontinence, dilated pupils, slowed reaction to light, slow heartbeat, arrhythmia, low blood pressure, a somber white facial complexion, reversal chilling of the four limbs, lowered body temperature, and circulatory collapse leading to death.

Xi Xin
(Herba Asari Cum Radice)

Standard daily dosage: 1-3g

AH: Do not use during pregnancy. Contains aristolochic acid (AA). Do not exceed recommended dose.

B&G: Nephrotoxic. Use with caution in patients with renal problems. According to some traditional sources, may antagonize *Shan Zhu Yu* (Fructus Corni Officinalis) and *Huang Qi* (Radix Astragali Membranacei).

PDR: Not to be used during pregnancy.

GLW: Symptoms of adverse reaction include headache, vomiting, vexation and agitation, sweating, stiffness of the neck, oral thirst, a rapid pulse, increased body temperature and blood pressure, slightly dilated pupils, a red flushed face, twitching muscles, generalized tension which may become convulsions, clenched teeth, arched-back rigidity, unclear thinking, cramping of the four limbs, dimming of consciousness, urinary block, and, eventually, death due to respiratory paralysis.

Xi Xin is on the FDA's "B List" of herbs which may potentially contain aristolochic acid (AA). *Xi Xin* is harvested in China mostly from *Asarum sieboldi* and *Asarum heteropoides*, neither of which have conclusively been shown to contain AA. However, other species of *Asarum* are sometimes substituted, and these may contain AA. As of this writing, the FDA has set no acceptable limit to AA consumption by humans.

DANG GUI SHAO YAO SAN
(Dang Gui & Peony Powder,
a.k.a. Tang-kuei & Peony Formula)

Category: Blood-supplementing
Functions: Harmonizes the liver and spleen, nourishes the blood and percolates dampness
Chinese medical indications: Liver-spleen disharmony with blood vacuity and dampness manifesting as continuous but not particularly severe abdominal cramping, slight edema of the lower extremities, possible difficulty urinating (especially during pregnancy), a pale, possibly enlarged tongue with thin, white fur, and a fine, bowstring or soggy, bowstring pulse
Contraindications: None listed
Western medical indications: Habitual or threatened miscarriage, primary dysmenorrhea, pelvic inflammatory disease, chronic nephritis, and beriberi
Potential formula toxicities & interactions: None listed

POTENTIAL MEDICINAL TOXICITIES & INTERACTIONS:

Dang Gui
(Radix Angelicae Sinensis)

Standard daily dosage: 3-15g
AH: Do not use during pregnancy. (This medicinal is routinely used in Chinese medical gynecology during pregnancy as part of formulas appropriately prescribed on the basis of pattern discrimination.)
B&G: Use with caution in patients with diarrhea or abdominal distention.
C&C: Contains potassium. Could possibly cause hyperkalemia when used with potassium-sparing diuretics. May exaggerate the anticoagulative effect of warfarin (Coumadin).

Bai Shao, Shao Yao
(Radix Albus Paeoniae Lactiflorae, white peony root)

Standard daily dosage: 6-30g
AH: Safe when used appropriately
B&G: Use with caution in debilitated patients with diarrhea. According to some traditional sources, antagonizes *Shi Hu* (Herba Dendrobii) and *Mang Xiao* (Mirabilitum), counteracts *Bie Jia* (Carapax Amydae Sinensis) and *Xiao Ji* (Herba Cephalanopoloris Segeti), and is incompatible with *Li Lu* (Rhizoma Et Radix Veratri).

C&C: Contains calcium, tannic acid, potassium, and glycosides. Could possibly cause hyperkalemia when used with potassium-sparing diuretics. Could possibly reduce the effect of most antibiotics, cause digitalis intoxication and heart arrhythmias, and Could possibly reduce the absorption and therapeutic effect of levadopa, isoniazid, chlorpromazine, calcium carbonate and gluconate, atropine, ephedrine, quinine, reserpine, vitamin B_1, trypsine, amylase, and pepsin. Vitamin C, nicotinic acid, glutamic acid, hydrochloric acid, and other highly acidic substances could possibly reduce the therapeutic effect of this medicinal.

Fu Ling, Bai Fu Ling, Yun Ling
(Sclerotium Poriae Cocos)

Standard daily dosage: 9-15g
B&G: Large doses or long-term use is discouraged. Contraindicated in patients with frequent, copious urination. According to traditional sources, may counteract *Di Yu* (Radix Sanguisorbae Officinalis), *Qin Jiao* (Radix Gentianae Qinjiao), and *Bie Jia* (Carapax Amydae Sinensis).
C&C: Contains potassium. Could possibly cause hyperkalemia when used with potassium-sparing diuretics.

Bai Zhu
(Rhizoma Atractylodis Macrocephalae)

Standard daily dosage: 4.5-9g
B&G: When rats were fed 0.5g/kg of this medicinal for two months, they developed a mild lymphopenia and anemia but suffered no damage to the brain, heart, or liver.

Ze Xie
(Rhizoma Alismatis Orientalis)

Standard daily dosage: 6-15g
AH: Prolonged use may cause gastrointestinal irritation.
B&G: Although considered safe, prolonged usage may irritate the intestinal tract and could possibly cause gastroenteritis.
C&C: Contains alkaloids and potassium. Could possibly cause hyperkalemia when used with potassium-sparing diuretics and reduce the absorption and therapeutic effect of potassium and sodium iodides, sodium bicarbonate, aluminum hydroxide, and magnesium sulfate.
PDR: Contains triterpenes, sesquiterpenes, flavone sulfate, and caffeic acid derivatives. No health hazards or side effects with proper administration of designated therapeutic dosages.

Chuan Xiong
(Radix Ligustici Wallichii)

Standard daily dosage: 3-9g (In China today, it is not uncommon for this medicinal to be prescribed up to 15 grams per day in decoction.)
AH: Do not use during pregnancy. (This medicinal is routinely used in Chinese medical gynecology during pregnancy as part of formulas appropriately prescribed on the basis of pattern discrimination.)
B&G: Not for patients with migraine headache or excessive menstrual bleeding. Overdosage causes vomiting and dizziness. According to some traditional texts, antagonizes *Shan Zhu Yu* (Fructus Corni Officinalis) and *Huang Qi* (Radix Astragali Membranacei), counteracts *Hua Shi* (Talcum) and *Huang Lian* (Rhizoma Coptidis Chinensis), and is incompatible with *Li Lu* (Rhizoma Et Radix Veratri).
C&C: Contains alkaloids and potassium. Could possibly cause hyperkalemia when used with potassium-sparing diuretics. Could possibly reduce the absorption and therapeutic effect of potassium and sodium iodides, sodium bicarbonate, aluminum hydroxide, and magnesium sulfate.

DAN SHEN YIN
(Salvia Beverage)

Category: Blood-quickening
Functions: Quickens the blood and dispels stasis, moves the qi and stops pain
Chinese medical indications: Blood stasis & qi stagnation with chest and stomach duct aching and pain
Contraindications: Yin vacuity
Western medical indications: Angina pectoris, hepatitis, pancreatitis, cholecystitis, chronic gastritis, peptic ulcer, and primary or secondary dysmenorrhea
Potential formula toxicities & interactions:
B&B: Contraindicated in pregnancy and in patients with any active hemorrhagic disorder.

POTENTIAL MEDICINAL TOXICITIES & INTERACTIONS:

Dan Shen
(Radix Salviae Miltiorrhizae)

Standard daily dosage: 6-60g
AH: Safe when used appropriately
BR: Possible additive effect to warfarin (Coumadin)
B&G: According to traditional texts, incompatible with *Li Lu* (Rhizoma Et Radix Veratri). Administration of tinctures of this herb can lead to pruritus, stomachache, or reduced appetite.
C&C: Contains potassium. Could possibly cause hyperkalemia when used with potassium-sparing diuretics. Increases the absorption and decreases the clearance of warfarin (Coumadin) which can adversely affect prothrombin time. Should not be used in cancer patients taking antineoplastic drugs, since this medicinal can hinder their therapeutic effect and promote tumor metastasis. Hinders the absorption of magnesium oxide, calcium carbonate, and aluminum hydroxide.
PDR: No health risks or side effects are known in conjunction with the proper administration of designated therapeutic dosages.

Tan Xiang, Bai Tan Xiang
(Lignum Santali Albi, sandlewood)

Standard daily dosage: 3-9g
AH: Contraindicated in kidney diseases involving the parenchyma of

the kidney. Do not use for more than six weeks without consultation with a physician.

PDR: Contraindicated in patients with kidney disease.

Sha Ren
(Fructus Amomi)

Standard daily dosage: 1.5-6g

AH: Safe when used appropriately

PDR: Use with caution in patients with gallstones since it can trigger colic due to its motility-enhancing effect.

COMMENTS

This formula is primarily used as a ready-made medicine. It is not commonly prescribed in decoction unless the ingredients in it are added to another, larger formula.

DANG GUI SI NI TANG
(Dang Gui Four Counterflows Decoction,
a.k.a. Tang-kuei & Jujube Combination)

Category: Interior-warming
Functions: Warms the channels and dissipates cold, nourishes
the blood and frees the flow of the vessels
Chinese medical indications: Cold in the channels in a patient
with blood vacuity manifesting as enduring cold hands and feet,
a pale tongue with white fur, and a fine, deep pulse
Contraindications: Effulgent fire due to yin vacuity
Western medical indications: Thromboangiitis obliterans, vari-
cose veins, frostbite, calluses and corns, dysmenorrhea, hernia,
colicky testalgia, chronic rheumatoid arthritis, Raynaud's phe-
nomenon or disease, fibromyalgia, sciatica, peptic ulcer, chronic
urticaria, midline pain, chilblains, and gangrene.
Potential formula toxicities & interactions: None listed

POTENTIAL MEDICINAL TOXICITIES & INTERACTIONS:

Dang Gui
(Radix Angelicae Sinensis)

Standard daily dosage: 3-15g
AH: Do not use during pregnancy. (This medicinal is routinely used in
Chinese medical gynecology during pregnancy as part of formulas
appropriately prescribed on the basis of pattern discrimination.)
B&G: Use with caution in patients with diarrhea or abdominal distention.
C&C: Contains potassium. Could possibly cause hyperkalemia when
used with potassium-sparing diuretics. May exaggerate the anticoagula-
tive effect of warfarin (Coumadin).

Bai Shao, Shao Yao
(Radix Albus Paeoniae Lactiflorae, white peony root)

Standard daily dosage: 6-30g
AH: Safe when used appropriately
B&G: Use with caution in debilitated patients with diarrhea. According to
some traditional sources, antagonizes *Shi Hu* (Herba Dendrobii) and *Mang
Xiao* (Mirabilitum), counteracts *Bie Jia* (Carapax Amydae Sinensis) and
Xiao Ji (Herba Cephalanopoloris Segeti), and is incompatible with *Li Lu*
(Rhizoma Et Radix Veratri).
C&C: Contains calcium, tannic acid, potassium, and glycosides. Could

possibly cause hyperkalemia when used with potassium-sparing diuretics. Could possibly reduce the effect of most antibiotics, cause digitalis intoxication and heart arrhythmias, and could possibly reduce the absorption and therapeutic effect of levadopa, isoniazid, chlorpromazine, calcium carbonate and gluconate, atropine, ephedrine, quinine, reserpine, vitamin B$_1$, trypsine, amylase, and pepsin. Vitamin C, nicotinic acid, glutamic acid, hydrochloric acid, and other highly acidic substances could possibly reduce the therapeutic effect of this medicinal.

Gui Zhi
(Ramulus Cinnamomi Cassiae, cinnamon twigs)

Standard daily dosage: 3-15g
AH: Safe when used appropriately
B&G: Use with caution in the presence of fever, during pregnancy, or during excessive menstruation.
PDR: Medicinal preparations are contraindicated during pregnancy.

Xi Xin
(Herba Asari Cum Radice)

Standard daily dosage: 1-3g
AH: Do not use during pregnancy. Contains aristolochic acid (AA). Do not exceed recommended dose.
B&G: Nephrotoxic. Use with caution in patients with renal problems. According to some traditional sources, may antagonize *Shan Zhu Yu* (Fructus Corni Officinalis) and *Huang Qi* (Radix Astragali Membranacei).
PDR: Not to be used during pregnancy.
GLW: Symptoms of adverse reaction include headache, vomiting, vexation and agitation, sweating, stiffness of the neck, oral thirst, a rapid pulse, increased body temperature and blood pressure, slightly dilated pupils, a red flushed face, twitching muscles, generalized tension which may become convulsions, clenched teeth, arched-back rigidity, unclear thinking, cramping of the four limbs, dimming of consciousness, urinary block, and, eventually, death due to respiratory paralysis.

Xi Xin is on the FDA's "B List" of herbs which may potentially contain aristolochic acid (AA). *Xi Xin* is harvested in China mostly from *Asarum sieboldi* and *Asarum heteropoides*, neither of which have conclusively been shown to contain AA. However, other species of *Asarum* are sometimes substituted, and these may contain AA. As of this writing, the FDA has set no acceptable limit to AA consumption by humans.

Gan Cao
(Radix Glycyrrhizae Uralensis, licorice)

Standard daily dosage: 2-12g
AH: Do not use during pregnancy. (This medicinal is routinely used in Chinese medical gynecology during pregnancy as part of formulas appropriately prescribed on the basis of pattern discrimination.) As a single herb in high doses, it is contraindicated in diabetes, hypertension, and liver disorders. Not for long-term use.
BR: May increase toxicity of cardiac glycosides. May increase potassium loss due to diuretics and laxatives. Possible additive effect to corticosteroids. May be synergistic with insulin in causing hypokalemia and sodium retention.
B&G: According to some traditional sources, incompatible with *Gan Sui* (Radix Euphorbiae Kansui), *Yuan Hua* (Flos Daphnes Genkwae), and *Yuan Zhi* (Radix Polygalae Tenuifoliae). If taken long-term, it may cause hypertension and/or edema. Contains glycyrrhetinic acid which could possibly cause a reduction in thyroid activity and basal metabolic rate.

The research on *Gan Cao* concurs that this medicinal is generally safe when used in small amounts as an envoy. It should not be taken long-term or as a single herb during pregnancy. When used as a single medicinal or in patients taking other potent Western pharmaceuticals, caution should be exercised to guard against potential toxicity and drug interaction.

Da Zao, Hong Zao
(Fructus Ziziphi Jujubae, red dates)

Standard daily dosage: 10-30g (3-12 pieces)
AH: Safe when used appropriately
PDR: No health risks or side effects are known in conjunction with the proper administration of designated therapeutic dosages.

Mu Tong
(Caulis Akebiae)

Standard daily dosage: 3-9g
B&G: Contraindicated during pregnancy. Could possibly cause dehydration and renal failure in large doses.
C&C: Contains potassium. Could possibly cause hyperkalemia when used with potassium-sparing diuretics.
PDR: Not to be administered during pregnancy. Large doses of the medicinal may lead to gastroenteritis, intestinal colic, and diarrhea due to saponin content.
GLW: Early stage symptoms of poisoning include upper abdominal dis-

comfort, vomiting, chest oppression, abdominal pain, and diarrhea. Secondarily, there is frequent urination, urgent urination, facial edema which gradually spreads to the entire body, inability to lie down, unclear consciousness, scanty urination or blocked urination, and increased blood pressure. Some patients present oily stools. In those with acute kidney failure, uremia leads to death.

This medicinal is often substituted with Caulis Aristolochiae Manchuriensis which contains aristolochic acid. Therefore, it is important that this medicinal only be prescribed in the form of Caulis Akebiae Trifoliatae or Akebiae Quinatae.

DAO CHI SAN
(Abduct the Red Powder,
a.k.a. Lead Out the Red Powder, Rehmannia & Akebia
Formula)

Category: Heat-clearing
Functions: Clears the heart and nourishes yin, disinhibits water
and frees the flow of strangury
Chinese medical indications: Heat in the heart & small intestine channels with easy anger, vexatious heat in the chest, dark,
scanty, astringent, and painful urination, possible hematuria,
thirst with a desire for cold drinks, a red facial complexion,
sores on the tip of the tongue, a red tongue, and a rapid pulse
Contraindications: Spleen vacuity
Western medical indications: Acute cystitis, urethritis, difficult
urination, glomerulonephritis, oral ulceration, glossitis, and
nightmares
Potential formula toxicities & interactions:
FL/B&B: Do not use in patients with diarrhea

POTENTIAL MEDICINAL TOXICITIES & INTERACTIONS:

Sheng Di, Sheng Di Huang
(uncooked Radix Rehmanniae Glutinosae)

Standard daily dosage: 9-30g
AH: Contraindicated in patients with diarrhea or lack of appetite
B&G: Contraindicated in pregnant women with anemias or digestive
weakness
C&C: Contains potassium. Could possibly cause hyperkalemia when
used with potassium-sparing diuretics.
PDR: No health risks or side effects are known in conjunction with the
proper administration of designated therapeutic dosages.

Mu Tong
(Caulis Akebiae)

Standard daily dosage: 3-9g
B&G: Contraindicated during pregnancy. Could possibly cause dehydration and renal failure in large doses.
C&C: Contains potassium. Could possibly cause hyperkalemia when
used with potassium-sparing diuretics.

PDR: Not to be administered during pregnancy. Large doses of the medicinal may lead to gastroenteritis, intestinal colic, and diarrhea due to saponin content.

GLW: Early stage symptoms of poisoning include upper abdominal discomfort, vomiting, chest oppression, abdominal pain, and diarrhea. Secondarily, there is frequent urination, urgent urination, facial edema which gradually spreads to the entire body, inability to lie down, unclear consciousness, scanty urination or blocked urination, and increased blood pressure. Some patients present oily stools. In those with acute kidney failure, uremia leads to death.

This medicinal is often substituted with Caulis Aristolochiae Manchuriensis which contains aristolochic acid. Therefore, it is important that this medicinal only be prescribed in the form of Caulis Akebiae Trifoliatae or Akebiae Quinatae.

Dan Zhu Ye
(Herba Lophatheri Gracilis)

Standard daily dosage: 6-9g
B&G: Use with caution in pregnancy.
C&C: Contains potassium. Could possibly cause hyperkalemia when used with potassium-sparing diuretics.

Gan Cao
(Radix Glycyrrhizae Uralensis, licorice)

Standard daily dosage: 2-12g
AH: Do not use during pregnancy. (This medicinal is routinely used in Chinese medical gynecology during pregnancy as part of formulas appropriately prescribed on the basis of pattern discrimination.) As a single herb in high doses, it is contraindicated in diabetes, hypertension, and liver disorders. Not for long-term use.
BR: May increase toxicity of cardiac glycosides. May increase potassium loss due to diuretics and laxatives. Possible additive effect to corticosteroids. May be synergistic with insulin in causing hypokalemia and sodium retention.
B&G: According to some traditional sources, incompatible with *Gan Sui* (Radix Euphorbiae Kansui), *Yuan Hua* (Flos Daphnes Genkwae), and *Yuan Zhi* (Radix Polygalae Tenuifoliae). If taken long-term, it may cause hypertension and/or edema. Contains glycyrrhetinic acid which could possibly cause a reduction in thyroid activity and basal metabolic rate.

The research on *Gan Cao* concurs that this medicinal is generally safe when used in small amounts as an envoy. It should not be taken long-term or as a single herb during pregnancy. When used as a single medicinal or in patients taking other potent Western pharmaceuticals, caution should be exercised to guard against potential toxicity and drug interaction.

COMMENTS

Although this formula, like *Ba Zheng San* (Eight [Ingredients] Correcting Powder) treats damp heat in the lower burner resulting in heat strangury difficult and/or painful urination, in this case, the heat has been transferred from the heart to the small intestine to the bladder. One of the keys to identifying and discriminating this pattern is the especially red tongue tip with possible/probable tongue sores. Since heart fire shifted to the bladder tends to be an acute exacerbation of depressive heat, this formula is typically only prescribed for a few days at a time. As soon as the heat has been cleared from the heart, one should switch to another formula to treat the underlying root.

DI HUANG YIN ZI
(Rehmannia Beverage)

Category: Wind-treating
Functions: Supplements and enriches kidney yin, supplements and invigorates kidney yang, opens the orifices and transforms phlegm
Chinese medical indications: Yin and yang dual vacuity with stiffness of the tongue and inability to speak, paralysis of the lower extremities, a dry mouth but no particular thirst, slimy, yellow tongue fur, and a deep, slow, fine, forceless pulse
Contraindications: Repletion disorders
Western medical indications: Amyotrophic lateral sclerosis, sequelae of cerebrovascular accident, acute transverse myelitis, hypertensive encephalopathy, cerebral arteriorsclerosis, and secondary hypertension associated with glomerulonephritis and pyelonephritis
Potential formula toxicities & interactions:
B&B: Should not be taken long-term. If taken for several weeks, *Xian Mao* (Rhizoma Curculiginis Orchioidis) and *Yin Yang Huo* (Herba Epimedii) should be substituted for *Fu Zi* (Radix Lateralis Praeparatus Aconiti Carmichaeli) and *Rou Gui* (Cortex Cinnamomi Cassiae).

POTENTIAL MEDICINAL TOXICITIES & INTERACTIONS:

Shu Di, Shu Di Huang
(cooked Radix Rehmanniae Glutinosae)

Standard daily dosage: 9-30g
AH: Contraindicated in patients with diarrhea or indigestion
B&G: Overuse can lead to abdominal distention and loose stools. Side effects include diarrhea, abdominal pain, dizziness, lethargy, and heart palpitations which often disappear upon continued administration of the herb.
PDR: No health risks or side effects are known in conjunction with the proper administration of designated therapeutic dosages.

Shan Zhu Yu, Shan Zhu Rou
(Fructus Corni Officinalis)

Standard daily dosage: 3-60g
AH: Contraindicated in patients with difficult or painful urination

B&G: Contraindicated in patients with difficult or painful urination. According to some traditional sources, antagonizes *Jie Geng* (Radix Platycodi Grandiflori), *Fang Feng* (Radix Ledebouriellae Divaricatae), and *Fang Ji* (Radix Aristolochiae Fangchi).

C&C: Contains tannic acid and glycosides. Could possibly reduce the absorption and biologic effect of most antibiotics, isoniazid, chlorpromazine, calcium carbonate and gluconate, atropine, ephedrine, quinine, reserpine, digitalis, vitamin B_1, trypsine, amylase, and pepsin. Vitamin C, nicotinic acid, glutamic acid, hydrochloric acid, and other highly acidic substances could possibly reduce the therapeutic effect of this medicinal.

PDR: No health hazards are known in conjunction with proper administration of designated therapeutic dosages.

Rou Cong Rong, Cong Rong
(Herba Cistanchis Deserticolae Seu Salsae)

Standard daily dosage: 9-21g
AH: Safe when used appropriately

Ba Ji Tian, Ba Ji Rou, Bai Ji
(Radix Morindae Officinalis)

Standard daily dosage: 6-15g
AH: Safe when used appropriately
B&G: According to some traditional sources, antagonizes *Dan Shen* (Radix Salviae Miltiorrhizae).
C&C: Highly acidic. Could possibly cause crystalluria and hematuria. Could possibly reduce the therapeutic effect of sodium bicarbonate, aluminum hydroxide, many antibiotics (especially aminoglycosides and sulfas), reserpine, caffeine, opiates, scopolamine, and berbamin.

Fu Zi, Shu Fu Zi, Fu Pian
(Radix Lateralis Praeparatus Aconiti Carmichaeli,
wolfsbane, monkshood)

Standard daily dosage: 1.5-15g
AH: To be used only under the supervision of an expert qualified in the appropriate use of this substance
B&G: Contraindicated during pregnancy. A very toxic medicinal which can be fatal if ingested in its uncooked form or in an inappropriate dose. It is generally combined with *Gan Cao* (Radix Glycyrhizae Uralensis) and *Gan Jiang* (dry Rhizoma Zingiberis Officinalis) in decoctions to

reduce its toxicity. Symptoms of toxicity include drooling, gastric upset, light-headedness, blurred vision, and numbness and tingling of the extremities. More severe symptoms include premature atrial contractions, dyspnea, and reduced temperature and blood pressure. Emergency measures include the administration of atropine.

C&C: Contains alkaloids. Could possibly reduce the absorption and therapeutic effect of potassium and sodium iodides, sodium bicarbonate, aluminum hydroxide, and magnesium sulfate.

PDR: Contains nor-diterpene alkaloids, including aconitine. Highly toxic; small doses can be fatal.

GLW: If mild poisoning, there is a burning hot sensation in the mouth and on the tongue, numbness, and pain which gradually spreads to the four limbs and then to the whole body, nausea, vomiting, dizziness, heart palpitations, rapid breathing, vexation, agitation, restlessness, drooling. If more severe poisoning, there may be generalized sweating, paralysis, convulsions, urinary incontinence, dilated pupils, slowed reaction to light, slow heartbeat, arrhythmia, low blood pressure, a somber white facial complexion, reversal chilling of the four limbs, lowered body temperature, and circulatory collapse leading to death.

Shi Hu
(Herba Dendrobii)

Standard daily dosage: 6-15g
AH: Safe when used appropriately
B&G: Retains and preserves disease evils and should not be used in patients with early stages of a warm disease. Also causes dampness and should not be used in patients with abdominal distention and thick, slimy tongue fur. Large doses had an inhibitory effect on the heart and lungs of experimental animals. Overdoses caused convulsions.

Mai Men Dong, Mai Dong
(Tuber Ophiopogoni Japonici)

Standard daily dosage: 6-15g
AH: Safe when used appropriately
B&G: According to some traditional sources, antagonizes *Kuan Dong Hua* (Flos Tussilaginis Farfarae) and counteracts *Ku Shen* (Radix Sophorae Flavescentis) and *Bai Mu Er* (Fructificatio Tremellae Fuciformis).
C&C: Contains glycosides. Vitamin C, nicotinic acid, glutamic acid, hydrochloric acid, and other highly acidic substances Could possibly reduce the therapeutic effect of this medicinal.

Shi Chang Pu, Chang Pu
(Rhizoma Acori Graminei, sweetflag rhizome)

Standard daily dosage: 3-9g
AH: Do not use during pregnancy.
B&G: According to some traditional sources, antagonizes *Ma Huang* (Herba Ephedrae). Massive overdose in mice led to convulsions, hypersensitivity to external stimuli, and death caused by stimulation of the spinal cord.
GLW: Symptoms of adverse reaction include headache, vomiting, vexation and agitation, sweating, stiffness of the neck, oral thirst, a rapid pulse, increased body temperature and blood pressure, slightly dilated pupils, a red flushed face, twitching muscles, generalized tension which may become convulsions, clenched teeth, arched-back rigidity, unclear thinking, cramping of the four limbs, dimming of consciousness, urinary block, and, eventually death due to respiratory paralysis.

Yuan Zhi
(Radix Polygalae Tenuifoliae)

Standard daily dosage: 3-9g
AH: Contraindicated in gastritis or when gastric ulcers are present.
B&G: Contraindicated in gastritis or when gastric ulcers are present. According to some traditional sources, counteracts *Zhen Zhu* (Margarita) and *Li Lu* (Rhizoma Et Radix Veratri).
C&C: Contains glycosides. Vitamin C, nicotinic acid, glutamic acid, hydrochloric acid, and other highly acidic substances could possibly reduce the therapeutic effect of this medicinal.

Fu Ling, Bai Fu Ling, Yun Ling
(Sclerotium Poriae Cocos)

Standard daily dosage: 9-15g
B&G: Large doses or long-term use is discouraged. Contraindicated in patients with frequent, copious urination. According to traditional sources, may counteract *Di Yu* (Radix Sanguisorbae Officinalis), *Qin Jiao* (Radix Gentianae Qinjiao), and *Bie Jia* (Carapax Amydae Sinensis).
C&C: Contains potassium. Could possibly cause hyperkalemia when used with potassium-sparing diuretics.

Wu Wei Zi
(Fructus Schisandrae Chinensis, schisandra)

Standard daily dosage: 1.5-9g

AH: Safe when used appropriately

B&G: Occasionally causes heartburn. In mice, toxic doses were 10-15g/kg. Symptoms of overdose included restlessness, insomnia, or dyspnea.

C&C: Contains potassium. Highly acidic. Could possibly cause crystalluria and hematuria. Could possibly cause hyperkalemia when used in large doses with potassium-sparing diuretics. Could possibly reduce the therapeutic effect of sodium bicarbonate, aluminum hydroxide, many antibiotics (especially aminoglycosides and sulfas), reserpine, caffeine, opiates, scopolamine, and berbamin.

PDR: No health risks or side effects are known in conjunction with the proper administration of designated therapeutic dosages.

Sheng Jiang
(uncooked Rhizoma Zingiberis Officinalis, fresh ginger)

Standard daily dose: 3-9g

AH: Safe when used appropriately

BR: Reduces vomiting caused by chemotherapeutic drugs. Increases absorption of oral drugs.

PDR: Recommended safe dosage limit is six grams (6g). Avoid larger doses if being used to treat morning sickness or if used in patients taking anticoagulants.

Da Zao, Hong Zao
(Fructus Zizyphi Jujubae, red dates)

Standard daily dosage: 10-30g (3-12 pieces)

AH: Safe when used appropriately

PDR: No health risks or side effects are known in conjunction with the proper administration of designated therapeutic dosages.

Bo He
(Herba Menthae Haplocalycis, field mint)

Standard daily dose: 1.5-6g

AH: Safe when used appropriately

B&G: Not recommended for nursing mothers as it may inhibit lactation.

Rou Gui, Gui Xin, Guan Gui
(Cortex Cinnamomi Cassiae, cinnamon bark)

Standard daily dosage: 1.5-4.5g

AH: Not to be used during pregnancy
BR: Reduces absorption of tetracyclines
B&G: Use with caution during pregnancy
C&C: Contains tannic acid and potassium. Could possibly cause hyper-kalemia when used with potassium-sparing diuretics. Could possibly reduce the absorption and biologic effect of most antibiotics, isoniazid, chlorpromazine, calcium carbonate and gluconate, atropine, ephedrine, quinine, reserpine, digitalis, vitamin B_1, trypsine, amylase, and pepsin.

DIE DA WAN
(Knock & Fall Pills)

Category: Blood-quickening
Functions: Quickens the blood and transforms stasis, harmonizes the constructive, disperses swelling, and stops pain
Chinese medical indications: Blood stasis after traumatic injury with bruising, swelling, distention, aching, and pain at a fixed location
Contraindications: Pregnancy
Western medical indications: Traumatic injury due to falls, fractures, contusions, and strains
Potential formula toxicities & interactions: None listed

POTENTIAL MEDICINAL TOXICITIES & INTERACTIONS:

Dang Gui
(Radix Angelicae Sinensis)

Standard daily dosage: 3-15g
AH: Do not use during pregnancy. (This medicinal is routinely used in Chinese medical gynecology during pregnancy as part of formulas appropriately prescribed on the basis of pattern discrimination.)
B&G: Use with caution in patients with diarrhea or abdominal distention.
C&C: Contains potassium. Could possibly cause hyperkalemia when used with potassium-sparing diuretics. May exaggerate the anticoagulative effect of warfarin (Coumadin).

Chuan Xiong
(Radix Ligustici Wallichii)

Standard daily dosage: 3-9g (In China today, it is not uncommon for this medicinal to be prescribed up to 15 grams per day in decoction.)
AH: Do not use during pregnancy. (This medicinal is routinely used in Chinese medical gynecology during pregnancy as part of formulas appropriately prescribed on the basis of pattern discrimination.)
B&G: Not for patients with migraine headache or excessive menstrual bleeding. Overdosage causes vomiting and dizziness. According to some traditional texts, antagonizes *Shan Zhu Yu* (Fructus Corni Officinalis) and *Huang Qi* (Radix Astragali Membranacei), counteracts *Hua Shi* (Talcum) and *Huang Lian* (Rhizoma Coptidis Chinensis), and is incompatible with *Li Lu* (Rhizoma Et Radix Veratri).
C&C: Contains alkaloids and potassium. Could possibly cause hyperkalemia when used with potassium-sparing diuretics. Could possibly

reduce the absorption and therapeutic effect of potassium and sodium iodides, sodium bicarbonate, aluminum hydroxide, and magnesium sulfate.

Ru Xiang
(Resina Olibani, frankincense)

Standard daily dosage: 3-9g
B&G: Contraindicated during pregnancy.

Mo Yao
(Resina Myrrhae, myrrh)

Standard daily dosage: 3-12g
B&G: Contraindicated during pregnancy and in patients with excessive uterine bleeding.
PDR: Not for use during pregnancy.

Xue Jie
(Sanguis Draconis)

Standard daily dosage: 0.3-1.5g as a powder or in a pill
AH: Safe when used appropriately
B&G: Contraindicated during pregnancy. Internal ingestion has been associated with one case of angioedema due to a hypersensitivity which was later reversed.

Tu Bie Chong, Di Bie Chong, Zhe Chong
(Eupolyphaga Seu Opisthoplatia)

Standard daily dosage: 3-6g
B&G: Contraindicated during pregnancy.

Ma Huang
(Herba Ephedrae, ephedra)

Standard daily dosage: 3-9g
AH: Not to be used during pregnancy. Contraindicated in anorexia, bulimia, and glaucoma. Not for long-term use.
BR: Increases thermogenesis when combined with methylxanthines in theophylline and caffeine. May induce toxicity with MAO-inhibitors. May reduce the effect of dexamethazone. Amytriptiline blocks its hypertensive effect. Antagonized by reserpine.
B&G: May raise blood pressure and cause tremors. As little as 15ml in

a 1% solution may be toxic to some individuals. May cause arrhythmias if used in conjunction with cardiac glycosides. Antidote for poisoning is atropine.

All research sources concur that *Ma Huang* is a very powerful herb with many potential side effects and interactions and, therefore, must be administered with care. It enhances digitalis, antagonizes barbiturates, and increases the effects of adrenergic agonists. It should only be pre-scribed by a properly trained practitioner and should not be given long-term or during pregnancy.

GLW: Initially after poisoning, there are central nervous and sympathet-ic nervous system symptoms, such as vexation, agitation, and restless-ness, extreme nerve reactivity, headache, dizziness, tinnitus, insomnia, nausea, vomiting, upper abdominal discomfort, dry mouth, sweating, increased blood pressure, dilated pupils, heart palpitations, shortness of breath, and precordial pain. Graver reactions include difficulty urinating, unclear vision, shock, syncope, difficulty breathing, fright reversal. If critical, there may be respiratory failure and death.

The U.S. FDA has banned the inclusion of this medicinal in all dietary supplements.

Zi Ran Tong
(Pyritum, native copper)

Standard daily dosage: 3-9g

No toxicity or interaction information listed in the sources

COMMENTS

This formula is usually administered in the form of a ready-made medicine.

DING CHUAN TANG
(Stabilize Panting Decoction, a.k.a.
Arrest Wheezing Decoction, Ma Huang & Ginkgo Combination)

Category: Qi-rectifying & counterflow-downbearing
Functions: Diffuses the lungs and downbears the qi, clears heat, transforms phlegm, and levels panting
Chinese medical indications: Wind cold depressed in the exterior and phlegm heat smoldering in the interior with coughing, panting, wheezing, profuse, thick, yellow phlegm, difficulty breathing, slimy, yellow tongue fur, and a slippery, rapid pulse
Contraindications: Wind cold external contraction without internal heat
Western medical indications: Chronic bronchitis, bronchial asthma, and bronchiolitis
Potential formula toxicities & interactions: None listed

POTENTIAL MEDICINAL TOXICITIES & INTERACTIONS:

Bai Guo, Yin Guo, Yin Xing
(Semen Ginkgo Bilobae, ginkgo seeds)

Standard daily dosage: 4.5-9g
AH: May potentiate MAO-inhibitors.
B&G: Slightly toxic and should not be taken long-term or in large quantities. Symptoms of overdose include headache, fever, tremors, irritability, and dyspnea. In serious cases, there is an increase in shedding of the mucus membranes. Antidote is 60 grams of boiled uncooked *Gan Cao* (Radix Glycyrrizae Uralensis) or 30 grams of boiled ginkgo shells.
C&C: Contains cyanophoric and other glycosides. If taken in large doses with codeine, morphine, or other opiates, hydrocyanic acid is produced which might lead to respiratory failure and death. Vitamin C, nicotinic acid, glutamic acid, hydrochloric acid, and other highly acidic substances could possibly reduce the therapeutic effect of this medicinal.
PDR: May cause cerebral hemorrhage in sensitive individuals. Avoid administering to patients on anticoagulant therapy. May cause infertility due to its adverse effect on oocytes.

Ma Huang
(Herba Ephedrae, ephedra)

Standard daily dosage: 3-9g
AH: Not to be used during pregnancy. Contraindicated in anorexia, bulimia, and glaucoma. Not for long-term use.
BR: Increases thermogenesis when combined with methylxanthines in theophylline and caffeine. May induce toxicity with MAO-inhibitors. May reduce the effect of dexamethazone. Amytriptiline blocks its hypertensive effect. Antagonized by reserpine.
B&G: May raise blood pressure and cause tremors. As little as 15ml in a 1% solution may be toxic to some individuals. May cause arrhythmias if used in conjunction with cardiac glycosides. Antidote for poisoning is atropine.

All research sources concur that *Ma Huang* is a very powerful herb with many potential side effects and interactions and, therefore, must be administered with care. It enhances digitalis, antagonizes barbiturates, and increases the effects of adrenergic agonists. It should only be prescribed by a properly trained practitioner and should not be given long-term or during pregnancy.

GLW: Initially after poisoning, there are central nervous and sympathetic nervous system symptoms, such as vexation, agitation, and restlessness, extreme nerve reactivity, headache, dizziness, tinnitus, insomnia, nausea, vomiting, upper abdominal discomfort, dry mouth, sweating, increased blood pressure, dilated pupils, heart palpitations, shortness of breath, and precordial pain. Graver reactions include difficulty urinating, unclear vision, shock, syncope, difficulty breathing, fright reversal. If critical, there may be respiratory failure and death.

The U.S. FDA has banned the inclusion of this medicinal in all dietary supplements.

Zi Su Zi, Su Zi
(Fructus Perillae Frutescentis)

Standard daily dosage: 4.5-9g
B&G: Contraindicated in cases of chronic diarrhea.

Gan Cao
(Radix Glycyrrhizae Uralensis, licorice)

Standard daily dosage: 2-12g

AH: Do not use during pregnancy. (This medicinal is routinely used in Chinese medical gynecology during pregnancy as part of formulas appropriately prescribed on the basis of pattern discrimination.) As a single herb in high doses, it is contraindicated in diabetes, hypertension, and liver disorders. Not for long-term use.

BR: May increase toxicity of cardiac glycosides. May increase potassium loss due to diuretics and laxatives. Possible additive effect to corticosteroids. May be synergistic with insulin in causing hypokalemia and sodium retention.

B&G: According to some traditional sources, incompatible with *Gan Sui* (Radix Euphorbiae Kansui), *Yuan Hua* (Flos Daphnes Genkwae), and *Yuan Zhi* (Radix Polygalae Tenuifoliae). If taken long-term, it may cause hypertension and/or edema. Contains glycyrrhetinic acid which could possibly cause a reduction in thyroid activity and basal metabolic rate.

The research on *Gan Cao* concurs that this medicinal is generally safe when used in small amounts as an envoy. It should not be taken long-term or as a single herb during pregnancy. When used as a single medicinal or in patients taking other potent Western pharmaceuticals, caution should be exercised to guard against potential toxicity and drug interaction.

Kuan Dong Hua
(Flos Tussilaginis Farfarae, coltsfoot flower)

Standard daily dosage: 1.5-9g
AH: Not to be used during pregnancy. Not for long-term use.
B&G: Large doses can lead to syncope and apnea. According to some traditional sources, antagonizes *Xuan Shen* (Radix Scrophulariae Ningpoensis) and counteracts *Bei Mu* (Bulbus Frittilariae), *Xin Yi Hua* (Flos Magnoliae), *Ma Huang* (Herba Ephedrae), *Huang Qin* (Radix Scutellariae Baicalensis), *Huang Lian* (Rhizoma Coptidis Chinensis), and *Huang Qi* (Radix Astragali Membranacei).
C&C: Vitamin C, nicotinic acid, glutamic acid, hydrochloric acid, and other highly acidic substances could possibly reduce the therapeutic effect of this medicinal.
PDR: Not for use during pregnancy or while nursing.

Xing Ren, Ku Xing Ren
(Semen Pruni Armenicae, apricot kernel)

Standard daily dosage: 3-9g
AH: To be used only under the supervision of an expert qualified in the appropriate use of this substance

B&G: Use with caution when treating infants or patients with diarrhea. Contains amygdalin and amygdalase which break down to hydrocyanic acid in the digestive tract. Lethal dosage in adults is 50-60 uncooked kernels, children 10 kernels. Eating this medicinal uncooked or in large quantities could possibly cause dizziness, nausea, vomiting, and headache, which can progress to dyspnea, spasms, dilated pupils, arrhythmias, and coma. In the advent of overdose, activated charcoal and syrup of ipacec should be administered orally.

C&C: Contains potassium and glycosides (including cyanophoric glycoside). If taken with codeine, morphine, or other opiates, hydrocyanic acid is produced, which can lead to respiratory failure and death. Could possibly cause hyperkalemia when used with potassium-sparing diuretics. Vitamin C, nicotinic acid, glutamic acid, hydrochloric acid, and other highly acidic substances will reduce the therapeutic effect of this medicinal.

GLW: Typically, 1-2 hours after ingestion of a poisonous amount, there is a bitter taste and astringent feeling within the mouth, drooling, headache, dizziness, nausea, vomiting accompanied by watery diarrhea, heart palpitations, and lack of strength. In more serious cases, there is difficulty breathing. Sometimes one can smell cyanide on the person's breath. Eventually, breathing becomes weak, consciousness becomes unclear, and the pupils of the eye dilate widely with loss of reactivity to light. The teeth become clenched, blood pressure drops, there are generalized convulsions, and respiratory paralysis leads to death.

The maximum concentration of toxins in this medicinal are in the skin and the tip. When used in Chinese medicine, the kernels are blanched to remove the skin and the tips are broken off.

Sang Bai Pi, Sang Gen Bai Pi
(Cortex Radicis Mori Albi, mulberry root bark)

Standard daily dosage: 6-15g
AH: Safe when used appropriately
B&G: Contraindicated in cases of excessive urination and for patients with cough due to the common cold.

Huang Qin, Tiao Qin
(Radix Scutellariae Baicalensis)

Standard daily dosage: 6-15g
AH: Safe when used appropriately
B&G: According to some traditional sources, counteracts *Dan Pi* (Cortex Radicis Moutan) and *Li Lu* (Rhizoma Et Radix Veratri).

C&C: Contains potassium and glycosides. Could possibly cause hyperkalemia when used with potassium-sparing diuretics. Vitamin C, nicotinic acid, glutamic acid, hydrochloric acid, and other highly acidic substances could possibly reduce the therapeutic effect of this medicinal.

Ban Xia
(Rhizoma Pinelliae Ternatae)

Standard daily dosage: 4.5-12g

AH: Do not use during pregnancy. (This medicinal is routinely used during pregnancy in China when indicated by disease and pattern discrimination.) Contraindicated in all hemorrhagic disorders.

B&G: Safe as long as it is properly prepared. Must be decocted with other herbs and not taken alone or uncooked. Toxic effects due to improper preparation or dosage include burning and numbness in throat and lips, nausea, and a feeling of pressure in the chest. Antidote is oral administration of raw ginger. Use with caution in patients with fever. According to some traditional sources, incompatible with *Wu Tou* (Radix Aconiti).

C&C: Contains alkaloids and glycosides. Could possibly reduce the absorption and therapeutic effect of potassium and sodium iodides, sodium bicarbonate, aluminum hydroxide, and magnesium sulfate. Vitamin C, nicotinic acid, glutamic acid, hydrochloric acid, and other highly acidic substances could possibly reduce the therapeutic effect of this medicinal.

GLW: Poisoning occurs within 15 minutes to three hours after ingestion of a suitable amount. Initially, there is burning pain in the mouth, tongue, and throat, and enlargement of the tongue. This is then followed by drooling, ulceration of the oral mucosa, unclear speech, difficulty swallowing, dizziness, low-grade fever, heart palpitations, numbness of the extremities, a somber white facial complexion, and a weak, forceless pulse. If severe, there may be convulsions and respiratory failure leading to death.

COMMENTS

The treatment of asthma in Chinese medicine is typically divided into two phases – acute attack phase and remission phase. During the acute attack phase, the pattern discrimination is basically divided between hot and cold patterns. This formula is for the hot pattern of acute, paroxysmal asthma. As soon as the acute attack is eliminated (meaning no more panting, wheezing, and coughing), this formula should be discontinued and the patient should be prescribed some other formula to treat the underlying roots of their condition. Therefore, this formula is not for long-term use.

Du Huo Ji Sheng Tang

(Angelica Pubescens & Loranthus Decoction,
a.k.a. Tuhuo & Vaeicum Combination)

Category: Dampness-dispelling
Functions: Dispels wind and eliminates dampness, frees the
flow of impediment and stops pain, boosts the liver and kidneys,
supplements the qi and blood
Chinese medical indications: Wind, damp, cold impediment
with liver-kidney vacuity manifesting as heaviness and pain at
fixed locations in the lower back and lower extremities accompanied stiffness, aversion to cold and a liking for warmth,
fatigue, lack of strength, a pale tongue with white fur, and a
fine, forceless, possibly slow pulse
Contraindications: Wind damp heat impediment
Western medical indications: Chronic rheumatoid arthritis,
osteoarthritis, rheumatic sciatica, lumbar strain, lumbar interver-
tebral disc herniation, pain in the midline and back during pregnancy, hemiplegia due to stroke, and the sequelae of
poliomyelitis
Potential formula toxicities & interactions: None listed

POTENTIAL MEDICINAL TOXICITIES & INTERACTIONS:

Du Huo
(Radix Angelicae Pubescentis)

Standard daily dosage: 3-9g
AH: Patients should avoid prolonged exposure to sunlight. (The authors
have never seen this reaction when this medicinal is used in the dosage
ranges commonly employed in Chinese medicine.)

Xi Xin
(Herba Asari Cum Radice)

Standard daily dosage: 1-3g
AH: Do not use during pregnancy. Contains aristolochic acid (AA). Do
not exceed recommended dose.
B&G: Nephrotoxic. Use with caution in patients with renal problems.
According to some traditional sources, may antagonize *Shan Zhu Yu*
(Fructus Corni Officinalis) and *Huang Qi* (Radix Astragali Membranacei).
PDR: Not to be used during pregnancy.

GLW: Symptoms of adverse reaction include headache, vomiting, vexation and agitation, sweating, stiffness of the neck, oral thirst, a rapid pulse, increased body temperature and blood pressure, slightly dilated pupils, a red flushed face, twitching muscles, generalized tension which may become convulsions, clenched teeth, arched-back rigidity, unclear thinking, cramping of the four limbs, dimming of consciousness, urinary block, and, eventually, death due to respiratory paralysis.

Xi Xin is on the FDA's "B List" of herbs which may potentially contain aristolochic acid (AA). *Xi Xin* is harvested in China mostly from *Asarum sieboldi* and *Asarum heteropoides*, neither of which have conclusively been shown to contain AA. However, other species of *Asarum* are sometimes substituted, and these may contain AA. As of this writing, the FDA has set no acceptable limit to AA consumption by humans.

Fang Feng
(Radix Ledebouriellae Divaricatae)

Standard daily dosage: 3-9g
AH: Safe when used appropriately
B&G: According to some traditional sources, may antagonize *Gan Jiang* (dry Rhizoma Zingiberis Officinalis), *Li Lu* (Rhizoma Et Radix Veratri) and counteracts *Bei Xie* (Rhizoma Dioscoreae Hypoglaucae).
C&C: Contains glycosides. Vitamin C, nicotinic acid, glutamic acid, hydrochloric acid, and other highly acidic substances could possibly reduce the therapeutic effect of this medicinal.

Qin Jiao
(Radix Gentianae Qinjiao)

Standard daily dosage: 4.5-12g
AH: Contraindicated in patients with diarrhea or lack of appetite
B&G: Contraindicated in cases with frequent urination or chronic pain with emaciation or diarrhea. Lethal dose in fifty percent of subjects (LD50) in mice is 480mg/kg. High dosages may cause nausea and vomiting.

Sang Ji Sheng, Sang Ji
(Ramulus Loranthi Seu Visci, mulberry mistletoe)

Standard daily dosage: 9-30g
B&G: Contains avicularin. Overdose has been shown to cause vomiting, diarrhea, and death in experimental animals.
C&C: Contains quercetin, potassium, and glycosides. Could possibly

cause hyperkalemia when used with potassium-sparing diuretics. Could possibly reduce the absorption of calcium gluconate, carbonate, and lactate, aluminum hydroxide, magnesium and ferrous sulfates, and bismuth subcarbonate. Vitamin C, nicotinic acid, glutamic acid, hydrochloric acid, and other highly acidic substances could possibly reduce the therapeutic effect of this medicinal.

Du Zhong
(Cortex Eucommiae Ulmoidis)

Standard daily dosage: 6-15g
AH: Safe when used appropriately
B&G: Has a mild sedative effect in large doses. According to some traditional sources, antagonizes *Xuan Shen* (Radix Scrophulariae Ningpoensis).
C&C: Contains tannic acid. Could possibly reduce the absorption and biologic effect of most antibiotics, isoniazid, chlorpromazine, calcium carbonate and gluconate, atropine, ephedrine, quinine, reserpine, digitalis, vitamin B_1, trypsine, amylase, and pepsin.

This medicinal contains latex. Therefore, some patients taking this medicinal may have an allergic reaction if they are allergic to latex.

Niu Xi, Huai Niu Xi, Tu Niu Xi
(Radix Achyranthis Bidentatae)

Standard daily dosage: 9-15g
AH: Not to be used during pregnancy. Contraindicated in menorrhagia.
B&G: Contraindicated during pregnancy, in debilitated patients with diarrhea, and in patients with excessive menstruation. According to some traditional sources, should not be used with *Bai Qian* (Radix Et Rhizoma Cynanchi Baiqian).
C&C: Contains alkaloids, potassium, and glycosides. Could possibly cause hyperkalemia when used with potassium-sparing diuretics. Could possibly reduce the absorption and therapeutic effect of potassium and sodium iodides, sodium bicarbonate, aluminum hydroxide, and magnesium sulfate. Vitamin C, nicotinic acid, glutamic acid, hydrochloric acid, and other highly acidic substances will reduce the therapeutic effect of this medicinal.

Rou Gui, Gui Xin, Guan Gui
(Cortex Cinnamomi Cassiae, cinnamon bark)

Standard daily dosage: 1.5-4.5g

AH: Not to be used during pregnancy

BR: Reduces absorption of tetracyclines

B&G: Use with caution during pregnancy

C&C: Contains tannic acid and potassium. Could possibly cause hyperkalemia when used with potassium-sparing diuretics. Could possibly reduce the absorption and biologic effect of most antibiotics, isoniazid, chlorpromazine, calcium carbonate and gluconate, atropine, ephedrine, quinine, reserpine, digitalis, vitamin B_1, trypsine, amylase, and pepsin.

Dang Gui
(Radix Angelicae Sinensis)

Standard daily dosage: 3-15g

AH: Do not use during pregnancy. (This medicinal is routinely used in Chinese medical gynecology during pregnancy as part of formulas appropriately prescribed on the basis of pattern discrimination.)

B&G: Use with caution in patients with diarrhea or abdominal distention.

C&C: Contains potassium. Could possibly cause hyperkalemia when used with potassium-sparing diuretics. May exaggerate the anticoagulative effect of warfarin (Coumadin).

Chuan Xiong
(Radix Ligustici Wallichii)

Standard daily dosage: 3-9g (In China today, it is not uncommon for this medicinal to be prescribed up to 15 grams per day in decoction.)

AH: Do not use during pregnancy. (This medicinal is routinely used in Chinese medical gynecology during pregnancy as part of formulas appropriately prescribed on the basis of pattern discrimination.)

B&G: Not for patients with migraine headache or excessive menstrual bleeding. Overdosage causes vomiting and dizziness. According to some traditional texts, antagonizes *Shan Zhu Yu* (Fructus Corni Officinalis) and *Huang Qi* (Radix Astragali Membranacei), counteracts *Hua Shi* (Talcum) and *Huang Lian* (Rhizoma Coptidis Chinensis), and is incompatible with *Li Lu* (Rhizoma Et Radix Veratri).

C&C: Contains alkaloids and potassium. Could possibly cause hyperkalemia when used with potassium-sparing diuretics. Could possibly reduce the absorption and therapeutic effect of potassium and sodium iodides, sodium bicarbonate, aluminum hydroxide, and magnesium sulfate.

Sheng Di, Sheng Di Huang
(uncooked Radix Rehmanniae Glutinosae)

Standard daily dosage: 9-30g
AH: Contraindicated in patients with diarrhea or lack of appetite
B&G: Contraindicated in pregnant women with anemias or digestive weakness
C&C: Contains potassium. Could possibly cause hyperkalemia when used with potassium-sparing diuretics.
PDR: No health risks or side effects are known in conjunction with the proper administration of designated therapeutic dosages.

Bai Shao, Shao Yao
(Radix Albus Paeoniae Lactiflorae, white peony root)

Standard daily dosage: 6-30g
AH: Safe when used appropriately
B&G: Use with caution in debilitated patients with diarrhea. According to some traditional sources, antagonizes *Shi Hu* (Herba Dendrobii) and *Mang Xiao* (Mirabilitum), counteracts *Bie Jia* (Carapax Amydae Sinensis) and *Xiao Ji* (Herba Cephalanopoloris Segeti), and is incompatible with *Li Lu* (Rhizoma Et Radix Veratri).
C&C: Contains calcium, tannic acid, potassium, and glycosides. Could possibly cause hyperkalemia when used with potassium-sparing diuretics. Could possibly reduce the effect of most antibiotics, cause digitalis intoxication and heart arrhythmias, and could possibly reduce the absorption and therapeutic effect of levadopa, isoniazid, chlorpromazine, calcium carbonate and gluconate, atropine, ephedrine, quinine, reserpine, vitamin B_1, trypsine, amylase, and pepsin. Vitamin C, nicotinic acid, glutamic acid, hydrochloric acid, and other highly acidic substances could possibly reduce the therapeutic effect of this medicinal.

Ren Shen
(Radix Panacis Ginseng, ginseng)

Standard daily dosage: 1-30g
AH: Contraindicated in hypertension
BR: May cause manic episodes in patients on MAO-inhibitors. May cause hypertension if consumed with caffeine. Possible additive effects to insulin. May reduce the anticoagulative effect of warfarin (Coumadin).
B&G: Contraindicated for hypertensive patients. Overdose can lead to headache, insomnia, heart palpitations, and a rise in blood pressure. A traditional antidote is mung bean soup.
C&C: Vitamin C, nicotinic acid, glutamic acid, hydrochloric acid, and

other highly acidic substances could possibly reduce the therapeutic effect of this medicinal.

PDR: Contraindicated in patients with hypertension. Not recommended in large doses during pregnancy or lactation due to potential neonatal androgenization. Enhances the effect of insulin and other antidiabetic agents. Use with MAO-inhibitors may cause headaches, tremors, and manias.

Fu Ling, Bai Fu Ling, Yun Ling
(Sclerotium Poriae Cocos)

Standard daily dosage: 9-15g

B&G: Large doses or long-term use is discouraged. Contraindicated in patients with frequent, copious urination. According to traditional sources, may counteract *Di Yu* (Radix Sanguisorbae Officinalis), *Qin Jiao* (Radix Gentianae Qinjiao), and *Bie Jia* (Carapax Amydae Sinensis).

C&C: Contains potassium. Could possibly cause hyperkalemia when used with potassium-sparing diuretics.

Gan Cao
(Radix Glycyrrhizae Uralensis, licorice)

Standard daily dosage: 2-12g

AH: Do not use during pregnancy. (This medicinal is routinely used in Chinese medical gynecology during pregnancy as part of formulas appropriately prescribed on the basis of pattern discrimination.) As a single herb in high doses, it is contraindicated in diabetes, hypertension, and liver disorders. Not for long-term use.

BR: May increase toxicity of cardiac glycosides. May increase potassium loss due to diuretics and laxatives. Possible additive effect to corticosteroids. May be synergistic with insulin in causing hypokalemia and sodium retention.

B&G: According to some traditional sources, incompatible with *Gan Sui* (Radix Euphorbiae Kansui), *Yuan Hua* (Flos Daphnes Genkwae), and *Yuan Zhi* (Radix Polygalae Tenuifoliae). If taken long-term, it may cause hypertension and/or edema. Contains glycyrrhetinic acid which could possibly cause a reduction in thyroid activity and basal metabolic rate.

The research on *Gan Cao* concurs that this medicinal is generally safe when used in small amounts as an envoy. It should not be taken long-term or as a single herb during pregnancy. When used as a single medicinal or in patients taking other potent Western pharmaceuticals, caution should be exercised to guard against potential toxicity and drug interaction.

AH= AHPA, B&B= Bensky & Barolet, B&G= Bensky & Gamble, Br= Brinker,
C&C= Chan & Cheung, Fl= Flaws, GLW= Gao Lu Wen, PDR= Physician's Desk Reference

ER CHEN TANG

(Two Aged [Ingredients] Decoction, a.k.a.
Two-Cured Decoction, Citrus & Pinellia Combination)

Category: Phlegm-transforming & dampness-drying
Functions: Dries dampness and transforms phlegm, rectifies the qi and harmonizes the center
Chinese medical indications: Phlegm dampness with cough with profuse, white phlegm, chest oppression, abdominal glomus, heart palpitations, nausea and vomiting, dizziness, an enlarged, fat tongue with teeth-marks on its edges and, thick, white, slimy fur, and a slippery pulse
Contraindications: Lung yin vacuity cough
Western medical indications: Meniere's disease, chronic tracheitis, chronic bronchitis, emphysema, goiter, chronic gastritis, peptic ulcer, eclampsia, hangover, gastroptis, and neurosis
Potential formula toxicities & interactions:
B&B: Improper use of this formula can lead to excessive thirst and a dry throat.

POTENTIAL MEDICINAL TOXICITIES & INTERACTIONS:

Ban Xia

(Rhizoma Pinelliae Ternatae)

Standard daily dosage: 4.5-12g
AH: Do not use during pregnancy. (This medicinal is routinely used during pregnancy in China when indicated by disease and pattern discrimination.) Contraindicated in all hemorrhagic disorders.
B&G: Safe as long as it is properly prepared. Must be decocted with other herbs and not taken alone or uncooked. Toxic effects due to improper preparation or dosage include burning and numbness in throat and lips, nausea, and a feeling of pressure in the chest. Antidote is oral administration of raw ginger. Use with caution in patients with fever. According to some traditional sources, incompatible with *Wu Tou* (Radix Aconiti).
C&C: Contains alkaloids and glycosides. Could possibly reduce the absorption and therapeutic effect of potassium and sodium iodides, sodium bicarbonate, aluminum hydroxide, and magnesium sulfate. Vitamin C, nicotinic acid, glutamic acid, hydrochloric acid, and other highly acidic substances could possibly reduce the therapeutic effect of this medicinal.

GLW: Poisoning occurs within 15 minutes to three hours after ingestion of a suitable amount. Initially, there is burning pain in the mouth, tongue, and throat, and enlargement of the tongue. This is then followed by drooling, ulceration of the oral mucosa, unclear speech, difficulty swallowing, dizziness, low-grade fever, heart palpitations, numbness of the extremities, a somber white facial complexion, and a weak, forceless pulse. If severe, there may be convulsions and respiratory failure leading to death.

Chen Pi, Ju Pi, Ju Hong
(Pericarpium Citri Reticulatae)

Standard daily dosage: 3-9g
AH: Safe when used appropriately
C&C: Contains potassium. Could possibly cause hyperkalemia when used with potassium-sparing diuretics.

Fu Ling, Bai Fu Ling, Yun Ling
(Sclerotium Poriae Cocos)

Standard daily dosage: 9-15g
B&G: Large doses or long-term use is discouraged. Contraindicated in patients with frequent, copious urination. According to traditional sources, may counteract *Di Yu* (Radix Sanguisorbae Officinalis), *Qin Jiao* (Radix Gentianae Qinjiao), and *Bie Jia* (Carapax Amydae Sinensis).
C&C: Contains potassium. Could possibly cause hyperkalemia when used with potassium-sparing diuretics.

Gan Cao
(Radix Glycyrrhizae Uralensis, licorice)

Standard daily dosage: 2-12g
AH: Do not use during pregnancy. (This medicinal is routinely used in Chinese medical gynecology during pregnancy as part of formulas appropriately prescribed on the basis of pattern discrimination.) As a single herb in high doses, it is contraindicated in diabetes, hypertension, and liver disorders. Not for long-term use.
BR: May increase toxicity of cardiac glycosides. May increase potassium loss due to diuretics and laxatives. Possible additive effect to corticosteroids. May be synergistic with insulin in causing hypokalemia and sodium retention.
B&G: According to some traditional sources, incompatible with *Gan Sui* (Radix Euphorbiae Kansui), *Yuan Hua* (Flos Daphnes Genkwae), and *Yuan Zhi* (Radix Polygalae Tenuifoliae). If taken long-term, it may

cause hypertension and/or edema. Contains glycyrrhetinic acid which could possibly cause a reduction in thyroid activity and basal metabolic rate.

The research on *Gan Cao* concurs that this medicinal is generally safe when used in small amounts as an envoy. It should not be taken long-term or as a single herb during pregnancy. When used as a single medicinal or in patients taking other potent Western pharmaceuticals, caution should be exercised to guard against potential toxicity and drug interaction.

Sheng Jiang
(uncooked Rhizoma Zingiberis Officinalis, fresh ginger)

Standard daily dose: 3-9g
AH: Safe when used appropriately
BR: Reduces vomiting caused by chemotherapeutic drugs. Increases absorption of oral drugs.
PDR: Recommended safe dosage limit is six grams (6g). Avoid larger doses if being used to treat morning sickness or if used in patients taking anticoagulants.

Wu Mei
(Frcutus Pruni Mume)

Standard daily dosage: 3-9g
AH: Safe when used appropriately
C&C: Highly acidic. Could possibly cause crystalluria and hematuria. Could possibly reduce the therapeutic effect of sodium bicarbonate, aluminum hydroxide, many antibiotics (especially aminoglycosides and sulfas), reserpine, caffeine, opiates, scopolamine, and berbamin.

COMMENTS

Wu Mei is often omitted from this formula. The three main ingredients in this formula (*Ban Xia, Chen Pi,* and *Fu Ling*) are also often added to other formulas whenever there is the need to transform phlegm and eliminate dampness.

ER XIAN TANG
(Two Immortals Decoction)

Category: Yang-supplementing
Functions: Enriches and supplements the liver and kidneys, warms yang but drains fire, regulates the chong and ren
Chinese medical indications: Liver blood-kidney yin & yang vacuity with internal heat manifesting as amenorrhea, night sweats, hot flashes, insomnia, dizziness, nervousness, fatigue, heart palpitations, and urinary frequency
Contraindications: None listed
Western medical indications: Menopausal complaints, amenorrhea, hypertension, nephritis, chronic pyelonephritis, chronic glomerulonephritis, polycystic kidneys, renal vascular disease, urinary tract infection, and hypofunction of the anterior pituitary
Potential formula toxicities & interactions:
Fl: Because this formula contains *Xian Mao* (Rhizoma Curculiginis Orchioidis) which is toxic, it should not be taken long-term.

POTENTIAL MEDICINAL TOXICITIES & INTERACTIONS:

Xian Mao
(Rhizoma Curculiginis Orchioidis)

Standard daily dosage: 3-9g
B&G: Not recommended for long-term use. Toxic reactions, such as swelling of the tongue, can occur. Antidote is a decoction of *Da Huang* (Radix Et Rhizoma Rhei), *Huang Lian* (Rhizoma Coptidis Chinensis), and *Huang Qin* (Radix Scutellariae Baicalensis).
C&C: Contains alkaloids & tannic acid. Could possibly reduce the absorption and therapeutic effect of potassium and sodium iodides, sodium bicarbonate, aluminum hydroxide, magnesium sulfate, most antibiotics, isoniazid, chlorpromazine, calcium carbonate and gluconate, atropine, ephedrine, quinine, reserpine, digitalis, vitamin B_1, trypsine, amylase, and pepsin.

Symptoms of overdose or toxicity from this medicinal commonly include the eruption of mouth and tongue sores.

Yin Yang Huo, Xian Ling Pi
(Herba Epimedii)

Standard daily dosage: 6-15g
AH: Not for long-term use
B&G: Not for long-term use. Japanese forms of this herb have caused hyper reflexia and spasms in mice. Large doses could possibly cause respiratory arrest.
C&C: Contains tannic acid, potassium, and glycosides. Could possibly cause hyperkalemia when used with potassium-sparing diuretics. Could possibly reduce the absorption and biologic effect of most antibiotics, isoniazid, chlorpromazine, calcium carbonate and gluconate, atropine, ephedrine, quinine, reserpine, digitalis, vitamin B_1, trypsine, amylase, and pepsin. Vitamin C, nicotinic acid, glutamic acid, hydrochloric acid, and other highly acidic substances could possibly reduce the therapeutic effect of this medicinal.

Ba Ji Tian, Ba Ji Rou, Ba Ji
(Radix Morindae Officinalis)

Standard daily dosage: 6-15g
AH: Safe when used appropriately
B&G: According to some traditional sources, antagonizes *Dan Shen* (Radix Salviae Miltiorrhizae).
C&C: Highly acidic. Could possibly cause crystalluria and hematuria. Could possibly reduce the therapeutic effect of sodium bicarbonate, aluminum hydroxide, many antibiotics (especially aminoglycosides and sulfas), reserpine, caffeine, opiates, scopolamine, and berbamin.

Huang Bai, Huang Bo
(Cortex Phellodendri)

Standard daily dosage: 3-12g
AH: Do not use during pregnancy. (This medicinal is commonly used during pregnancy in China.)
B&G: Chinese literature reports one case of a patient who developed a skin rash after ingestion.
C&C: Contains alkaloids & quercetin. Could possibly reduce the absorption and therapeutic effect of potassium and sodium iodides, sodium bicarbonate, calcium gluconate, carbonate, and lactate, aluminum hydroxide, magnesium and ferrous sulfates, and bismuth subcarbonate.

Zhi Mu
(Rhizoma Anemarrhenae Aspheloidis)

Standard daily dosage: 6-12g
AH: Safe when used appropriately.
B&G: May cause diarrhea in some patients.
C&C: Contains potassium and glycosides. Could possibly cause hyperkalemia when used with potassium-sparing diuretics. Vitamin C, nicotinic acid, glutamic acid, hydrochloric acid, and other highly acidic substances could possibly reduce the therapeutic effect of this medicinal.
PDR: No health hazards are known in conjunction with the proper administration of designated therapeutic dosages.

Dang Gui
(Radix Angelicae Sinensis)

Standard daily dosage: 3-15g
AH: Do not use during pregnancy. (This medicinal is routinely used in Chinese medical gynecology during pregnancy as part of formulas appropriately prescribed on the basis of pattern discrimination.)
B&G: Use with caution in patients with diarrhea or abdominal distention.
C&C: Contains potassium. Could possibly cause hyperkalemia when used with potassium-sparing diuretics. May exaggerate the anticoagulative effect of warfarin (Coumadin).

COMMENTS

While this formula was originally created to treat perimenopausal hypertension, it has become a very popular one for treating perimenopausal syndrome in general. However, it is rarely prescribed in its simple, discrete form. Often *Yin Yang Huo* is deleted from this formula for fear of its toxicity resulting in the engenderment of internal heat.

GAN MAI DA ZAO TANG

(Licorice, Wheat & Red Date Decoction,
a.k.a. Licorice & Jujube Combination)

Category: Spirit-quieting
Functions: Nourishes the heart, calms the spirit, and harmonizes
the middle burner
Chinese medical indications: Visceral agitation due to mal-
nourishment of the heart spirit with loss of constancy of crying
and laughing, inability to control oneself, insomnia, frequent
yawning, a red tongue with scanty fur, and a fine, rapid, commonly bowstring pulse
Contraindications: None listed
Western medical indications: Hysteria, neurosis, menopausal
syndrome, autonomic dystonia, enuresis, and fever of unknown
etiology
Potential formula toxicities & interactions: None listed

POTENTIAL MEDICINAL TOXICITIES & INTERACTIONS:

Gan Cao

(Radix Glycyrrhizae Uralensis, licorice)

Standard daily dosage: 2-12g
AH: Do not use during pregnancy. (This medicinal is routinely used in
Chinese medical gynecology during pregnancy as part of formulas
appropriately prescribed on the basis of pattern discrimination.) As a
single herb in high doses, it is contraindicated in diabetes, hypertension,
and liver disorders. Not for long-term use.
BR: May increase toxicity of cardiac glycosides. May increase potassium loss due to diuretics and laxatives. Possible additive effect to corticosteroids. May be synergistic with insulin in causing hypokalemia and
sodium retention.
B&G: According to some traditional sources, incompatible with *Gan Sui*
(Radix Euphorbiae Kansui), *Yuan Hua* (Flos Daphnes Genkwae), and
Yuan Zhi (Radix Polygalae Tenuifoliae). If taken long-term, it may cause
hypertension and/or edema. Contains glycyrrhetinic acid which could possibly cause a reduction in thyroid activity and basal metabolic rate.

The research on *Gan Cao* concurs that this medicinal is generally safe
when used in small amounts as an envoy. It should not be taken long-term
or as a single herb during pregnancy. When used as a single medicinal or

in patients taking other potent Western pharmaceuticals, caution should be exercised to guard against potential toxicity and drug interaction.

Xiao Mai, Huai Xiao Mai, Fu Xiao Mai

(*Fu Xiao Mai* is the blighted form of this seed. It is used especially when there are spontaneous perspiration and/or night sweats. A portion of this seed floats when thrown into water.)

(Semen Tritici Aestivi, wheat)

Standard daily dosage: 9-15g (It is common for this medicinal to be prescribed in China in doses of up to 60 grams per day.)

PDR: No health risks or side effects are known in conjunction with the proper administration, of designated therapeutic dosages.

Da Zao, Hong Zao

(Fructus Zizyphi Jujubae, red dates)

Standard daily dosage: 10-30g (3-12 pieces)

AH: Safe when used appropriately

PDR: No health risks or side effects are known in conjunction with the proper administration of designated therapeutic dosages.

COMMENTS

Unless administered in some ready-made form, this formula is rarely prescribed in its simple, discrete form. More commonly, these three ingredients are added to other formulas when there is spirit disquietude due to lack of nourishment and construction.

GE GEN TANG
(Pueraria Decoction, a.k.a. Pueraria Combination)

Category: Exterior-resolving
Functions: Resolves the exterior, resolves the muscles, and engenders fluids
Chinese medical indications: External contraction of wind cold accompanied by fever, aversion to wind, no sweating, a sore, stiff neck and upper back, thin, white tongue fur, and a floating, tight or bowstring pulse
Contraindications: Wind heat external contraction
Western medical indications: Upper respiratory tract infection, influenza, stomach flu, acute cervical myositis, tendinitis, or bursitis of the shoulder, urticaria, allergic rhinitis, and early stage poliomyelitis or encephalitis, chronic pediatric diarrhea
Potential formula toxicities & interactions: None listed

POTENTIAL MEDICINAL TOXICITIES & INTERACTIONS:

Ge Gen
(Radix Puerariae, kudzu root)

Standard daily dosage: 6-12g (For the treatment of upper back and nape of the neck stiffness and tension, this medicinal is commonly prescribed up to 18 grams per day.)
AH: Safe when used appropriately

Ma Huang
(Herba Ephedrae, ephedra)

Standard daily dosage: 3-9g
AH: Not to be used during pregnancy. Contraindicated in anorexia, bulimia, and glaucoma. Not for long-term use.
BR: Increases thermogenesis when combined with methylxanthines in theophylline and caffeine. May induce toxicity with MAO-inhibitors. May reduce the effect of dexamethazone. Amytriptiline blocks its hypertensive effect. Antagonized by reserpine.
B&G: May raise blood pressure and cause tremors. As little as 15ml in a 1% solution may be toxic to some individuals. May cause arrhythmias if used in conjunction with cardiac glycosides. Antidote for poisoning is atropine.

All research sources concurs that *Ma Huang* is a very powerful herb with many potential side effects and interactions and, therefore, must be administered with care. It enhances digitalis, antagonizes barbiturates, and increases the effects of adrenergic agonists. It should only be prescribed by a properly trained practitioner and should not be given long-term or during pregnancy.

GLW: Initially after poisoning, there are central nervous and sympathetic nervous system symptoms, such as vexation, agitation, and restlessness, extreme nerve reactivity, headache, dizziness, tinnitus, insomnia, nausea, vomiting, upper abdominal discomfort, dry mouth, sweating, increased blood pressure, dilated pupils, heart palpitations, shortness of breath, and precordial pain. Graver reactions include difficulty urinating, unclear vision, shock, syncope, difficulty breathing, fright reversal. If critical, there may be respiratory failure and death.

The U.S. FDA has banned the inclusion of this medicinal in all dietary supplements.

Gui Zhi
(Ramulus Cinnamomi Cassiae, cinnamon twigs)

Standard daily dosage: 3-15g
AH: Safe when used appropriately
B&G: Use with caution in the presence of fever, during pregnancy, or during excessive menstruation.
PDR: Contraindicated during pregnancy.

Bai Shao, Shao Yao
(Radix Albus Paeoniae Lactiflorae, white peony root)

Standard daily dosage: 6-30g
AH: Safe when used appropriately
B&G: Use with caution in debilitated patients with diarrhea. According to some traditional sources, antagonizes *Shi Hu* (Herba Dendrobii) and *Mang Xiao* (Mirabilitum), counteracts *Bie Jia* (Carapax Amydae Sinensis) and *Xiao Ji* (Herba Cephalanopoloris Segeti), and is incompatible with *Li Lu* (Rhizoma Et Radix Veratri).
C&C: Contains calcium, tannic acid, potassium, and glycosides. Could possibly cause hyperkalemia when used with potassium-sparing diuretics. Could possibly reduce the effect of most antibiotics, cause digitalis intoxication and heart arrhythmias, and could possibly reduce the absorption and therapeutic effect of levadopa, isoniazid, chlorpromazine, calcium carbonate and gluconate, atropine, ephedrine, quinine, reserpine, vitamin B_1, trypsine, amylase, and pepsin. Vitamin C, nicotinic acid, glutamic acid, hydrochloric acid, and other highly acidic substances could possibly reduce the therapeutic effect of this medicinal.

Sheng Jiang
(uncooked Rhizoma Zingiberis Officinalis, fresh ginger)

Standard daily dose: 3-9g
AH: Safe when used appropriately
BR: Reduces vomiting caused by chemotherapeutic drugs. Increases absorption of oral drugs.
PDR: Recommended safe dosage limit is six grams (6g). Avoid larger doses if being used to treat morning sickness or if used in patients taking anticoagulants.

Da Zao, Hong Zao
(Fructus Zizyphi Jujubae, red dates)

Standard daily dosage: 10-30g (3-12 pieces)
AH: Safe when used appropriately
PDR: No health risks or side effects are known in conjunction with the proper administration of designated therapeutic dosages.

Gan Cao
(Radix Glycyrrhizae Uralensis, licorice)

Standard daily dosage: 2-12g
AH: Do not use during pregnancy. (This medicinal is routinely used in Chinese medical gynecology during pregnancy as part of formulas appropriately prescribed on the basis of pattern discrimination.) As a single herb in high doses, it is contraindicated in diabetes, hypertension, and liver disorders. Not for long-term use.
BR: May increase toxicity of cardiac glycosides. May increase potassium loss due to diuretics and laxatives. Possible additive effect to corticosteroids. May be synergistic with insulin in causing hypokalemia and sodium retention.
B&G: According to some traditional sources, incompatible with *Gan Sui* (Radix Euphorbiae Kansui), *Yuan Hua* (Flos Daphnes Genkwae), and *Yuan Zhi* (Radix Polygalae Tenuifoliae). If taken long-term, it may cause hypertension and/or edema. Contains glycyrrhetinic acid which Could possibly cause a reduction in thyroid activity and basal metabolic rate.

The research on *Gan Cao* concurs that this medicinal is generally safe when used in small amounts as an envoy. It should not be taken long-term or as a single herb during pregnancy. When used as a single medicinal or in patients taking other potent Western pharmaceuticals, caution should be exercised to guard against potential toxicity and drug interaction.

GU CHONG TANG
(Secure the Chong Decoction)

Category: Securing & astringing
Functions: Boosts the qi and fortifies the spleen, secures the
chong and stops bleeding
Chinese medical indications: Uterine bleeding or menorrhagia
due to spleen-kidney qi vacuity with either profuse, pale, thin
blood or a continuous trickle, heart palpitations, shortness of
breath, a pale tongue, and fine, forceless pulse
Contraindications: Blood heat bleeding or vacuity desertion
Western medical indications: Functional uterine bleeding,
excessive lochiorrhea, bleeding peptic ulcers
Potential formula toxicities & interactions:
FL/B&B: Not for patients with severe bleeding accompanied by
profuse sweating, cold limbs, and a faint pulse.

POTENTIAL MEDICINAL TOXICITIES & INTERACTIONS:

Bai Zhu
(Rhizoma Atractylodis Macrocephalae)

Standard daily dosage: 4.5-9g
AH: Safe when used appropriately
B&G: When rats were fed 0.5g/kg of this medicinal for two months,
they developed a mild lymphopenia and anemia but suffered no damage
to the brain, heart, or liver.

Huang Qi, Bei Qi
(Radix Astragali Membranacei, astragalus)

Standard daily dosage: 9-60g
AH: Safe when used appropriately
C&C: Contains alkaloids and potassium. Could possibly cause hyperkalemia when used with potassium-sparing diuretics. Could possibly
reduce the absorption and therapeutic effect of potassium and sodium
iodides, sodium bicarbonate, aluminum hydroxide, and magnesium sulfate.
PDR: Caution should be taken with patients receiving immunosuppressive therapy, such as transplant patients or patients with autoimmune
disorders. May cause neurological dysfunction in high doses. May
potentiate the risk of bleeding when used concomitantly with anticoagulants, antiplatelets, or antithrombotic agents.

Shan Zhu Yu, Shan Zhu Rou
(Fructus Corni Officinalis)

Standard daily dosage: 3-60g
AH: Contraindicated in patients with difficult or painful urination
B&G: Contraindicated in patients with difficult or painful urination.
According to some traditional sources, antagonizes *Jie Geng* (Radix
Platycodi Grandiflori), *Fang Feng* (Radix Ledebouriellae Divaricatae),
and *Fang Ji* (Radix Aristolochiae Fangchi).
C&C: Contains tannic acid and glycosides. Could possibly reduce the
absorption and biologic effect of most antibiotics, isoniazid, chlorpromazine, calcium carbonate and gluconate, atropine, ephedrine, quinine,
reserpine, digitalis, vitamin B$_1$, trypsine, amylase, and pepsin. Vitamin C,
nicotinic acid, glutamic acid, hydrochloric acid, and other highly acidic
substances could possibly reduce the therapeutic effect of this medicinal.
PDR: No health hazards are known in conjunction with proper administration of designated therapeutic dosages.

Bai Shao, Shao Yao
(Radix Albus Paeoniae Lactiflorae, white peony root)

Standard daily dosage: 6-30g
AH: Safe when used appropriately
B&G: Use with caution in debilitated patients with diarrhea. According
to some traditional sources, antagonizes *Shi Hu* (Herba Dendrobii) and
Mang Xiao (Mirabilitum), counteracts *Bie Jia* (Carapax Amydae
Sinensis) and *Xiao Ji* (Herba Cephalanopoloris Segeti), and is incompatible with *Li Lu* (Rhizoma Et Radix Veratri).
C&C: Contains calcium, tannic acid, potassium, and glycosides. Could
possibly cause hyperkalemia when used with potassium-sparing diuretics. Could possibly reduce the effect of most antibiotics, cause digitalis
intoxication and heart arrhythmias, and could possibly reduce the
absorption and therapeutic effect of levadopa, isoniazid, chlorpromazine,
calcium carbonate and gluconate, atropine, ephedrine, quinine, reserpine, vitamin B$_1$, trypsine, amylase, and pepsin. Vitamin C, nicotinic
acid, glutamic acid, hydrochloric acid, and other highly acidic substances could possibly reduce the therapeutic effect of this medicinal.

Long Gu
(Os Draconis, fossilized bone)

Standard daily dosage: 15-30g
B&G: According to some traditional sources, counteracts *Shi Gao*
(Gypsum Fibrosum) and should not be mixed with fish.

C&C: Contains calcium, iron, magnesium, aluminum, and potassium. Could possibly cause hyperkalemia when used with potassium-sparing diuretics. Could possibly reduce the effect of most antibiotics, levadopa, and prednisolone, cause digitalis intoxication and heart arrhythmias, and hinder the absorption of isoniazid.

Mu Li
(Concha Ostreae, oyster shell)

Standard daily dosage: 15-30g
B&G: Contraindicated when the patient has high fever without sweating. Overdose may lead to indigestion or constipation. According to some traditional sources, works synergistically with *Bei Mu* (Bulbus Fritillariae), *Gan Cao* (Radix Glycyrrizae Uralensis), *Niu Xi* (Radix Achyranthis Bidentatae), and *Yuan Zhi* (Radix Polygalae Tenuifoliae), and has adverse effects when combined with *Ma Huang* (Herba Ephedrae), *Wu Zhu Yu* (Fructus Evodiae Rutecarpae), and *Xi Xin* (Herba Asari Cum Radice).
C&C: Contains calcium, iron, magnesium, and aluminum. Could possibly reduce the effects of most antibiotics, levadopa, and prednisolone, cause digitalis intoxication and heart arrhythmias, and hinder the absorption of isoniazid.

Hai Piao Xiao, Wu Zei Gu
(Os Sepiae Seu Sepiellae, cuttlefish bone)

Standard daily dosage: 4.5-12g
B&G: If used too long, may lead to constipation. According to some traditional sources, antagonizes *Fu Zi* (Radix Lateralis Praeparatus Aconiti Carmichaeli) and *Bai Ji* (Rhizoma Bletillae Striatae).
C&C: Contains calcium and magnesium. Could possibly reduce the effect of most antibiotics, levadopa, and prednisolone, cause digitalis intoxication and heart arrhythmias, and hinder the absorption of isoniazid.

Lu Zong Tan
(carbonized Fibra Stipulae Trachycarpi)

Standard daily dosage: 9-15g

No toxicity or interaction information listed in the sources

Wu Bei Zi
(Galla Rhois Chinensis, sumac nutgall)

Standard daily dosage: 1.5-6g

No toxicity or interaction information listed in the sources

Qian Cao, Qian Cao Gen
(Radix Rubiae Cordifoliae)

Standard daily dosage: 6-9g

No toxicity or interaction information listed in the sources

COMMENTS

The spleen, as the latter heaven root, and the kidneys, as the former heaven root, are mutually rooted. Therefore, enduring spleen disease may eventually reach the kidneys resulting in kidney qi not securing. This is exactly the type of uterine bleeding this formula addresses, a spleen-kidney qi vacuity. In its unmodified form, it is not for the treatment of blood heat bleeding nor does it address the common complication of blood stasis.

GUI PI TANG
(Return the Spleen Decoction, a.k.a. Ginseng & Longan
Combination)

Category: Qi & blood supplementing
Functions: Boosts the qi and supplements the blood, fortifies the
spleen and nourishes the heart
Chinese medical indications: Heart-spleen dual vacuity with
impaired memory, heart palpitations, insomnia, profuse dreams,
anxiety and worry, fatigue, lack of strength, poor appetite, a sallow yellow facial complexion, pale lips and nails, a pale,
enlarged tongue with teeth-marks on its edges and thin, white
fur, and a fine, forceless pulse
Contraindications: None listed
Western medical indications: Insomnia, sleep disturbances,
mood and personality disorders, functional uterine bleeding,
thrombocytic or allergic purpura, superventricular tachycardia,
congestive heart disease, postconcussion syndrome, and myasthenia gravis
Potential formula toxicities & interactions: None listed

POTENTIAL MEDICINAL TOXICITIES & INTERACTIONS:

Ren Shen
(Radix Panacis Ginseng, ginseng)

Standard daily dosage: 1-30g
AH: Contraindicated in hypertension
BR: May cause manic episodes in patients on MAO-inhibitors. May
cause hypertension if consumed with caffeine. Possible additive effects
to insulin. May reduce the anticoagulative effect of warfarin
(Coumadin).
B&G: Contraindicated for hypertensive patients. Overdose can lead to
headache, insomnia, heart palpitations, and a rise in blood pressure. A
traditional antidote is mung bean soup.
C&C: Vitamin C, nicotinic acid, glutamic acid, hydrochloric acid, and
other highly acidic substances could possibly reduce the therapeutic
effect of this medicinal.
PDR: Contraindicated in patients with hypertension. Not recommended in
large doses during pregnancy or lactation due to potential neonatal andro-

genization. Enhances the effect of insulin and other antidiabetic agents. Use with MAO-inhibitors may cause headaches, tremors, and manias.

Huang Qi, Bei Qi
(Radix Astragali Membranacei, astragalus)

Standard daily dosage: 9-60g
AH: Safe when used appropriately
C&C: Contains alkaloids and potassium. Could possibly cause hyperkalemia when used with potassium-sparing diuretics. Could possibly reduce the absorption and therapeutic effect of potassium and sodium iodides, sodium bicarbonate, aluminum hydroxide, magnesium sulfate.
PDR: Caution should be taken with patients receiving immunosuppressive therapy, such as transplant patients or patients with autoimmune disorders. May cause neurological dysfunction in high doses. May potentiate the risk of bleeding when used concomitantly with anticoagulants, antiplatelets, or antithrombotic agents.

Bai Zhu
(Rhizoma Atractylodis Macrocephalae)

Standard daily dosage: 4.5-9g
AH: Safe when used appropriately
B&G: When rats were fed 0.5g/kg of this medicinal for two months, they developed a mild lymphopenia and anemia but suffered no damage to the brain, heart, or liver.

Fu Ling, Bai Fu Ling, Yun Ling
(Sclerotium Poriae Cocos)

Standard daily dosage: 9-15g
B&G: Large doses or long-term use is discouraged. Contraindicated in patients with frequent, copious urination. According to traditional sources, may counteract *Di Yu* (Radix Sanguisorbae Officinalis), *Qin Jiao* (Radix Gentianae Qinjiao), and *Bie Jia* (Carapax Amydae Sinensis).
C&C: Contains potassium. Could possibly cause hyperkalemia when used with potassium-sparing diuretics.

Suan Zao Ren
(Semen Zizyphi Spinosae)

Standard daily dosage: 9-18g
AH: Not to be used during pregnancy. (No such prohibition exists for this medicinal in traditional Chinese medicine.)

Long Yan Rou, Yuan Rou
(Arillus Euphoriae Longanae, longan fruit)

Standard daily dosage: 6-30g

No toxicity or interaction information listed in the sources

Mu Xiang
(Radix Aucklandiae Lappae)

Standard daily dosage: 1.5-9g
AH: Safe when used appropriately
PDR: No health risks or side effects are known in conjunction with the proper administration of designated therapeutic dosages.

Gan Cao
(Radix Glycyrrhizae Uralensis, licorice root)

Standard daily dosage: 2-12g
AH: Do not use during pregnancy. (This medicinal is routinely used in Chinese medical gynecology during pregnancy as part of formulas appropriately prescribed on the basis of pattern discrimination.) As a single herb in high doses, it is contraindicated in diabetes, hypertension, and liver disorders. Not for long-term use.
BR: May increase toxicity of cardiac glycosides. May increase potassium loss due to diuretics and laxatives. Possible additive effect to corticosteroids. May be synergistic with insulin in causing hypokalemia and sodium retention.
B&G: According to some traditional sources, incompatible with *Gan Sui* (Radix Euphorbiae Kansui), *Yuan Hua* (Flos Daphnes Genkwae), and *Yuan Zhi* (Radix Polygalae Tenuifoliae). If taken long-term, it may cause hypertension and/or edema. Contains glycyrrhetinic acid which could possibly cause a reduction in thyroid activity and basal metabolic rate.

The research on *Gan Cao* concurs that this medicinal is generally safe when used in small amounts as an envoy. It should not be taken long-term or as a single herb during pregnancy. When used as a single medicinal or in patients taking other potent Western pharmaceuticals, caution should be exercised to guard against potential toxicity and drug interaction.

Dang Gui
(Radix Angelicae Sinensis)

Standard daily dosage: 3-15g
AH: Do not use during pregnancy. (This medicinal is routinely used in Chinese medical gynecology during pregnancy as part of formulas

appropriately prescribed on the basis of pattern discrimination.)
B&G: Use with caution in patients with diarrhea or abdominal distention.
C&C: Contains potassium. Could possibly cause hyperkalemia when used with potassium-sparing diuretics. May exaggerate the anticoagulative effect of warfarin (Coumadin).

Yuan Zhi
(Radix Polygalae Tenuifoliae)

Standard daily dosage: 3-9g
AH: Contraindicated in gastritis or when gastric ulcers are present.
B&G: Contraindicated in gastritis or when gastric ulcers are present. According to some traditional sources, counteracts *Zhen Zhu* (Margarita) and *Li Lu* (Rhizoma Et Radix Veratri).
C&C: Contains glycosides. Vitamin C, nicotinic acid, glutamic acid, hydrochloric acid, and other highly acidic substances could possibly reduce the therapeutic effect of this medicinal.

Sheng Jiang
(uncooked Rhizoma Zingiberis Officinalis, fresh ginger)

Standard daily dose: 3-9g
AH: Safe when used appropriately
BR: Reduces vomiting caused by chemotherapeutic drugs. Increases absorption of oral drugs.
PDR: Recommended safe dosage limit is six grams (6g). Avoid larger doses if being used to treat morning sickness or if used in patients taking anticoagulants.

Da Zao, Hong Zao
(Fructus Zizyphi Jujubae, red dates)

Standard daily dosage: 10-30g (3-12 pieces)
AH: Safe when used appropriately
PDR: No health risks or side effects are known in conjunction with the proper administration of designated therapeutic dosages.

COMMENTS

This formula does address an element of liver depression which commonly complicates a heart-spleen dual vacuity. In case of even more pronounced liver depression, one or more other qi-rectifying agents may be added.

Chapter 4
Toxicities & Drug Interaction • 133

GUI ZHI FU LING WAN
(Cinnamon Twig & Poria Pills, a.k.a. Cinnamon & Hoelen Formula)

Category: Blood-quickening
Functions: Quickens the blood and transforms stasis, disperses concretions and gatherings
Chinese medical indications: Uterine blood stasis with mild, ceaseless uterine bleeding during pregnancy which is dark and purplish, abdominal pain that refuses pressure, blocked menstruation with distention and pain, painful menstruation, nonprecipitation of the lochia, a dark, purplish tongue or possible static macules and/or speckles, and a choppy pulse
Contraindications: Use with caution during pregnancy and postpartum and only if there is the confirmed presence of blood stasis.
Western medical indications: Primary dysmenorrhea, uterine fibroids, endometriosis, ovarian cysts, chronic salpingitis, chronic pelvic inflammatory disease, lochioschesis, and cervical erosion
Potential formula toxicities & interactions:
B&B: Although this formula is designed to treat patients with uterine bleeding during pregnancy, it should be used with great caution due to the potential harming of the fetus.

POTENTIAL MEDICINAL TOXICITIES & INTERACTIONS:

Gui Zhi
(Ramulus Cinnamomi Cassiae, cinnamon twigs)

Standard daily dosage: 3-15g
AH: Safe when used appropriately
B&G: Use with caution in the presence of fever, during pregnancy, or during excessive menstruation.
PDR: Contraindicated during pregnancy.

Fu Ling, Bai Fu Ling, Yun Ling
(Sclerotium Poriae Cocos)

Standard daily dosage: 9-15g
B&G: Large doses or long-term use is discouraged. Contraindicated in patients with frequent, copious urination. According to traditional

sources, may counteract *Di Yu* (Radix Sanguisorbae Officinalis), *Qin Jiao* (Radix Gentianae Qinjiao), and *Bie Jia* (Carapax Amydae Sinensis).
C&C: Contains potassium. Could possibly cause hyperkalemia when used with potassium-sparing diuretics.

Bai Shao, Shao Yao
(Radix Albus Paeoniae Lactiflorae, white peony root)

Standard daily dosage: 6-30g
AH: Safe when used appropriately
B&G: Use with caution in debilitated patients with diarrhea. According to some traditional sources, antagonizes *Shi Hu* (Herba Dendrobii) and *Mang Xiao* (Mirabilitum), counteracts *Bie Jia* (Carapax Amydae Sinensis) and *Xiao Ji* (Herba Cephalanopoloris Segeti), and is incompatible with *Li Lu* (Rhizoma Et Radix Veratri).
C&C: Contains calcium, tannic acid, potassium, and glycosides. Could possibly cause hyperkalemia when used with potassium-sparing diuretics. Could possibly reduce the effect of most antibiotics, cause digitalis intoxication and heart arrhythmias, and could possibly reduce the absorption and therapeutic effect of levadopa, isoniazid, chlorpromazine, calcium carbonate and gluconate, atropine, ephedrine, quinine, reserpine, vitamin B_1, trypsine, amylase, and pepsin. Vitamin C, nicotinic acid, glutamic acid, hydrochloric acid, and other highly acidic substances could possibly reduce the therapeutic effect of this medicinal.

Dan Pi, Mu Dan Pi
(Cortex Radicis Moutan, tree peony root bark)

Standard daily dosage: 6-12g
AH: Not to be used during pregnancy. (This ingredient is commonly used in China during pregnancy to treat heat in the blood and/or blood stasis.)
B&G: Should not be used during pregnancy or in patients with excessive sweating or profuse menstruation. Avoid using with garlic.
According to some traditional sources, may counteract the effect of *Tu Si Zi* (Semen Cuscutae Chinensis), *Bei Mu* (Bulbus Fritillariae), and *Da Huang* (Radix Et Rhizoma Rhei).
C&C: Contains tannic acid, potassium, and glycosides. Could possibly cause hyperkalemia when used with potassium-sparing diuretics. Could possibly reduce the absorption and biologic effect of most antibiotics, isoniazid, chlorpromazine, calcium carbonate and gluconate, atropine, ephedrine, quinine, reserpine, digitalis, vitamin B_1, trypsine, amylase, and pepsin. Vitamin C, nicotinic acid, glutamic acid, hydrochloric acid, and other highly acidic substances could possibly reduce the therapeutic effect of this medicinal.

Tao Ren
(Semen Pruni Persicae, peach kernel)

Standard daily dosage: 4.5-9g
AH: Not to be used during pregnancy
B&G: Contraindicated during pregnancy
C&C: Contains potassium and glycosides (including cyanophoric glycosides). If taken with codeine, morphine, or other opiates, hydrocyanic acid is produced which can lead to respiratory failure and death. Could possibly cause hyperkalemia when used with potassium-sparing diuretics. Vitamin C, nicotinic acid, glutamic acid, hydrochloric acid, and other highly acidic substances could possibly reduce the therapeutic effect of this medicinal.
GLW: If use has caused poisioning, typically, 1-2 hours after ingestion, there is a bitter taste and astringent feeling within the mouth, drooling, headache, dizziness, nausea, vomiting accompanied by watery diarrhea, heart palpitations, and lack of strength. In more serious cases, there is difficulty breathing. Sometimes one can smell cyanide on the person's breath. Eventually, breathing becomes weak, consciousness becomes unclear, and the pupils of the eye dilate widely with loss of reactivity to light. The teeth become clenched, blood pressure drops, there are generalized convulsions, and respiratory paralysis leads to death.

Most of the toxins in this medicinal reside in the skin and tip. Therefore, this medicinal is blanched before using and its tip is broken off in order to make it less or non-toxic.

COMMENTS

This formula is only appropriate for the treatment of uterine fibroids when there are clear signs and symptoms of blood stasis, and such is not always the case. Because uterine fibroids tend to occur in women between 35-55 years of age, there is usually a pronounced element of spleen vacuity and there may also be an element of kidney vacuity as well. In such cases, this formula would need to be modified with spleen and kidney supplements or another formula chosen altogether.

GUI ZHI TANG
(Cinnamon Twig Decoction, a.k.a. Cinnamon Combination)

Category: Exterior-resolving
Functions: Resolves the muscles and effuses the exterior, regulates and harmonizes the constructive and defensive
Chinese medical indications: Externally contracted wind cold with an exterior cold and vacuous condition manifesting fever and aversion to wind unrelieved by sweating, stiff neck, nasal congestion, thin, white, moist tongue fur, and a floating, forceless pulse
Contraindications: Exterior cold and interior heat
Western medical indications: Common cold, neuralgia, headache, abdominal pain due to chills, bodily weakness and vacuity, eclampsia, and neurasthenia
Potential formula toxicities & interactions:
FL: Contraindicated in hemorrhagic conditions.
B&B: Large doses may cause profuse sweating, high fever, severe thirst, heart palpitations, and irritability. Antidote is *Bai Hu Jia Ren Shen Tang* (White Tiger Plus Ginseng Decoction).

POTENTIAL MEDICINAL TOXICITIES & INTERACTIONS:

Gui Zhi
(Ramulus Cinnamomi Cassiae, cinnamon twigs)

Standard daily dosage: 3-15g
AH: Safe when used appropriately
B&G: Use with caution in the presence of fever, during pregnancy, or during excessive menstruation.
PDR: Contraindicated during pregnancy.

Bai Shao, Shao Yao
(Radix Albus Paeoniae Lactiflorae, white peony root)

Standard daily dosage: 6-30g
AH: Safe when used appropriately
B&G: Use with caution in debilitated patients with diarrhea. According to some traditional sources, antagonizes *Shi Hu* (Herba Dendrobii) and *Mang Xiao* (Mirabilitum), counteracts *Bie Jia* (Carapax Amydae Sinensis) and *Xiao Ji* (Herba Cephalanopoloris Segeti), and is incompatible with *Li Lu* (Rhizoma Et Radix Veratri).
C&C: Contains calcium, tannic acid, potassium, and glycosides. Could

possibly cause hyperkalemia when used with potassium-sparing diuretics. Could possibly reduce the effect of most antibiotics, cause digitalis intoxication and heart arrhythmias, and could possibly reduce the absorption and therapeutic effect of levadopa, isoniazid, chlorpromazine, calcium carbonate and gluconate, atropine, ephedrine, quinine, reserpine, vitamin B_1, trypsine, amylase, and pepsin. Vitamin C, nicotinic acid, glutamic acid, hydrochloric acid, and other highly acidic substances could possibly reduce the therapeutic effect of this medicinal.

Sheng Jiang
(uncooked Rhizoma Zingiberis Officinalis, fresh ginger)

Standard daily dose: 3-9g
AH: Safe when used appropriately
BR: Reduces vomiting caused by chemotherapeutic drugs. Increases absorption of oral drugs.
PDR: Recommended safe dosage limit is six grams (6g). Avoid larger doses if being used to treat morning sickness or if used in patients taking anticoagulants.

Da Zao, Hong Zao
(Fructus Zizyphi Jujubae, red dates)

Standard daily dosage: 10-30g (3-12 pieces)
AH: Safe when used appropriately
PDR: No health risks or side effects are known in conjunction with the proper administration of designated therapeutic dosages.

Gan Cao
(Radix Glycyrrhizae Uralensis, licorice root)

Standard daily dosage: 2-12g
AH: Do not use during pregnancy. (This medicinal is routinely used in Chinese medical gynecology during pregnancy as part of formulas appropriately prescribed on the basis of pattern discrimination.) As a single herb in high doses, it is contraindicated in diabetes, hypertension, and liver disorders. Not for long-term use.
BR: May increase toxicity of cardiac glycosides. May increase potassium loss due to diuretics and laxatives. Possible additive effect to corticosteroids. May be synergistic with insulin in causing hypokalemia and sodium retention.
B&G: According to some traditional sources, incompatible with *Gan Sui* (Radix Euphorbiae Kansui), *Yuan Hua* (Flos Daphnes Genkwae), and *Yuan Zhi* (Radix Polygalae Tenuifoliae). If taken long-term, it may cause hypertension and/or edema. Contains glycyrrhetinic acid which

could possibly cause a reduction in thyroid activity and basal metabolic rate.

The research on *Gan Cao* concurs that this medicinal is generally safe when used in small amounts as an envoy. It should not be taken long-term or as a single herb during pregnancy. When used as a single medicinal or in patients taking other potent Western pharmaceuticals, caution should be exercised to guard against potential toxicity and drug interaction.

COMMENTS

This is another classic formula which is rarely prescribed in its textbook standard form today.

GUN TAN WAN
(Phlegm-rolling Pills, a.k.a. Vaporize Phlegm Pills)

Category: Orifice-opening
Functions: Drains fire, transforms phlegm, and opens the orifices
Chinese medical indications: Phlegm fire resulting in mania and withdrawal, heart palpitations, coughing and wheezing with thick, sticky phlegm, chest oppression and ductal glomus, dizziness, tinnitus, insomnia, thick, slimy, yellow tongue fur, and a slippery, rapid, forceful pulse
Contraindications: Pregnancy, postpartum, and vacuity weakness
Western medical indications: Hysteria, anxiety neurosis, manic-depression, schizophrenia, seizure disorder, Meniere's disease, benign positional vertigo, bronchial asthma, acute bronchitis, and chronic obstructive pulmonary disease
Potential formula toxicities & interactions: None listed

POTENTIAL MEDICINAL TOXICITIES & INTERACTIONS:

Meng Shi
(Lapis Micae Seu Chloriti, mica schist)

Standard daily dosage: 9-15g in decoction; 1.5-3g in pills and powders
B&G: Contraindicated in pregnancy and for the debilitated.

Da Huang, Dai Huang, Chuan Jun, Jun
(Radix Et Rhizoma Rhei, rhubarb root)

Standard daily dosage: 3-12g
AH: Do not use during pregnancy. Not to be used while nursing. Contraindicated in intestinal obstruction, abdominal pain of unknown origin, or any inflammatory condition of the intestines.
BR: Reduces absorption of oral drugs. Overuse may cause hypokalemia and increased toxicity of cardiac glycosides. May aggravate potassium loss from diuretics.
B&G: Use with extreme caution during pregnancy, menstruation, or postpartum. Contraindicated for nursing mothers since active ingredients enter the milk.
C&C: Contains alkaloids, tannic acid, potassium, and glycosides. Could possibly cause hyperkalemia when used with potassium-sparing diuretics. Vitamin C, nicotinic acid, glutamic acid, hydrochloric acid, and

other highly acidic substances could possibly reduce the therapeutic effect of this medicinal.

PDR: Consult a physician before using this medicinal during pregnancy or while nursing. Contraindicated in cases of intestinal obstruction, acute inflammatory intestinal disease, appendicitis and abdominal pain of unknown origin.

Huang Qin, Tiao Qin
(Radix Scutellariae Baicalensis)

Standard daily dosage: 6-15g
AH: Safe when used appropriately
B&G: According to some traditional sources, counteracts *Dan Pi* (Cortex Radicis Moutan) and *Li Lu* (Rhizoma Et Radix Veratri).
C&C: Contains potassium and glycosides. Could possibly cause hyperkalemia when used with potassium-sparing diuretics. Vitamin C, nicotinic acid, glutamic acid, hydrochloric acid, and other highly acidic substances could possibly reduce the therapeutic effect of this medicinal.

Chen Xiang
(Lignum Aquilariae, aloeswood)

Standard daily dosage: 1.5-3g as a powder

No toxicity or interaction information listed in the sources

COMMENTS

The main ingredients in this formula are often used for the treatment of phlegm heat associated with mental-emotional problems. This formula is not commonly used as the base prescription for phlegm heat respiratory problems.

HAI ZAO YU HU TANG
(Sargassium Jade Flask Decoction)

Category: Phlegm-transforming
Functions: Tranforms phlegm and softens the hard, dissipates binding and disperses goiter
Chinese medical indications: Qi goiter due to stagnation and binding of the qi, dampness, phlegm, and blood between the skin and flesh of the neck with hard, fixed masses in the center of the neck which do not change the color of the overlying skin and do not ulcerate, thin, slimy tongue fur, and a bowstring, slippery pulse
Contraindications: None listed
Western medical indications: Goiter, thyroid adenoma, and hyperthyroidism
Potential formula toxicities & interactions:
B&B: Must be taken for 3-6 months to be effective.

POTENTIAL MEDICINAL TOXICITIES & INTERACTIONS:

Hai Zao
(Herba Sargassii)

Standard daily dosage: 4.5-15g
B&G: According to traditional sources, incompatible with *Gan Cao* (Radix Glycerrhizae Uralensis).
C&C: Contains potassium. Could possibly cause hyperkalemia when used with potassium-sparing diuretics.

Kun Bu
(Thallus Algae)

Standard daily dosage: 4.5-15g
C&C: Contains potassium. Could possibly cause hyperkalemia when used with potassium-sparing diuretics.

Hai Dai
(Thallus Laminariae)

Standard daily dosage: 6-9g

PDR: No health risks or side effects are known in conjunction with the proper administration of designated therapeutic dosages.

Zhe Bei Mu
(Bulbus Fritillariae Thunbergii)

Standard daily dosage: 3-9g
AH: Not to be used during pregnancy
C&C: Contains alkaloids. Could possibly reduce the absorption and therapeutic effect of potassium and sodium iodides, sodium bicarbonate, aluminum hydroxide, and magnesium sulfate.

This medicinal should never be used internally uncooked since it is very toxic when uncooked.

Ban Xia
(Rhizoma Pinelliae Ternatae)

Standard daily dosage: 4.5-12g
AH: Do not use during pregnancy. (This medicinal is routinely used during pregnancy in China when indicated by disease and pattern discrimination.) Contraindicated in all hemorrhagic disorders.
B&G: Safe as long as it is properly prepared. Must be decocted with other herbs and not taken alone or uncooked. Toxic effects due to improper preparation or dosage include burning and numbness in throat and lips, nausea, and a feeling of pressure in the chest. Antidote is oral administration of raw ginger. Use with caution in patients with fever. According to some traditional sources, incompatible with *Wu Tou* (Radix Aconiti).
C&C: Contains alkaloids and glycosides. Could possibly reduce the absorption and therapeutic effect of potassium and sodium iodides, sodium bicarbonate, aluminum hydroxide, and magnesium sulfate. Vitamin C, nicotinic acid, glutamic acid, hydrochloric acid, and other highly acidic substances could possibly reduce the therapeutic effect of this medicinal.
GLW: Poisoning occurs within 15 minutes to three hours after ingestion of a suitable amount. Initially, there is burning pain in the mouth, tongue, and throat, and enlargement of the tongue. This is then followed by drooling, ulceration of the oral mucosa, unclear speech, difficulty swallowing, dizziness, low-grade fever, heart palpitations, numbness of the extremities, a somber white facial complexion, and a weak, forceless pulse. If severe, there may be convulsions and respiratory failure leading to death.

Du Huo
(Radix Angelicae Pubescentis)

Standard daily dosage: 3-9g
AH: Patients should avoid prolonged exposure to sunlight.(The authors have never seen this reaction when this medicinal is used in the dosage ranges commonly employed in Chinese medicine.)

Chuan Xiong
(Radix Ligustici Wallichii)

Standard daily dosage: 3-9g (In China today, it is not uncommon for this medicinal to be prescribed up to 15 grams per day in decoction.)
AH: Do not use during pregnancy. (This medicinal is routinely used in Chinese medical gynecology during pregnancy as part of formulas appropriately prescribed on the basis of pattern discrimination.)
B&G: Not for patients with migraine headache or excessive menstrual bleeding. Overdosage causes vomiting and dizziness. According to some traditional texts, antagonizes *Shan Zhu Yu* (Fructus Corni Officinalis) and *Huang Qi* (Radix Astragali Membranacei), counteracts *Hua Shi* (Talcum) and *Huang Lian* (Rhizoma Coptidis Chinensis), and is incompatible with *Li Lu* (Rhizoma Et Radix Veratri).
C&C: Contains alkaloids and potassium. Could possibly cause hyperkalemia when used with potassium-sparing diuretics. Could possibly reduce the absorption and therapeutic effect of potassium and sodium iodides, sodium bicarbonate, aluminum hydroxide, and magnesium sulfate.

Dang Gui
(Radix Angelicae Sinensis)

Standard daily dosage: 3-15g
AH: Do not use during pregnancy. (This medicinal is routinely used in Chinese medical gynecology during pregnancy as part of formulas appropriately prescribed on the basis of pattern discrimination.)
B&G: Use with caution in patients with diarrhea or abdominal distention.
C&C: Contains potassium. Could possibly cause hyperkalemia when used with potassium-sparing diuretics. May exaggerate the anticoagulative effect of warfarin (Coumadin).

Qing Pi
(Pericarpium Citri Reticulatae Viride)

Standard daily dosage: 3-6g
AH: Safe when used appropriately

Chen Pi, Ju Pi, Ju Hong
(Pericarpium Citri Reticulatae, tangerine peel)

Standard daily dosage: 3-9g

AH: Safe when used appropriately
C&C: Contains potassium. Could possibly cause hyperkalemia when used with potassium-sparing diuretics.

Lian Qiao
(Fructus Forsythiae Suspensae, dried forsythia fruit pods)

Standard daily dosage: 6-15g
AH: Not to be used during pregnancy (This medicinal is commonly used in China during pregnancy to treat wind heat external contractions and heat toxins.)
B&G: Contraindicated in patients with diarrhea, carbuncles that have already ulcerated, and skin ulcers.
C&C: Contains potassium and glycosides. Could possibly cause hyper-kalemia when used with potassium-sparing diuretics. Vitamin C, nicotinic acid, glutamic acid, hydrochloric acid, and other highly acidic substances could possibly reduce the therapeutic effect of this medicinal.

Gan Cao
(Radix Glycyrrhizae Uralensis, licorice root)

Standard daily dosage: 2-12g
AH: Do not use during pregnancy. (This medicinal is routinely used in Chinese medical gynecology during pregnancy as part of formulas appropriately prescribed on the basis of pattern discrimination.) As a single herb in high doses, it is contraindicated in diabetes, hypertension, and liver disorders. Not for long-term use.
BR: May increase toxicity of cardiac glycosides. May increase potassium loss due to diuretics and laxatives. Possible additive effect to corticosteroids. May be synergistic with insulin in causing hypokalemia and sodium retention.
B&G: According to some traditional sources, incompatible with *Gan Sui* (Radix Euphorbiae Kansui), *Yuan Hua* (Flos Daphnes Genkwae), and *Yuan Zhi* (Radix Polygalae Tenuifoliae). If taken long-term, it may cause hypertension and/or edema. Contains glycyrrhetinic acid which could possibly cause a reduction in thyroid activity and basal metabolic rate.

The research on *Gan Cao* concurs that this medicinal is generally safe when used in small amounts as an envoy. It should not be taken long-term or as a single herb during pregnancy. When used as a single medicinal or in patients taking other potent Western pharmaceuticals, caution should be exercised to guard against potential toxicity and drug interaction.

COMMENTS

The first five ingredients in this formula plus *Chen Pi* are commonly used to treat many different types of phlegm binding or nodulation. Depending on complicating patterns and where the phlegm bindings are located, these ingredients are combined with various other Chinese medicinals.

HUAI HUA SAN
(Sophora Flower Powder)

Category: Bleeding-stopping
Functions: Cools the intestines and stops bleeding, dispels wind and moves the qi
Chinese medical indications: Wind heat or damp heat in the intestines and stomach with bright red bleeding from the anus during or before defecation, bleeding hemorrhoids, a red tongue, and a bowstring, rapid or soggy, rapid pulse
Contraindications: Bleeding due to qi vacuity
Western medical indications: Hemorrhoids, anal fissure, rectal prolapse, ulcerative colitis, amoebic dysentery
Potential formula toxicities & interactions:
B&B: Not for long-term use.

POTENTIAL MEDICINAL TOXICITIES & INTERACTIONS:

Huai Hua, Huai Hua Mi
(Flos Immaturus Sophorae Japonicae)

Standard daily dosage: 6-15g
B&G: Research notes one case of anaphylatic reaction in a child.
C&C: Contains alkaloids, tannic acid, quercetin, and glycosides. Could possibly reduce the absorption and therapeutic effect of potassium and sodium iodides, sodium bicarbonate, aluminum hydroxide, most antibiotics, isoniazid, chlorpromazine, calcium carbonate, gluconate and lactate, atropine, ephedrine, quinine, reserpine, digitalis, vitamin B_1, trypsine, amylase, and pepsin, magnesium and ferrous sulfates, and bismuth subcarbonate. Vitamin C, nicotinic acid, glutamic acid, hydrochloric acid, and other highly acidic substances could possibly reduce the therapeutic effect of this medicinal.

Ce Bai Ye
(Cacumen Biotae Orientalis)

Standard daily dosage: 6-15g
B&G: Long-term use or a large dose may cause dizziness and gastric upset.

Jing Jie Sui, Jing Jie
(Herba Seu Flos Schizonepetae Tenuifoliae)

Standard daily dosage: 3-9g
AH: No toxicity information listed in current sources.

Zhi Ke, Zhi Qiao
(Fructus Citri Aurantii, bitter orange)

Standard daily dose: 3-9g
B&G: Use with caution during pregnancy.
C&C: Contains tannic acid. Highly acidic. Could possibly cause crystalluria and hematuria. Could possibly reduce the absorption and biologic effect of most antibiotics, isoniazid, chlorpromazine, calcium carbonate and gluconate, atropine, ephedrine, quinine, reserpine, digitalis, vitamin B$_1$, trypsine, amylase, and pepsin, sodium bicarbonate, aluminum hydroxide, reserpine, caffeine, opiates, scopolamine, and berbamin.
PDR: May cause UV-sensitivity in light-skinned individuals. Otherwise no health hazards are known in conjunction with the proper administration of designated therapeutic dosages.

COMMENTS

This formula is specifically for the treatment of heat pattern bleeding hemorrhoids for which it is extremely effective.

AH= AHPA, B&B= Bensky & Barolet, B&G= Bensky & Gamble, Br= Brinker, C&C= Chan & Cheung, Fl= Flaws, GLW= Gao Lu Wen, PDR= Physician's Desk Reference

HUANG LIAN E JIAO TANG
(Coptis & Donkey Skin Glue Decoction, a.k.a.
Coptis & Gelatin Combination)

Category: Spirit-quieting
Functions: Enriches the yin and descends fire, eliminates vexation and quiets the spirit
Chinese medical indications: Noninteraction of the heart and kidneys due to yin vacuity and fire blazing with vexatious heat in the chest, easy anger, insomnia, heart palpitations, a red tongue with dry, yellow fur, and a fine, rapid pulse
Contraindications: Noninteraction of the heart and kidneys with kidney yang vacuity below
Western medical indications: Mood and anxiety disorders, the recuperative stage of an infectious disease, apthous ulcers, and dysentery
Potential formula toxicities & interactions: None listed

POTENTIAL MEDICINAL TOXICITIES & INTERACTIONS:

Huang Lian
(Rhizoma Coptidis Chinensis)

Standard daily dosage: 1.5-9g
AH: Not to be used during pregnancy (This medicinal is commonly used during pregnancy in China when indicated by disease and pattern discrimination.)
B&G: Contains berberine. Long-term use may damage the digestive system. According to some traditional sources, antagonizes *Ju Hua* (Flos Chrysanthemi Morifolii), *Xuan Shen* (Radix Scrophulariae Ningpoensis), *Bai Xian Pi* (Cortex Radicis Dictamni Dasycarpi), and *Jiang Can* (Bombyx Batryticatus). According to some traditional sources, counteracts *Kuan Dong Hua* (Flos Tussilaginis Farfarae) and *Niu Xi* (Radix Achyranthis Bidentatae). Some traditional sources say it should not be taken with pork.
C&C: Contains alkaloids, quercetin, and potassium. Could possibly cause hyperkalemia when used with potassium-sparing diuretics. Could possibly reduce the absorption and therapeutic effect of potassium and sodium iodides, sodium bicarbonate, calcium gluconate, carbonate, and lactate, aluminum hydroxide, magnesium and ferrous sulfates, and bismuth subcarbonate.

Huang Qin, Tiao Qin
(Radix Scutellariae Baicalensis)

Standard daily dosage: 6-15g
AH: Safe when used appropriately
B&G: According to some traditional sources, counteracts *Dan Pi* (Cortex Radicis Moutan) and *Li Lu* (Rhizoma Et Radix Veratri).
C&C: Contains potassium and glycosides. Could possibly cause hyperkalemia when used with potassium-sparing diuretics. Vitamin C, nicotinic acid, glutamic acid, hydrochloric acid, and other highly acidic substances could possibly reduce the therapeutic effect of this medicinal.

E Jiao
(Gelatinum Corii Asini, donkey skin glue)

Standard daily dosage: 3-15g
B&G: According to some traditional sources counteracts *Da Huang* (Radix Et Rhizoma Rhei).

Bai Shao, Shao Yao
(Radix Albus Paeoniae Lactiflorae, white peony root)

Standard daily dosage: 6-30g
B&G: Use with caution in debilitated patients with diarrhea. According to some traditional sources, antagonizes *Shi Hu* (Herba Dendrobii) and *Mang Xiao* (Mirabilitum), counteracts *Bie Jia* (Carapax Amydae Sinensis), and *Xiao Ji* (Herba Cephalanopoloris Segeti), and is incompatible with *Li Lu* (Rhizoma Et Radix Veratri).
C&C: Contains calcium, tannic acid, potassium, and glycosides. Could possibly cause hyperkalemia when used with potassium-sparing diuretics. Could possibly reduce the effect of most antibiotics, cause digitalis intoxication and heart arrhythmias, and Could possibly reduce the absorption and therapeutic effect of levadopa, isoniazid, chlorpromazine, calcium carbonate and gluconate, atropine, ephedrine, quinine, reserpine, vitamin B_1, trypsine, amylase, and pepsin. Vitamin C, nicotinic acid, glutamic acid, hydrochloric acid, and other highly acidic substances could possibly reduce the therapeutic effect of this medicinal.

Ji Zi Huang
(Egg yolk)

Standard daily dosage: No standard daily dose

No toxicity or interaction information listed in the sources

HUANG LIAN JIE DU TANG
(Coptis Resolve Toxins Decoction, a.k.a.
Coptis & Scute Combination)

Category: Heat-clearing & toxin-resolving
Functions: Drains fire and resolves toxins
Chinese medical indications: Fire toxins in the three burners
with high fever, easy anger, a dry mouth and parched throat,
deranged speech, insomnia, dark urine, a red tongue with yellow
fur, and a rapid, forceful pulse
Contraindications: Vacuity weakness
Western medical indications: Serious infections including septicemia, dysentery, pneumonia, urinary tract infections, carbuncles, furuncles, boils, acute enteritis, acute icteric hepatitis, acute
cholecystitis, encephalitis, acute conjunctivitis, acute pelvic
inflammatory diseases, erysipelas, cellulitis. Also useful in treating skin ulcers, hemoptysis, epistaxis, urticaria, pruritus, cerebral hemorrhage, hypertension, and a variety of neurological and
emotional disorders including anxiety, heart palpitations, insomnia, hysteria, and neurasthenia.
Potential formula toxicities & interactions:
FL/B&B: Not for prolonged use or with weakened patients.

POTENTIAL MEDICINAL TOXICITIES & INTERACTIONS:

Huang Lian
(Rhizoma Coptidis Chinensis)

Standard daily dosage: 1.5-9g
AH: Not to be used during pregnancy. (This medicinal is commonly used dur-
ing pregnancy in China when indicated by disease and pattern discrimination.)
B&G: Contains berberine. Long-term use may damage the digestive
system. According to some traditional sources, antagonizes *Ju Hua*
(Flos Chrysanthemi Morifolii), *Xuan Shen* (Radix Scrophulariae
Ningpoensis), *Bai Xian Pi* (Cortex Radicis Dictamni Dasycarpi), and
Jiang Can (Bombyx Batryticatus). According to some traditional
sources, counteracts *Kuan Dong Hua* (Flos Tussilaginis Farfarae) and
Niu Xi (Radix Achyranthis Bidentatae). Some traditional sources say it
should not be taken with pork.
C&C: Contains alkaloids, quercetin, and potassium. Could possibly
cause hyperkalemia when used with potassium-sparing diuretics. Could
possibly reduce the absorption and therapeutic effect of potassium and
sodium iodides, sodium bicarbonate, calcium gluconate, carbonate, and

lactate, aluminum hydroxide, magnesium and ferrous sulfates, and bismuth subcarbonate.

Huang Qin, Tiao Qin
(Radix Scutellariae Baicalensis)

Standard daily dosage: 6-15g
AH: Safe when used appropriately
B&G: According to some traditional sources, counteracts *Dan Pi* (Cortex Radicis Moutan) and *Li Lu* (Rhizoma Et Radix Veratri).
C&C: Contains potassium and glycosides. Could possibly cause hyperkalemia when used with potassium-sparing diuretics. Vitamin C, nicotinic acid, glutamic acid, hydrochloric acid, and other highly acidic substances could possibly reduce the therapeutic effect of this medicinal.

Huang Bai, Huang Bo
(Cortex Phellodendri)

Standard daily dosage: 3-12g
AH: Not to be used during pregnancy. (This medicinal is commonly used during pregnancy in China.)
B&G: Chinese literature reports one case of a patient who developed a skin rash after ingestion.
C&C: Contains alkaloids and quercetin. Could possibly reduce the absorption and therapeutic effect of potassium and sodium iodides, sodium bicarbonate, calcium gluconate, carbonate, and lactate, aluminum hydroxide, magnesium and ferrous sulfates, and bismuth subcarbonate.

Zhi Zi, Shan Zhi, Shan Zhi Zi
(Fructus Gardeniae Jasminoidis, dried gardenia fruit pod)

Standard daily dosage: 3-12g
B&G: Contains geniposide which caused diarrhea in mice.
C&C: Contains potassium and glycosides. Could possibly cause hyperkalemia when used with potassium-sparing diuretics. Vitamin C, nicotinic acid, glutamic acid, hydrochloric acid, and other highly acidic substances could possibly reduce the therapeutic effect of this medicinal.

COMMENTS

This formula is for the treatment of acute heat toxins. Because its ingredients are so bitter, cold, attacking, and draining, it may cause diarrhea. In a robust patient with a replete constitution, this side effect is considered acceptable for a while if the medicinals result in speedy eradication of the heat and toxins.

HUANG TU TANG
(Yellow Earth Decoction)

Category: Bleeding-stopping
Functions: Warms yang and fortifies the spleen, nourishes the blood and stops bleeding
Chinese medical indications: Spleen yang vacuity with spleen qi not containing the blood resulting in hemafecia, hematemesis, hemoptysis, epistaxis, or abnormal uterine bleeding with pale red blood, cold extremities, a sallow yellow or somber white facial complexion, a pale tongue with white fur, and a deep, fine, forceless pulse
Contraindications: Bleeding due to heat
Western medical indications: Chronic hemorrhagic gastritis, bleeding peptic ulcer, functional uterine bleeding
Potential formula toxicities & interactions: None listed

POTENTIAL MEDICINAL TOXICITIES & INTERACTIONS:

Fu Long Gan, Zao Xin Tu
(Terra Flava Usta)

Standard daily dosage: 15-60g

No toxicity or interaction information listed in the sources

Sheng Di, Sheng Di Huang
(uncooked Radix Rehmanniae Glutinosae)

Standard daily dosage: 9-30g
AH: Contraindicated in patients with diarrhea or lack of appetite
B&G: Contraindicated in pregnant women with anemias or digestive weakness
C&C: Contains potassium. Could possibly cause hyperkalemia when used with potassium-sparing diuretics.
PDR: No health risks or side effects are known in conjunction with the proper administration of designated therapeutic dosages.

E Jiao
(Gelatinum Corii Asini, donkey skin glue)

Standard daily dosage: 3-15g
B&G: According to some traditional sources, counteracts *Da Huang* (Radix Et Rhizoma Rhei).

Bai Zhu
(Rhizoma Atractylodis Macrocephalae)

Standard daily dosage: 4.5-9g
B&G: When rats were fed 0.5g/kg of this medicinal for two months, they developed a mild lymphopenia and anemia but suffered no damage to the brain, heart, or liver.

Gan Cao
(Radix Glycyrrhizae Uralensis, licorice root)

Standard daily dosage: 2-12g
AH: Do not use during pregnancy. (This medicinal is routinely used in Chinese medical gynecology during pregnancy as part of formulas appropriately prescribed on the basis of pattern discrimination.) As a single herb in high doses, it is contraindicated in diabetes, hypertension, and liver disorders. Not for long-term use.
BR: May increase toxicity of cardiac glycosides. May increase potassium loss due to diuretics and laxatives. Possible additive effect to corticosteroids. May be synergistic with insulin in causing hypokalemia and sodium retention.
B&G: According to some traditional sources, incompatible with *Gan Sui* (Radix Euphorbiae Kansui), *Yuan Hua* (Flos Daphnes Genkwae), and *Yuan Zhi* (Radix Polygalae Tenuifoliae). If taken long-term, it may cause hypertension and/or edema. Contains glycyrrhetinic acid which could possibly cause a reduction in thyroid activity and basal metabolic rate.

The research on *Gan Cao* concurs that this medicinal is generally safe when used in small amounts as an envoy. It should not be taken long-term or as a single herb during pregnancy. When used as a single medicinal or in patients taking other potent Western pharmaceuticals, caution should be exercised to guard against potential toxicity and drug interaction.

Fu Zi, Shu Fu Zi, Fu Pian
(Radix Lateralis Praeparatus Aconiti Carmichaeli, wolfsbane, monkshood)

Standard daily dosage: 1.5-15g
AH: To be used only under the supervision of an expert qualified in the appropriate use of this substance.
B&G: Contraindicated during pregnancy. A very toxic medicinal which can be fatal if ingested in its uncooked form or in an inappropriate dose. It is generally combined with *Gan Cao* (Radix Glycyrhizae Uralensis) and *Gan Jiang* (dry Rhizoma Zingiberis Officinalis) in decoctions to reduce its toxicity. Symptoms of toxicity include drooling, gastric upset,

light-headedness, blurred vision, and numbness and tingling of the extremities. More severe symptoms include premature atrial contractions, dyspnea, and reduced temperature and blood pressure. Emergency measures include the administration of atropine.

C&C: Contains alkaloids. Could possibly reduce the absorption and therapeutic effect of potassium and sodium iodides, sodium bicarbonate, aluminum hydroxide, and magnesium sulfate.

PDR: Contains nor-diterpene alkaloids, including aconitine. Highly toxic; small doses can be fatal.

GLW: If mild poisoning, there is a burning hot sensation in the mouth and on the tongue, numbness, and pain which gradually spreads to the four limbs and then to the whole body, nausea, vomiting, dizziness, heart palpitations, rapid breathing, vexation, agitation, restlessness, drooling. If more severe poisoning, there may be generalized sweating, paralysis, convulsions, urinary incontinence, dilated pupils, slowed reaction to light, slow heartbeat, arrhythmia, low blood pressure, a somber white facial complexion, reversal chilling of the four limbs, lowered body temperature, and circulatory collapse leading to death.

Huang Qin, Tiao Qin
(Radix Scutellariae Baicalensis)

Standard daily dosage: 6-15g

AH: Safe when used appropriately

B&G: According to some traditional sources, counteracts *Dan Pi* (Cortex Radicis Moutan) and *Li Lu* (Rhizoma Et Radix Veratri).

C&C: Contains potassium and glycosides. Could possibly cause hyperkalemia when used with potassium-sparing diuretics. Vitamin C, nicotinic acid, glutamic acid, hydrochloric acid, and other highly acidic substances could possibly reduce the therapeutic effect of this medicinal.

COMMENTS

Although this formula includes *Huang Qin*, it is not indicated for the treatment of heat pattern bleeding. In this case, *Huang Qin* is acting as a harmonizing agent to moderate the warmth and acridity of the other ingredients, especially *Fu Zi*. Today, *Chi Shi Zhi* (Hallyositum Rubrum) is commonly substituted for *Fu Long Gan*.

HUO LUO XIAO LING DAN
(Network Vessel Quickening Miraculously Effective Elixir)

Category: Blood-quickening
Functions: Quickens the blood and dispels stasis, frees the flow of the network vessels and stops pain
Chinese medical indications: Qi stagnation and blood stasis in the network vessels causing pain in various locations, such as the heart, stomach, abdomen, back, or arms and legs, bruising and swelling due to traumatic injury, a dark, purplish tongue or possible static macules or speckles, and a bowstring pulse
Contraindications: Pregnancy
Western medical indications: Angina pectoris, cerebral thrombosis, sciatica, pelvic inflammatory disease, arthritis, traumatic injury, and ectopic pregnancy
Potential formula toxicities & interactions:
B&B: Not for use during pregnancy

POTENTIAL MEDICINAL TOXICITIES & INTERACTIONS:

Dang Gui
(Radix Angelicae Sinensis)

Standard daily dosage: 3-15g
AH: Do not use during pregnancy. (This medicinal is routinely used in Chinese medical gynecology during pregnancy as part of formulas appropriately prescribed on the basis of pattern discrimination.)
B&G: Use with caution in patients with diarrhea or abdominal distention.
C&C: Contains potassium. Could possibly cause hyperkalemia when used with potassium-sparing diuretics. May exaggerate the anticoagulative effect of warfarin (Coumadin).

Dang Shen
(Radix Codonopsitis Pilosulae)

Standard daily dosage: 9-30g
AH: Safe when used appropriately
B&G: According to some traditional sources, incompatible with *Li Lu* (Rhizoma Et Radix Veratri).
C&C: Contains alkaloids, potassium, and glycosides. Could possibly cause hyperkalemia when used with potassium-sparing diuretics. Could possibly reduce the absorption and therapeutic effect of potassium and sodium iodides, sodium bicarbonate, aluminum hydroxide, magnesium

sulfate. Vitamin C, nicotinic acid, glutamic acid, hydrochloric acid, and other highly acidic substances could possibly reduce the therapeutic effect of this medicinal.

Ru Xiang
(Resina Olibani, frankincense)

Standard daily dosage: 3-9g
B&G: Contraindicated during pregnancy

Mo Yao
(Resina Myrrhae, myrrh)

Standard daily dose: 3-12g
B&G: Contraindicated during pregnancy and in patients with excessive uterine bleeding.
PDR: Not for use during pregnancy.

COMMENTS

This formula is most commonly administered as a ready-made medicine. In that case, it is often administered with other formulas designed to treat the root, while this formula treats the tip or branch of blood stasis having entered the network vessels. When taken in decoction, *Ru Xiang* and *Mo Yao* often cause indigestion. This side effect is commonly avoided when these medicinals are taken in pill form and the pills are taken with meals.

JI CHUAN JIAN
(Flow of the River Brew, a.k.a.
Ferry Brew, Benefit the River [Flow] Decoction)

Category: Draining and precipitating
Functions: Warms the kidneys, moistens the intestines, and frees the flow of the stools
Chinese medical indications: Chronic constipation due to yang, qi, and blood vacuity complicated by qi stagnation
Contraindication: Replete heat constipation
Western medical indications: Atonic constipation, degenerative joint disease, chronic arthritis
Potential formula toxicities & interactions: None listed

POTENTIAL MEDICINAL TOXICITIES & INTERACTIONS:

Rou Cong Rong, Cong Rong
(Herba Cistanchis Deserticolae Seu Salsae)

Standard daily dosage: 9-21g
AH: Safe when used appropriately

Dang Gui
(Radix Angelicae Sinensis)

Standard daily dosage: 3-15g
AH: Do not use during pregnancy. (This medicinal is routinely used in Chinese medical gynecology during pregnancy as part of formulas appropriately prescribed on the basis of pattern discrimination.)
B&G: Use with caution in patients with diarrhea or abdominal distention.
C&C: Contains potassium. Could possibly cause hyperkalemia when used with potassium-sparing diuretics. May exaggerate the anticoagulative effect of warfarin (Coumadin).

Niu Xi, Huai Niu Xi, Tu Niu Xi
(Radix Achyranthis Bidentatae)

Standard daily dosage: 9-15g
AH: Not to be used during pregnancy. Contraindicated in menorrhagia.
B&G: Contraindicated during pregnancy, in debilitated patients with diarrhea, and in patients with excessive menstruation. According to some traditional sources, should not be used with *Bai Qian* (Radix Et Rhizoma Cynanchi Baiqian).
C&C: Contains alkaloids, potassium, and glycosides. Could possibly cause

hyperkalemia when used with potassium-sparing diuretics. Could possibly reduce the absorption and therapeutic effect of potassium and sodium iodides, sodium bicarbonate, aluminum hydroxide, and magnesium sulfate. Vitamin C, nicotinic acid, glutamic acid, hydrochloric acid, and other highly acidic substances will reduce the therapeutic effect of this medicinal.

Ze Xie
(Rhizoma Alismatis Orientalis)

Standard daily dosage: 6-15g
AH: Prolonged use may cause gastrointestinal irritation.
B&G: Although considered safe, prolonged usage may irritate the intestinal tract and could possibly cause gastroenteritis.
C&C: Contains alkaloids and potassium. Could possibly cause hyperkalemia when used with potassium-sparing diuretics and reduce the absorption and therapeutic effect of potassium and sodium iodides, sodium bicarbonate, aluminum hydroxide, magnesium sulfate.
PDR: Contains triterpenes, sesquiterpenes, flavone sulfate, and caffeic acid derivatives. No health hazards or side effects with proper administration of designated therapeutic dosages.

Zhi Ke, Zhi Qiao
(Fructus Citri Aurantii, bitter orange)

Standard daily dose: 3-9g
AH: Safe when used appropriately
B&G: Use with caution during pregnancy.
C&C: Contains tannic acid. Highly acidic. Could possibly cause crystalluria and hematuria. Could possibly reduce the absorption and biologic effect of most antibiotics, isoniazid, chlorpromazine, calcium carbonate and gluconate, atropine, ephedrine, quinine, reserpine, digitalis, vitamin B_1, trypsine, amylase, and pepsin, sodium bicarbonate, aluminum hydroxide, caffeine, opiates, scopolamine, and berbamin.
PDR: May cause UV-sensitivity in light-skinned individuals. Otherwise no health hazards are known in conjunction with the proper administration of designated therapeutic dosages.

Sheng Ma
(Rhizoma Cimicifugae, black cohosh)

Standard daily dosage: 1.5-9g
AH: Not to be used during pregnancy. (This medicinal is commonly used during pregnancy in China.) Not to be used while nursing.
B&G: Contraindicated in cases of fully erupted measles and in patients

with breathing difficulties. Overdose causes headaches, dizziness, vomiting, tremors, gastroenteritis, and pathogenic erections.

C&C: Vitamin C, nicotinic acid, glutamic acid, hydrochloric acid, and other highly acidic substances could possibly reduce the therapeutic effect of this medicinal.

PDR: Not for use during pregnancy due to an increased risk of spontaneous abortion. Contains glycosides which may potentiate the effect of antihypertensive medications and result in hypotension.

COMMENTS

While this formula does nourish the blood and moisten the intestines, it also frees the flow of the stools by rectifying the qi and invigorating yang. Only if the intestines are steamed and warmed by lifegate fire can their qi function correctly. Therefore, this formula is quite different from *Run Chang Wan* (Moisten the Intestines Pills) and *Ma Zi Ren Wan* (Cannabis Seed Pills) which also moisten the intestines.

JIN GUI SHEN QI WAN
(*Golden Cabinet* Kidney Qi Pills,
a.k.a. *Ba Wei Wan*, Eight Flavors Pills)

Category: Yang-supplementing
Functions: Warms and supplements kidney yang
Chinese medical indications: Kidney yang vacuity with low back and knee soreness and limpness, tinnitus, dizziness, deafness, possible edema, a cold sensation in the lower half of the body, lower abdominal tension, polyuria, nocturia, a pale, swollen tongue with thin, white, moist fur, and a deep, weak pulse
Contraindications: Yin vacuity without yang vacuity
Western medical indications: Nephritis, nephrosclerosis, kidney stones, renal tuberculosis, pyelitis, albuminuria, edema, cystitis, chronic urethritis, prostatic hypertrophy, urinary incontinence, primary hyperaldosteronism, Addison's disease, hypothyroidism, postpartum urinary retention, arthritis, diabetes, cerebral hemorrhage, hyper/hypotension, spermatorrhea, impotence, lumbago, sciatica, glaucoma, keratitis, senile pruritus, vaginal itching, urticaria, chronic gonorrhea, rectal prolapse, menopausal complaints, and chronic bronchial asthma
Potential formula toxicities & interactions:
FL: Do not use in patients with chronic gastrointestinal weakness and diarrhea.

POTENTIAL MEDICINAL TOXICITIES & INTERACTIONS:

Shu Di, Shu Di Huang
(cooked Radix Rehmanniae Glutinosae)

Standard daily dosage: 9-30g
AH: Contraindicated in patients with diarrhea or indigestion
B&G: Overuse can lead to abdominal distention and loose stools. Side effects include diarrhea, abdominal pain, dizziness, lethargy, and heart palpitations which often disappear upon continued administration of the herb.
PDR: No health risks or side effects are known in conjunction with the proper administration of designated therapeutic dosages.

Shan Zhu Yu, Shan Zhu Rou
(Fructus Corni Officinalis)

Standard daily dosage: 3-60g
AH: Contraindicated in patients with difficult or painful urination
B&G: Contraindicated in patients with difficult or painful urination.
According to some traditional sources, antagonizes *Jie Geng* (Radix
Platycodi Grandiflori), *Fang Feng* (Radix Ledebouriellae Divaricatae),
and *Fang Ji* (Radix Aristolochiae Fangchi).
C&C: Contains tannic acid and glycosides. Could possibly reduce the
absorption and biologic effect of most antibiotics, isoniazid, chlorpromazine, calcium carbonate and gluconate, atropine, ephedrine, quinine,
reserpine, digitalis, vitamin B_1, trypsine, amylase, and pepsin. Vitamin C,
nicotinic acid, glutamic acid, hydrochloric acid, and other highly acidic
substances could possibly reduce the therapeutic effect of this medicinal.
PDR: No health hazards are known in conjunction with proper administration of designated therapeutic dosages.

Shan Yao
(Radix Dioscoreae Oppositae)

Standard daily dosage: 9-30g
AH: Safe when used appropriately
B&G: According to some traditional sources, antagonizes *Gan Sui*
(Radix Euphorbiae Kansui).
C&C: Contains alkaloids, potassium, amylase, and glycosides. Could
possibly cause hyperkalemia when used with potassium-sparing diuretics.
Could possibly reduce the absorption and therapeutic effect of potassium
and sodium iodides, sodium bicarbonate, aluminum hydroxide, magnesium sulfate, tetracyclines, sulphanomides, and aspirin. Vitamin C, nicotinic acid, glutamic acid, hydrochloric acid, and other highly acidic substances could possibly reduce the therapeutic effect of this medicinal.
PDR: Use of this medicinal may reduce the antiinflammatory effect of
indomethacin. May have an additive estrogenic effect when administered
with estrogen-containing drugs. Poisoning in overdosages may occur
from the picrotoxin-like effect of dioscorin.

Fu Zi, Shu Fu Zi, Fu Pian
(Radix Lateralis Praeparatus Aconiti Carmichaeli,
wolfsbane, monkshood)

Standard daily dosage: 1.5-15g
AH: To be used only under the supervision of an expert qualified in the
appropriate use of this substance

B&G: Contraindicated during pregnancy. A very toxic medicinal which can be fatal if ingested in its uncooked form or in an inappropriate dose. It is generally combined with *Gan Cao* (Radix Glycyrhizae Uralensis) and *Gan Jiang* (dry Rhizoma Zingiberis Officinalis) in decoctions to reduce its toxicity. Symptoms of toxicity include drooling, gastric upset, light-headedness, blurred vision, and numbness and tingling of the extremities. More severe symptoms include premature atrial contractions, dyspnea, and reduced temperature and blood pressure. Emergency measures include the administration of atropine.

C&C: Contains alkaloids. Could possibly reduce the absorption and therapeutic effect of potassium and sodium iodides, sodium bicarbonate, aluminum hydroxide, and magnesium sulfate.

PDR: Contains nor-diterpene alkaloids, including aconitine. Highly toxic; small doses can be fatal.

GLW: If mild poisoning, there is a burning hot sensation in the mouth and on the tongue, numbness, and pain which gradually spreads to the four limbs and then to the whole body, nausea, vomiting, dizziness, heart palpitations, rapid breathing, vexation, agitation, restlessness, drooling. If more severe poisoning, there may be generalized sweating, paralysis, convulsions, urinary incontinence, dilated pupils, slowed reaction to light, slow heartbeat, arrhythmia, low blood pressure, a somber white facial complexion, reversal chilling of the four limbs, lowered body temperature, and circulatory collapse leading to death.

Gui Zhi
(Ramulus Cinnamomi Cassiae, cinnamon twigs)

Standard daily dosage: 3-15g
AH: Safe when used appropriately
B&G: Use with caution in the presence of fever, during pregnancy, or during excessive menstruation.
PDR: Contraindicated during pregnancy.

Ze Xie
(Rhizoma Alismatis Orientalis)

Standard daily dosage: 6-15g
AH: Prolonged use may cause gastrointestinal irritation.
B&G: Although considered safe, prolonged usage may irritate the intestinal tract and Could possibly cause gastroenteritis.
C&C: Contains alkaloids and potassium. Could possibly cause hyperkalemia when used with potassium-sparing diuretics and reduce the absorption and therapeutic effect of potassium and sodium iodides, sodium bicarbonate, aluminum hydroxide, magnesium sulfate.

PDR: Contains triterpenes, sesquiterpenes, flavone sulfate, and caffeic acid derivatives. No health hazards or side effects with proper administration of designated therapeutic dosages.

Fu Ling, Bai Fu Ling, Yun Ling
(Sclerotium Poriae Cocos)

Standard daily dosage: 9-15g
B&G: Large doses or long-term use is discouraged. Contraindicated in patients with frequent, copious urination. According to traditional sources, may counteract *Di Yu* (Radix Sanguisorbae Officinalis), *Qin Jiao* (Radix Gentianae Qinjiao), and *Bie Jia* (Carapax Amydae Sinensis).
C&C: Contains potassium. Could possibly cause hyperkalemia when used with potassium-sparing diuretics.

Dan Pi, Mu Dan Pi
(Cortex Radicis Moutan, tree peony root bark)

Standard daily dosage: 6-12g
AH: Not to be used during pregnancy. (This ingredient is commonly used in China during pregnancy to treat heat in the blood and/or blood stasis.)
B&G: Should not be used during pregnancy or in patients with excessive sweating or menstruation. Avoid using with garlic. According to some traditional sources, may counteract the effect of *Tu Si Zi* (Semen Cuscutae Chinensis), *Bei Mu* (Bulbus Fritillariae), and *Da Huang* (Radix Et Rhizoma Rhei).
C&C: Contains tannic acid, potassium, and glycosides. Could possibly cause hyperkalemia when used with potassium-sparing diuretics. Could possibly reduce the absorption and biologic effect of most antibiotics, isoniazid, chlorpromazine, calcium carbonate and gluconate, atropine, ephedrine, quinine, reserpine, digitalis, vitamin B_1, trypsine, amylase, and pepsin. Vitamin C, nicotinic acid, glutamic acid, hydrochloric acid, and other highly acidic substances could possibly reduce the therapeutic effect of this medicinal.

COMMENTS

This is the form of this formula found originally in the *Jin Gui Yao Lue (Essentials [Worth] A Thousand [Pieces of] Gold)*. Today, the more common version substitutes *Rou Gui* (Cortex Cinnamomi Cassiae) for *Gui Zhi*. Because of the interdependence of the spleen and kidneys, this formula must commonly be modified by the addition of more spleen-supplements or this formula combined with a spleen-supplementing one.

AH= AHPA, B&B= BENSKY & BAROLET, B&G= BENSKY & GAMBLE, BR= BRINKER, C&C= CHAN & CHEUNG, FL= FLAWS, GLW= GAO LU WEN, PDR= PHYSICIAN'S DESK REFERENCE

JU HE WAN
(Tangerine Seed Pills)

Category: Qi-rectifying
Functions: Moves the qi and stops pain, softens the hard and dissipates binding
Chinese medical indications: Damp cold invading the liver channel with unilateral testicular swelling, colicky pain possibly reaching to the umbilicus, rock-like hardness and swelling of the scrotum, oozing of yellow fluid from the scrotum
Contraindications: None listed
Western medical indications: Hydrocoele, orchitis, epididymitis
Potential formula toxicities & interactions: None listed

POTENTIAL MEDICINAL TOXICITIES & INTERACTIONS:

Ju He
(Semen Citri Reticulate)

Standard daily dosage: 3-9g

No toxicity or interaction information listed in the sources

Chuan Lian Zi, Jin Ling Zi
(Fructus Meliae Toosendan)

Standard daily dosage: 3-9g
AH: Safe when used appropriately
GLW: Symptoms of adverse reaction include abdominal distention, abdominal pain, vomiting, diarrhea, poor appetite, dizziness, headache, a red facial complexion, blurred vision, inhibited speech, uneasy respiration, epistaxis, hemorrhage of the liver, kidney, and/or intestines, mania and agitation, convulsions, numbness of the four extremities, heart arrhythmia, shrunken pupils. Poisoning can lead to toxic hepatitis and red blood cells in the urine. In grave conditions, there may be atrial fibrillation, frequent premature beats, and atrioventricular conduction block, low blood pressure, syncope, shock, and even death.

Mu Xiang
(Radix Aucklandiae Lappae)

Standard daily dosage: 1.5-9g

AH: Safe when used appropriately
PDR: No health risks or side effects are known in conjunction with the proper administration of designated therapeutic dosages.

Tao Ren
(Semen Pruni Persicae, peach kernel)

Standard daily dosage: 4.5-9g
B&G: Contraindicated during pregnancy.
C&C: Contains potassium and glycosides (including cyanophoric glycosides). If taken with codeine, morphine, or other opiates, hydrocyanic acid is produced which can lead to respiratory failure and death. Could possibly cause hyperkalemia when used with potassium-sparing diuretics. Vitamin C, nicotinic acid, glutamic acid, hydrochloric acid, and other highly acidic substances could possibly reduce the therapeutic effect of this medicinal.
GLW: In case of poisoning, typically, 1-2 hours after ingestion, there is a bitter taste and astringent feeling within the mouth, drooling, headache, dizziness, nausea, vomiting accompanied by watery diarrhea, heart palpitations, and lack of strength. In more serious cases, there is difficulty breathing. Sometimes one can smell cyanide on the person's breath. Eventually, breathing becomes weak, consciousness becomes unclear, and the pupils of the eye dilate widely with loss of reactivity to light. The teeth become clenched, blood pressure drops, there are generalized convulsions, and respiratory paralysis leads to death.

Most of the toxins in this medicinal reside in the skin and tip. Therefore, this medicinal is blanched before using and its tip is broken off in order to make it less or non-toxic.

Yan Hu Suo, Yan Hu, Yuan Hu, Yuan Hu Suo, Xuan Hu, Xuan Hu Suo
(Rhizoma Corydalis Yanhusuo)

Standard daily dosage: 4.5-12g
AH: Not to be used during pregnancy.
B&G: Contraindicated during pregnancy. LD50 in mice varies from 125.3g/kg to 36.6g/kg depending upon preparation and purity.
C&C: Contains alkaloids. Highly alkaline. Toxic when taken with some antibiotics (aminoglycosides) and quinidine. Could possibly cause hyperkalemia when taken with potassium-sparing diuretics and reduce the absorption and therapeutic effect of most antibiotics, potassium and sodium iodides, sodium bicarbonate, aluminum hydroxide, and magnesium sulfate.

PDR: Overdose may result in clonic spasms with muscle tremor.
GLW: Symptoms of adverse reaction include dizziness, somnolence, abdominal distention. Prolonged ingestion may cause elevations in SGPT and drug-induced fever. Ingestion of 60-120g per time may cause a somber white facial complexion, lack of strength in the four limbs, difficulty breathing, convulsions, low blood pressure, decreased heart strength, and, if severe, fright reversal, shock, and respiratory failure.

Rou Gui, Gui Xin, Guan Gui
(Cortex Cinnamomi Cassiae, cinnamon bark)

Standard daily dosage: 1.5-4.5g
AH: Not to be used during pregnancy.
BR: Reduces absorption of tetracyclines
B&G: Use with caution during pregnancy.
C&C: Contains tannic acid and potassium. Could possibly cause hyperkalemia when used with potassium-sparing diuretics. Could possibly reduce the absorption and biologic effect of most antibiotics, isoniazid, chlorpromazine, calcium carbonate and gluconate, atropine, ephedrine, quinine, reserpine, digitalis, vitamin B_1, trypsine, amylase, and pepsin.

Mu Tong
(Caulis Akebiae)

Standard daily dosage: 3-9g
B&G: Contraindicated during pregnancy. Could possibly cause dehydration and renal failure in large doses.
C&C: Contains potassium. Could possibly cause hyperkalemia when used with potassium-sparing diuretics.
PDR: Not to be administered during pregnancy. Large doses of the medicinal may lead to gastroenteritis, intestinal colic and diarrhea, due to saponin content.
GLW: Early stage symptoms of poisoning include upper abdominal discomfort, vomiting, chest oppression, abdominal pain, and diarrhea. Secondarily, there is frequent urination, urgent urination, facial edema which gradually spreads to the entire body, inability to lie down, unclear consciousness, scanty urination or blocked urination, and increased blood pressure. Some patients present oily stools. In those with acute kidney failure, uremia leads to death.

This medicinal is often substituted with Caulis Aristolochiae Manchuriensis which contains aristolochic acid. Therefore, it is important that this medicinal only be prescribed in the form of Caulis Akebiae Trifoliatae or Akebiae Quinatae.

Hou Po, Chuan Po
(Cortex Magnoliae Officinalis)

Standard daily dosage: 3-9g
AH: Not to be used during pregnancy (This medicinal is commonly used in China during pregnancy, especially for the treatment of nausea and vomiting.)
B&G: Use with caution during pregnancy. According to some traditional sources, antagonizes *Ze Xie* (Rhizoma Alismatis Orientalis) and *Han Shui Shi* (Calcitum).
C&C: Contains tannic acid and potassium. Could possibly cause hyperkalemia when used with potassium-sparing diuretics and reduce the absorption and biologic effect of most antibiotics, isoniazid, chlorpromazine, calcium carbonate and gluconate, atropine, ephedrine, quinine, reserpine, digitalis, vitamin B_1, trypsine, amylase, and pepsin.
PDR: No health risks or side effects are known in conjunction with the proper administration of designated therapeutic dosages.

Zhi Shi
(Fructus Immaturus Citri Aurantii, immature bitter orange)

Standard daily dosage: 3-9
B&G: Use with caution during pregnancy or in debilitated patients.
C&C: Contains tannic acid. Highly acidic. Could possibly cause crystalluria and hematuria and reduce the absorption and biologic effect of most antibiotics, isoniazid, chlorpromazine, calcium carbonate and gluconate, atropine, ephedrine, quinine, reserpine, digitalis, vitamin B_1, trypsine, amylase, and pepsin, sodium bicarbonate, aluminum hydroxide, reserpine, caffeine, opiates, scopolamine, and berbamin.

Hai Zao
(Herba Sargassii)

Standard daily dosage: 4.5-15g
B&G: According to traditional sources, incompatible with *Gan Cao* (Radix Glycerrhizae Uralensis).
C&C: Contains potassium. Could possibly cause hyperkalemia when used with potassium-sparing diuretics.

Kun Bu
(Thallus Algae)

Standard daily dosage: 4.5-15g
C&C: Contains potassium. Could possibly cause hyperkalemia when used with potassium-sparing diuretics.

Hai Dai
(Thallus Laminariae)

Standard daily dosage: 6-9g

PDR: No health risks or side effects are known in conjunction with the proper administration of designated therapeutic dosages.

COMMENTS

Although this formula can eliminate the discomfort of inguinal hernia and may arrest the progression of this disorder, this is a surgical condition which cannot be cured by the internal administration of medicinals, Chinese or otherwise.

Ju Pi Zhu Ru Tang
(Tangerine Peel & Bamboo Shavings Decoction,
a.k.a. Aurantium & Bamboo Combination)

Category: Qi-rectifying
Functions: Downbears counterflow and stops hiccup, boosts the qi and clears heat
Chinese medical indications: Stomach heat and disharmony resulting in hiccup, nausea, dry heaves, or retching accompanied by a tender, red tongue and a rapid, forceless pulse
Contraindications: Replete heat or vacuity cold
Western medical indications: Hiccup, nausea and vomiting, morning sickness, postsurgical persistent hiccup, chronic gastric diseases, and incomplete pyloric obstruction
Potential formula toxicities & interactions: None listed

POTENTIAL MEDICINAL TOXICITIES & INTERACTIONS:

Chen Pi, Ju Pi, Ju Hong
(Pericarpium Citri Reticulatae, tangerine peel)

Standard daily dosage: 3-9g
AH: Safe when used appropriately
C&C: Contains potassium. Could possibly cause hyperkalemia when used with potassium-sparing diuretics.

Zhu Rhu
(Caulis Bambusae In Taeniis, bamboo shavings)

Standard daily dosage: 4.5-9g
C&C: Contains potassium. Could possibly cause hyperkalemia when used with potassium-sparing diuretics.

Ren Shen
(Radix Panacis Ginseng, ginseng)

Standard daily dosage: 1-30g
AH: Contraindicated in hypertension
BR: May cause manic episodes in patients on MAO-inhibitors. May cause hypertension if consumed with caffeine. Possible additive effects to insulin. May reduce the anticoagulative effect of warfarin (Coumadin).
B&G: Contraindicated for hypertensive patients. Overdose can lead to

headache, insomnia, heart palpitations, and a rise in blood pressure. A traditional antidote is mung bean soup.

C&C: Vitamin C, nicotinic acid, glutamic acid, hydrochloric acid, and other highly acidic substances could possibly reduce the therapeutic effect of this medicinal.

PDR: Contraindicated in patients with hypertension. Not recommended in large doses during pregnancy or lactation due to potential neonatal androgenization. Enhances the effect of insulin and other antidiabetic agents. Use with MAO-inhibitors may cause headaches, tremors, and manias.

Sheng Jiang
(uncooked Rhizoma Zingiberis Officinalis, fresh ginger)

Standard daily dose: 3-9g
AH: Safe when used appropriately
BR: Reduces vomiting caused by chemotherapeutic drugs. Increases absorption of oral drugs.
PDR: Recommended safe dosage limit is six grams (6g). Avoid larger doses if being used to treat morning sickness or if used in patients taking anticoagulants.

Gan Cao
(Radix Glycyrrhizae Uralensis, licorice root)

Standard daily dosage: 2-12g
AH: Do not use during pregnancy. (This medicinal is routinely used in Chinese medical gynecology during pregnancy as part of formulas appropriately prescribed on the basis of pattern discrimination.) As a single herb in high doses, it is contraindicated in diabetes, hypertension, and liver disorders. Not for long-term use.

BR: May increase toxicity of cardiac glycosides. May increase potassium loss due to diuretics and laxatives. Possible additive effect to corticosteroids. May be synergistic with insulin in causing hypokalemia and sodium retention.

B&G: According to some traditional sources, incompatible with *Gan Sui* (Radix Euphorbiae Kansui), *Yuan Hua* (Flos Daphnes Genkwae), and *Yuan Zhi* (Radix Polygalae Tenuifoliae). If taken long-term, it may cause hypertension and/or edema. Contains glycyrrhetinic acid which could possibly cause a reduction in thyroid activity and basal metabolic rate.

The research on *Gan Cao* concurs that this medicinal is generally safe when used in small amounts as an envoy. It should not be taken long-term or as a single herb during pregnancy. When used as a single medicinal or

in patients taking other potent Western pharmaceuticals, caution should be exercised to guard against potential toxicity and drug interaction.

Da Zao, Hong Zao
(Fructus Zizyphi Jujubae, red dates)

Standard daily dosage: 10-30g (3-12 pieces)
AH: Safe when used appropriately
PDR: No health risks or side effects are known in conjunction with the proper administration of designated therapeutic dosages.

COMMENTS

This formula is commonly used for the treatment of nausea and vomiting during pregnancy when there is a combination of liver-spleen-stomach disharmony with some depressive heat.

Juan Bi Tang
(Assuage Impediment Decoction, a.k.a.
Impediment-alleviating Decoction, Chianghuo & Turmeric
Combination)

Category: Dampness-dispelling
Functions: Dispels wind and eliminates dampness, supplements the qi and nourishes the blood, assuages impediment
Chinese medical indications: Wind damp cold impediment complicated by qi and blood vacuity with generalized heaviness of the body, stiff neck, shoulder, and upper back, numbness in the extremities, difficulty moving, white tongue fur, and a soggy, moderate pulse
Contraindications: Wind damp heat impediment
Western medical indications: Osteoarthritis, rheumatoid arthritis, gouty arthritis, and bursitis
Potential formula toxicities & interactions: None listed

Potential Medicinal Toxicities & Interactions:

Qiang Huo
(Rhizoma Seu Radix Notopterygii)

Standard daily dosage: 6-15g
AH: Safe when used appropriately

Du Huo
(Radix Angelicae Pubescentis)

Standard daily dosage: 3-9g
AH: Patients should avoid prolonged exposure to sunlight. The authors have never seen this reaction when this medicinal is used in the dosage ranges commonly employed in Chinese medicine.)

Qin Jiao
(Radix Gentianae Qinjiao)

Standard daily dosage: 4.5-12g
AH: Safe when used appropriately. High doses may cause nausea and vomiting.
B&G: Contraindicated in cases with frequent urination, chronic pain with emaciation, or diarrhea. LD50 in mice is 480mg/kg. High dosages may cause nausea and vomiting.

Sang Zhi
(Ramulus Mori Albi, mulberry twigs)

Standard daily dosage: 10-30g
AH: Not to be used during pregnancy. As a single herb in high doses, it is contraindicated in diabetes, hypertension, and liver disorders. Not for long-term use.

Hai Feng Teng
(Caulis Piperis Futokadsurae)

Standard daily dosage: 6-15g

No toxicity or interaction information listed in the sources

Dang Gui
(Radix Angelicae Sinensis)

Standard daily dosage: 3-15g
AH: Do not use during pregnancy. (This medicinal is routinely used in Chinese medical gynecology during pregnancy as part of formulas appropriately prescribed on the basis of pattern discrimination.)
B&G: Use with caution in patients with diarrhea or abdominal distention.
C&C: Contains potassium. Could possibly cause hyperkalemia when used with potassium-sparing diuretics. May exaggerate the anticoagulative effect of warfarin (Coumadin).

Chuan Xiong
(Radix Ligustici Wallichii)

Standard daily dosage: 3-9g (In China today, it is not uncommon for this medicinal to be prescribed up to 15 grams per day in decoction.)
AH: Do not use during pregnancy. (This medicinal is routinely used in Chinese medical gynecology during pregnancy as part of formulas appropriately prescribed on the basis of pattern discrimination.)
B&G: Not for patients with migraine headache or excessive menstrual bleeding. Overdosage causes vomiting and dizziness. According to some traditional texts, antagonizes *Shan Zhu Yu* (Fructus Corni Officinalis) and *Huang Qi* (Radix Astragali Membranacei), counteracts *Hua Shi* (Talcum) and *Huang Lian* (Rhizoma Coptidis Chinensis), and is incompatible with *Li Lu* (Rhizoma Et Radix Veratri).
C&C: Contains alkaloids and potassium. Could possibly cause hyperkalemia when used with potassium-sparing diuretics. Could possibly reduce the absorption and therapeutic effect of potassium and sodium iodides, sodium bicarbonate, aluminum hydroxide, and magnesium sulfate.

Ru Xiang
(Resina Olibani, frankincense)

Standard daily dosage: 3-9g
B&G: Contraindicated during pregnancy

Mu Xiang
(Radix Aucklandiae Lappae)

Standard daily dosage: 1.5-9g
AH: Safe when used appropriately
PDR: No health risks or side effects are known in conjunction with the proper administration of designated therapeutic dosages.

Rou Gui, Gui Xin, Guan Gui
(Cortex Cinnamomi Cassiae, cinnamon bark)

Standard daily dosage: 1.5-4.5g
AH: Not to be used during pregnancy
BR: Reduces absorption of tetracyclines
B&G: Use with caution during pregnancy
C&C: Contains tannic acid and potassium. Could possibly cause hyperkalemia when used with potassium-sparing diuretics. Could possibly reduce the absorption and biologic effect of most antibiotics, isoniazid, chlorpromazine, calcium carbonate and gluconate, atropine, ephedrine, quinine, reserpine, digitalis, vitamin B_1, trypsine, amylase, and pepsin.

Gan Cao
(Radix Glycyrrhizae Uralensis, licorice root)

Standard daily dosage: 2-12g
AH: Do not use during pregnancy. (This medicinal is routinely used in Chinese medical gynecology during pregnancy as part of formulas appropriately prescribed on the basis of pattern discrimination.) As a single herb in high doses, it is contraindicated in diabetes, hypertension, and liver disorders. Not for long-term use.
BR: May increase toxicity of cardiac glycosides. May increase potassium loss due to diuretics and laxatives. Possible additive effect to corticosteroids. May be synergistic with insulin in causing hypokalemia and sodium retention.
B&G: According to some traditional sources, incompatible with *Gan Sui* (Radix Euphorbiae Kansui), *Yuan Hua* (Flos Daphnes Genkwae), and *Yuan Zhi* (Radix Polygalae Tenuifoliae). If taken long-term, it may cause hypertension and/or edema. Contains glycyrrhetinic acid which

could possibly cause a reduction in thyroid activity and basal metabolic rate.

The research on *Gan Cao* concurs that this medicinal is generally safe when used in small amounts as an envoy. It should not be taken long-term or as a single herb during pregnancy. When used as a single medicinal or in patients taking other potent Western pharmaceuticals, caution should be exercised to guard against potential toxicity and drug interaction.

COMMENTS

Unlike *Du Huo Ji Sheng Wan* (Angelica Pubescens & Loranthus Pills), this formula does not address a concomitant liver-kidney vacuity nor a spleen qi vacuity. However, it does address concomitant blood stasis in the network vessels.

LI ZHONG WAN
(Rectify the Center Pills)

Category: Interior-warming
Functions: Warms the center and dispels cold, fortifies the spleen and supplements the qi
Chinese medical indications: Spleen-stomach yang vacuity with diarrhea, watery stools, nausea and vomiting, torpid intake, insidious abdominal pain and discomfort, a pale tongue with white fur, and a deep, fine pulse
Contraindications: Externally contracted conditions with fever or yin vacuity
Western medical indications: Acute and chronic gastritis, gastric or duodenal ulcers, irritable bowel syndrome, chronic colitis, cholera-like disorders, chronic bronchitis, oral herpes, functional uterine bleeding, bloody stools due to gastroduodenal ulcer, angina pectoris, and anemia
Potential formula toxicities & interactions: None listed

POTENTIAL MEDICINAL TOXICITIES & INTERACTIONS:

Gan Jiang
(dry Rhizoma Zingiberis Officinalis, dry ginger)

Standard daily dosage: 3-12g
AH: Not to be used during pregnancy. Patients with gallstones should consult a practitioner prior to use.
B&G: Use with caution during pregnancy.

Ren Shen
(Radix Panacis Ginseng, ginseng)

Standard daily dosage: 1-30g
AH: Contraindicated in hypertension
BR: May cause manic episodes in patients on MAO-inhibitors. May cause hypertension if consumed with caffeine. Possible additive effects to insulin. May reduce the anticoagulative effect of warfarin (Coumadin).
B&G: Contraindicated for hypertensive patients. Overdose can lead to headache, insomnia, heart palpitations, and a rise in blood pressure. A traditional antidote is mung bean soup.
C&C: Vitamin C, nicotinic acid, glutamic acid, hydrochloric acid, and

other highly acidic substances could possibly reduce the therapeutic effect of this medicinal.

PDR: Contraindicated in patients with hypertension. Not recommended in large doses during pregnancy or lactation due to potential neonatal androgenization. Enhances the effect of insulin and other antidiabetic agents. Use with MAO-inhibitors may cause headaches, tremors, and manias.

Bai Zhu
(Rhizoma Atractylodis Macrocephalae)

Standard daily dosage: 4.5-9g
AH: Safe when used appropriately
B&G: When rats were fed 0.5g/kg of this medicinal for two months, they developed a mild lymphopenia and anemia but suffered no damage to the brain, heart, or liver.

Gan Cao
(Radix Glycyrrhizae Uralensis, licorice root)

Standard daily dosage: 2-12g
AH: Do not use during pregnancy. (This medicinal is routinely used in Chinese medical gynecology during pregnancy as part of formulas appropriately prescribed on the basis of pattern discrimination.) As a single herb in high doses, it is contraindicated in diabetes, hypertension, and liver disorders. Not for long-term use.
BR: May increase toxicity of cardiac glycosides. May increase potassium loss due to diuretics and laxatives. Possible additive effect to corticosteroids. May be synergistic with insulin in causing hypokalemia and sodium retention.
B&G: According to some traditional sources, incompatible with *Gan Sui* (Radix Euphorbiae Kansui), *Yuan Hua* (Flos Daphnes Genkwae), and *Yuan Zhi* (Radix Polygalae Tenuifoliae). If taken long-term, it may cause hypertension and/or edema. Contains glycyrrhetinic acid which could possibly cause a reduction in thyroid activity and basal metabolic rate.

The research on *Gan Cao* concurs that this medicinal is generally safe when used in small amounts as an envoy. It should not be taken long-term or as a single herb during pregnancy. When used as a single medicinal or in patients taking other potent Western pharmaceuticals, caution should be exercised to guard against potential toxicity and drug interaction.

COMMENTS

Dang Shen (Radix Codonopsitis Pilosulae) is commonly substituted for *Ren Shen* in this formula. However, except in pill form and when combined with other formulas, it is not that commonly used in Western clinical practice.

Liu Wei Di Huang Wan
(Six Flavors Rehmannia Pills, a.k.a. Rehmannia Six Formula)

Category: Yin-supplementing
Functions: Enriches the yin and nourishes the kidneys
Chinese medical indications: Kidney yin vacuity with dizziness, tinnitus, decrease in auditory acuity, low back and knee soreness and limpness, night sweats, nocturia, a red tongue with scanty fur, and a fine, rapid pulse
Contraindications: Spleen qi vacuity with dampness
Western medical indications: Neurasthenia, pulmonary tuberculosis, diabetes mellitus, hyperthyroidism, chronic nephritis, chronic glomerulonephritis, urinary tract infection, hypertension, failure to thrive, functional uterine bleeding, optic neuritis, optic nerve atrophy, and central retinitis
Potential formula toxicities & interactions:
FL/B&B: This formula should be used with caution in patients with indigestion or diarrhea.

POTENTIAL MEDICINAL TOXICITIES & INTERACTIONS:

Shu Di, Shu Di Huang
(cooked Radix Rehmanniae Glutinosae)

Standard daily dosage: 9-30g
AH: Contraindicated in patients with diarrhea or indigestion
B&G: Overuse can lead to abdominal distention and loose stools. Side effects include diarrhea, abdominal pain, dizziness, lethargy, and heart palpitations which often disappear upon continued administration of the herb.
PDR: No health risks or side effects are known in conjunction with the proper administration of designated therapeutic dosages.

Shan Zhu Yu, Shan Zhu Rou
(Fructus Corni Officinalis)

Standard daily dosage: 3-60g
AH: Contraindicated in patients with difficult or painful urination
B&G: Contraindicated in patients with difficult or painful urination. According to some traditional sources, antagonizes *Jie Geng* (Radix Platycodi Grandiflori), *Fang Feng* (Radix Ledebouriellae Divaricatae), and *Fang Ji* (Radix Aristolochiae Fangchi).

C&C: Contains tannic acid and glycosides. Could possibly reduce the absorption and biologic effect of most antibiotics, isoniazid, chlorpromazine, calcium carbonate and gluconate, atropine, ephedrine, quinine, reserpine, digitalis, vitamin B_1, trypsine, amylase, and pepsin. Vitamin C, nicotinic acid, glutamic acid, hydrochloric acid, and other highly acidic substances could possibly reduce the therapeutic effect of this medicinal.

PDR: No health hazards are known in conjunction with proper administration of designated therapeutic dosages.

Shan Yao
(Radix Dioscoreae Oppositae)

Standard daily dosage: 9-30g
AH: Safe when used appropriately
B&G: According to some traditional sources, antagonizes *Gan Sui* (Radix Euphorbiae Kansui).
C&C: Contains alkaloids, potassium, amylase, and glycosides. Could possibly cause hyperkalemia when used with potassium-sparing diuretics. Could possibly reduce the absorption and therapeutic effect of potassium and sodium iodides, sodium bicarbonate, aluminum hydroxide, magnesium sulfate, tetracyclines, sulphanomides, and aspirin. Vitamin C, nicotinic acid, glutamic acid, hydrochloric acid, and other highly acidic substances could possibly reduce the therapeutic effect of this medicinal.
PDR: Use of this medicinal may reduce the antiinflammatory effect of indomethacin. May have an additive estrogenic effect when administered with estrogen-containing drugs. Poisoning in overdosages may occur from the picrotoxin-like effect of dioscorin.

Fu Ling, Bai Fu Ling, Yun Ling
(Sclerotium Poriae Cocos)

Standard daily dosage: 9-15g
B&G: Large doses or long-term use is discouraged. Contraindicated in patients with frequent, copious urination. According to traditional sources, may counteract *Di Yu* (Radix Sanguisorbae Officinalis), *Qin Jiao* (Radix Gentianae Qinjiao), and *Bie Jia* (Carapax Amydae Sinensis).
C&C: Contains potassium. Could possibly cause hyperkalemia when used with potassium-sparing diuretics.

Dan Pi, Mu Dan Pi
(Cortex Radicis Moutan, tree peony root bark)

Standard daily dosage: 6-12g
AH: Not to be used during pregnancy. (This ingredient is commonly used in China during pregnancy to treat heat in the blood and/or blood stasis.)
B&G: Should not be used during pregnancy or in patients with excessive sweating or profuse menstruation. Avoid using with garlic.
According to some traditional sources, may counteract the effect of *Tu Si Zi* (Semen Cuscutae Chinensis), *Bei Mu* (Bulbus Fritillariae), and *Da Huang* (Radix Et Rhizoma Rhei).
C&C: Contains tannic acid, potassium, and glycosides. Could possibly cause hyperkalemia when used with potassium-sparing diuretics. Could possibly reduce the absorption and biologic effect of most antibiotics, isoniazid, chlorpromazine, calcium carbonate and gluconate, atropine, ephedrine, quinine, reserpine, digitalis, vitamin B_1, trypsine, amylase, and pepsin. Vitamin C, nicotinic acid, glutamic acid, hydrochloric acid, and other highly acidic substances could possibly reduce the therapeutic effect of this medicinal.

Ze Xie
(Rhizoma Alismatis Orientalis)

Standard daily dosage: 6-15g
AH: Prolonged use may cause gastrointestinal irritation.
B&G: Although considered safe, prolonged usage may irritate the intestinal tract and could possibly cause gastroenteritis.
C&C: Contains alkaloids and potassium. Could possibly cause hyperkalemia when used with potassium-sparing diuretics and reduce the absorption and therapeutic effect of potassium and sodium iodides, sodium bicarbonate, aluminum hydroxide, magnesium sulfate.
PDR: Contains triterpenes, sesquiterpenes, flavone sulfate, and caffeic acid derivatives. No health hazards or side effects with proper administration of designated therapeutic dosages.

COMMENTS

As with many other famous formulas, this formula is not commonly indicated in its simple, textbook form. However, when taken in pill form, it is commonly combined with other formulas, and it is often modified extensively when taken in decoction. In fact, Chinese doctors still say the patient is taking the base of this formula as long as their prescription contains as few of its ingredients as *Shu Di, Shan Zhu Yu,* and *Shan Yao.*

LONG DAN XIE GAN TANG
(Gentiana Drain the Liver Decoction, a.k.a. Gentiana Combination)

Category: Heat-clearing and dampness-eliminating
Functions: Drains liver-gallbladder replete heat, clears lower burner damp heat
Chinese medical indications: Replete heat in the liver and gall-bladder channels with rib-side pain, headache, dizziness, red, painful eyes, hearing loss, pain and swelling in the ears, a bitter taste in the mouth, easy anger, a red tongue with yellow fur, and a bowstring, rapid, forceful pulse
Contraindications: Spleen vacuity or damaged fluids
Western medical indications: Acute cholecystitis, herpes infections, eye infections, ear infections, hypertension, acute icteric hepatitis, acute cystitis and urethritis, pyelonephritis, male and female genital infections (prostatitis, orchitis, epididymitis, vaginitis, vaginal itching, pelvic inflammatory disease), migraine headache, eczema, and intercostal neuralgia
Potential formula toxicities & interactions:
FL/B&B: Not to be used in large doses or for long periods of time in patients with digestive weakness.

POTENTIAL MEDICINAL TOXICITIES & INTERACTIONS:

Long Dan Cao
(Radix Gentianae Longdancao)

Standard daily dosage: 3-9g
AH: Safe when used appropriately
B&G: Contraindicated in patients with diarrhea
C&C: Contains glycosides. Vitamin C, nicotinic acid, glutamic acid, hydrochloric acid, and other highly acidic substances could possibly reduce the therapeutic effect of this medicinal.

Huang Qin, Tiao Qin
(Radix Scutellariae Baicalensis)

Standard daily dosage: 6-15g
AH: Safe when used appropriately
B&G: According to some traditional sources, counteracts *Dan Pi* (Cortex Radicis Moutan) and *Li Lu* (Rhizoma Et Radix Veratri).

C&C: Contains potassium and glycosides. Could possibly cause hyperkalemia when used with potassium-sparing diuretics. Vitamin C, nicotinic acid, glutamic acid, hydrochloric acid, and other highly acidic substances could possibly reduce the therapeutic effect of this medicinal.

Zhi Zi, Shan Zhi, Shan Zhi Zi
(Fructus Gardeniae Jasminoidis, dried gardenia fruit pod)

Standard daily dosage: 3-12g
AH: Safe when used appropriately
B&G: Contains geniposide which caused diarrhea in mice.
C&C: Contains potassium and glycosides. Could possibly cause hyperkalemia when used with potassium-sparing diuretics. Vitamin C, nicotinic acid, glutamic acid, hydrochloric acid, and other highly acidic substances could possibly reduce the therapeutic effect of this medicinal.

Mu Tong
(Caulis Akebiae)

Standard daily dosage: 3-9g
B&G: Contraindicated during pregnancy. Could possibly cause dehydration and renal failure in large doses.
C&C: Contains potassium. Could possibly cause hyperkalemia when used with potassium-sparing diuretics.
PDR: Not to be administered during pregnancy. Large doses of the medicinal may lead to gastroenteritis, intestinal colic, and diarrhea due to saponin content.
GLW: Early stage symptoms of poisoning include upper abdominal discomfort, vomiting, chest oppression, abdominal pain, and diarrhea. Secondarily, there is frequent urination, urgent urination, facial edema which gradually spreads to the entire body, inability to lie down, unclear consciousness, scanty urination or blocked urination, and increased blood pressure. Some patients present oily stools. In those with acute kidney failure, uremia leads to death.

This medicinal is often substituted with Caulis Aristolochiae Manchuriensis which contains aristolochic acid. Therefore, it is important that this medicinal only be prescribed in the form of Caulis Akebiae Trifoliatae or Akebiae Quinatae.

Che Qian Zi, Che Qian Ren
(Semen Plantaginis, plantain seeds)

Standard daily dosage: 4.5-9g
B&G: Contraindicated during pregnancy

C&C: Contains glycosides. Highly acidic. Could possibly cause crystalluria and hematuria and reduce the therapeutic effect of sodium bicarbonate, aluminum hydroxide, many antibiotics (especially aminoglycosides and sulfas), reserpine, caffeine, opiates, scopolamine, and berbamin. Vitamin C, nicotinic acid, glutamic acid, hydrochloric acid, and other highly acidic substances could possibly reduce the therapeutic effect of this medicinal.

Ze Xie
(Rhizoma Alismatis Orientalis)

Standard daily dosage: 6-15g
AH: Prolonged use may cause gastrointestinal irritation.
B&G: Although considered safe, prolonged usage may irritate the intestinal tract and could possibly cause gastroenteritis.
C&C: Contains alkaloids and potassium. Could possibly cause hyperkalemia when used with potassium-sparing diuretics and reduce the absorption and therapeutic effect of potassium and sodium iodides, sodium bicarbonate, aluminum hydroxide, and magnesium sulfate.
PDR: Contains triterpenes, sesquiterpenes, flavone sulfate, caffeic acid derivatives. No health hazards or side effects with proper administration of designated therapeutic dosages.

Chai Hu
(Radix Bupleuri)

Standard daily dosage: 3-12g
AH: Safe when used appropriately
B&G: May occasionally cause nausea and vomiting, in which case the dose should then be reduced significantly.
C&C: Vitamin C, nicotinic acid, glutamic acid, hydrochloric acid, and other highly acidic substances could possibly reduce the therapeutic effect of this medicinal.
PDR: Not to be administered during pregnancy. (This medicinal is routinely used in Chinese medical gynecology during pregnancy as part of formulas appropriately prescribed on the basis of pattern discrimination.) Overdose may lead to gastroenteritis, intestinal colic, and diarrhea due to saponin content.

Sheng Di, Sheng Di Huang
(uncooked Radix Rehmanniae Glutinosae)

Standard daily dosage: 9-30g
AH: Contraindicated in patients with diarrhea or lack of appetite
B&G: Contraindicated in pregnant women with anemias or digestive weakness

C&C: Contains potassium. Could possibly cause hyperkalemia when used with potassium-sparing diuretics.

PDR: No health risks or side effects are known in conjunction with the proper administration of designated therapeutic dosages.

Dang Gui
(Radix Angelicae Sinensis)

Standard daily dosage: 3-15g

AH: Do not use during pregnancy. (This medicinal is routinely used in Chinese medical gynecology during pregnancy as part of formulas appropriately prescribed on the basis of pattern discrimination.)

B&G: Use with caution in patients with diarrhea or abdominal distention.

C&C: Contains potassium. Could possibly cause hyperkalemia when used with potassium-sparing diuretics. May exaggerate the anticoagulative effect of warfarin (Coumadin).

Gan Cao
(Radix Glycyrrhizae Uralensis, licorice root)

Standard daily dosage: 2-12g

AH: Do not use during pregnancy. (This medicinal is routinely used in Chinese medical gynecology during pregnancy as part of formulas appropriately prescribed on the basis of pattern discrimination.) As a single herb in high doses, it is contraindicated in diabetes, hypertension, and liver disorders. Not for long-term use.

BR: May increase toxicity of cardiac glycosides. May increase potassium loss due to diuretics and laxatives. Possible additive effect to corticosteroids. May be synergistic with insulin in causing hypokalemia and sodium retention.

B&G: According to some traditional sources, incompatible with *Gan Sui* (Radix Euphorbiae Kansui), *Yuan Hua* (Flos Daphnes Genkwae), and *Yuan Zhi* (Radix Polygalae Tenuifoliae). If taken long-term, it may cause hypertension and/or edema. Contains glycyrrhetinic acid which Could possibly cause a reduction in thyroid activity and basal metabolic rate.

The research on *Gan Cao* concurs that this medicinal is generally safe when used in small amounts as an envoy. It should not be taken long-term or as a single herb during pregnancy. When used as a single medicinal or in patients taking other potent Western pharmaceuticals, caution should be exercised to guard against potential toxicity and drug interaction.

COMMENTS

This formula tends to be overprescribed in the West. It is indicated for solely replete conditions, and few Western patients are solely replete.

Some practitioners employ this formula nevertheless on the basis of "in acute [conditions], treat the tip [or branch]," administering this formula for only a couple of days or so until the heat evils have been cleared. Even so, this formula may cause diarrhea due to its bitter, cold nature.

MA HUANG TANG
(Ephedra Decoction, a.k.a. Ma-huang Combination)

Standard daily dosage: 3-9g
Category: Exterior-resolving
Functions: Out-thrusts sweat and resolves the exterior, diffuses the lungs and levels panting
Chinese medical indications: Wind cold external contraction with fever, aversion to wind, no sweating, headache, generalized body aches, wheezing and panting, thin, white tongue fur, and a floating, tight or bowstring pulse
Contraindications: Vacuity weakness
Western medical indications: Common cold, cough, asthma, typhoid fever, pneumonia, bronchitis, measles, rhinitis, stuffy nose
Potential formula toxicities & interactions:
B&B: Contraindicated in patients with copious urination and those prone to nosebleeds. Use with caution in patients with hypertension.

POTENTIAL MEDICINAL TOXICITIES & INTERACTIONS:

Ma Huang
(Herba Ephedrae, ephedra)

Standard daily dosage: 3-9g
AH: Not to be used during pregnancy. Contraindicated in anorexia, bulimia, and glaucoma. Not for long-term use.
BR: Increases thermogenesis when combined with methylxanthines in theophylline and caffeine. May induce toxicity with MAO-inhibitors. May reduce the effect of dexamethasone. Amytriptiline blocks its hypertensive effect. Antagonized by reserpine.
B&G: May raise blood pressure and cause tremors. As little as 15ml in a 1% solution may be toxic to some individuals. May cause arrhythmias if used in conjunction with cardiac glycosides. Antidote for poisoning is atropine.

All research sources concur that *Ma Huang* is a very powerful herb with many potential side effects and interactions and, therefore, must be administered with care. It enhances digitalis, antagonizes barbiturates, and increases the effects of adrenergic agonists. It should only be prescribed by a properly trained practitioner and should not be given long-term or during pregnancy.

GLW: Initially after poisoning, there are central nervous and sympathetic nervous system symptoms, such as vexation, agitation, and restlessness, extreme nerve reactivity, headache, dizziness, tinnitus, insomnia, nausea, vomiting, upper abdominal discomfort, dry mouth, sweating, increased blood pressure, dilated pupils, heart palpitations, shortness of breath, and precordial pain. Graver reactions include difficulty urinating, unclear vision, shock, syncope, difficulty breathing, fright reversal. If critical, there may be respiratory failure and death.

The U.S. FDA has banned the inclusion of this medicinal in all dietary supplements.

Gui Zhi
(Ramulus Cinnamomi Cassiae, cinnamon twigs)

Standard daily dosage: 3-15g
AH: Safe when used appropriately
B&G: Use with caution in the presence of fever, during pregnancy, or during excessive menstruation.
PDR: Contraindicated during pregnancy.

Xing Ren, Ku Xing Ren
(Semen Pruni Armenicae, apricot kernel)

Standard daily dosage: 3-9g
AH: To be used only under the supervision of an expert qualified in the appropriate use of this substance
B&G: Use with caution when treating infants or patients with diarrhea. Contains amygdalin and amygdalase which break down to hydrocyanic acid in the digestive tract. Lethal dosage in adults is 50-60 uncooked kernels; children 10 kernels. Eating this medicinal uncooked or in large quantities could possibly cause dizziness, nausea, vomiting, and headache which can progress to dyspnea, spasms, dilated pupils, arrhythmias, and coma. In the event of overdosage, activated charcoal and syrup of ipecac should be administered orally.
C&C: Contains potassium and glycosides (including cyanophoric glycoside). If taken with codeine, morphine, or other opiates, hydrocyanic acid is produced which can lead to respiratory failure and death. Could possibly cause hyperkalemia when used with potassium-sparing diuretics. Vitamin C, nicotinic acid, glutamic acid, hydrochloric acid, and other highly acidic substances will reduce the therapeutic effect of this medicinal.
GLW: In the case of poisoning, typically, 1-2 hours after ingestion there is a bitter taste and astringent feeling within the mouth, drooling,

headache, dizziness, nausea, vomiting accompanied by watery diarrhea, heart palpitations, and lack of strength. In more serious cases, there is difficulty breathing. Sometimes one can smell cyanide on the person's breath. Eventually, breathing becomes weak, consciousness becomes unclear, and the pupils of the eye dilate widely with loss of reactivity to light. The teeth become clenched, blood pressure drops, there are generalized convulsions, and respiratory paralysis leads to death.

The maximum concentration of toxins in this medicinal are in the skin and the tip. When used in Chinese medicine, the kernels are blanched to remove the skin and the tips are broken off.

Gan Cao
(Radix Glycyrrhizae Uralensis, licorice root)

Standard daily dosage: 2-12g
AH: Do not use during pregnancy. (This medicinal is routinely used in Chinese medical gynecology during pregnancy as part of formulas appropriately prescribed on the basis of pattern discrimination.) As a single herb in high doses, it is contraindicated in diabetes, hypertension, and liver disorders. Not for long-term use.
BR: May increase toxicity of cardiac glycosides. May increase potassium loss due to diuretics and laxatives. Possible additive effect to corticosteroids. May be synergistic with insulin in causing hypokalemia and sodium retention.
B&G: According to some traditional sources, incompatible with *Gan Sui* (Radix Euphorbiae Kansui), *Yuan Hua* (Flos Daphnes Genkwae), and *Yuan Zhi* (Radix Polygalae Tenuifoliae). If taken long-term, it may cause hypertension and/or edema. Contains glycyrrhetinic acid which could possibly cause a reduction in thyroid activity and basal metabolic rate.

The research on *Gan Cao* concurs that this medicinal is generally safe when used in small amounts as an envoy. It should not be taken long-term or as a single herb during pregnancy. When used as a single medicinal or in patients taking other potent Western pharmaceuticals, caution should be exercised to guard against potential toxicity and drug interaction.

COMMENTS

Except for the treatment of acute wind cold asthma, this formula is rarely appropriate for Western patients.

MA XING SHI GAN TANG
(Ephedra, Apricot Kernel, Gypsum & Licorice Decoction,
a.k.a. Ma-huang & Apricot Seed Combination)

Category: Heat-clearing
Functions: Clears heat and diffuses the lungs, downbears counterflow and levels panting
Chinese medical indications: Lung heat with fever with or without sweating, thirst, panting and wheezing, cough, difficulty breathing, nasal flaring with breathing, yellow tongue fur, and a slippery, rapid pulse
Contraindications: Cold panting or qi vacuity enduring cough
Western medical indications: Respiratory tract infection, lobar pneumonia, bronchial pneumonia, bronchial asthma, measles-caused pneumonitis, bronchiolitis, pertussis, and diphtheria
Potential formula toxicities & interactions: None listed

POTENTIAL MEDICINAL TOXICITIES & INTERACTIONS:

Ma Huang
(Herba Ephedrae, ephedra)

Standard daily dosage: 3-9g
AH: Not to be used during pregnancy. Contraindicated in anorexia, bulimia, and glaucoma. Not for long-term use.
BR: Increases thermogenesis when combined with methylxanthines in theophylline and caffeine. May induce toxicity with MAO-inhibitors. May reduce the effect of dexamethazone. Amytriptiline blocks its hypertensive effect. Antagonized by reserpine.
B&G: May raise blood pressure and cause tremors. As little as 15ml in a 1% solution may be toxic to some individuals. May cause arrhythmias if used in conjunction with cardiac glycosides. Antidote for poisoning is atropine.

All research sources concur that *Ma Huang* is a very powerful herb with many potential side effects and interactions and, therefore, must be administered with care. It enhances digitalis, antagonizes barbiturates, and increases the effects of adrenergic agonists. It should only be prescribed by a properly trained practitioner and should not be given long-term or during pregnancy.

GLW: Initially after poisoning, there are central nervous and sympathetic nervous system symptoms, such as vexation, agitation, and restlessness, extreme nerve reactivity, headache, dizziness, tinnitus, insomnia, nausea, vomiting, upper abdominal discomfort, dry mouth, sweating, increased blood pressure, dilated pupils, heart palpitations, shortness of breath, and precordial pain. Graver reactions include difficulty urinating, unclear vision, shock, syncope, difficulty breathing, fright reversal. If critical, there may be respiratory failure and death.

The U.S. FDA has banned the inclusion of this medicinal in all dietary supplements.

Shi Gao
(Gypsum Fibrosum)

Standard daily dosage: 9-30g
B&G: Could possibly cause gastric upset in some patients.
C&C: Contains calcium. Could possibly reduce the effect of most antibiotics and levadopa, cause digitalis intoxication and heart arrhythmias, and hinder the absorption of isoniazid.

Xing Ren, Ku Xing Ren
(Semen Pruni Armenicae, apricot kernel)

Standard daily dosage: 3-9g
AH: To be used only under the supervision of an expert qualified in the appropriate use of this substance.
B&G: Use with caution when treating infants or patients with diarrhea. Contains amygdalin and amygdalase which break down to hydrocyanic acid in the digestive tract. Lethal dosage in adults is 50-60 uncooked kernels; children 10 kernels. Eating this medicinal uncooked or in large quantities Could possibly cause dizziness, nausea, vomiting, and headache, which can progress to dyspnea, spasms, dilated pupils, arrhythmias, and coma. In the event of overdosage, activated charcoal and syrup of ipecac should be administered orally.
C&C: Contains potassium and glycosides (including cyanophoric glycoside). If taken with codeine, morphine, or other opiates, hydrocyanic acid is produced which can lead to respiratory failure and death. Could possibly cause hyperkalemia when used with potassium-sparing diuretics. Vitamin C, nicotinic acid, glutamic acid, hydrochloric acid, and other highly acidic substances could possibly reduce the therapeutic effect of this medicinal.
GLW: In case of poisoning, typically, 1-2 hours after ingestion there is a bitter taste and astringent feeling within the mouth, drooling,

headache, dizziness, nausea, vomiting accompanied by watery diarrhea, heart palpitations, and lack of strength. In more serious cases, there is difficulty breathing. Sometimes one can smell cyanide on the person's breath. Eventually, breathing becomes weak, consciousness becomes unclear, and the pupils of the eye dilate widely with loss of reactivity to light. The teeth become clenched, blood pressure drops, there are generalized convulsions, and respiratory paralysis leads to death.

The maximum concentration of toxins in this medicinal are in the skin and the tip. When used in Chinese medicine, the kernels are blanched to remove the skin and the tips are broken off.

Gan Cao
(Radix Glycyrrhizae Uralensis, licorice root)

Standard daily dosage: 2-12g
AH: Do not use during pregnancy. (This medicinal is routinely used in Chinese medical gynecology during pregnancy as part of formulas appropriately prescribed on the basis of pattern discrimination.) As a single herb in high doses, it is contraindicated in diabetes, hypertension, and liver disorders. Not for long-term use.
BR: May increase toxicity of cardiac glycosides. May increase potassium loss due to diuretics and laxatives. Possible additive effect to corticosteroids. May be synergistic with insulin in causing hypokalemia and sodium retention.
B&G: According to some traditional sources, incompatible with *Gan Sui* (Radix Euphorbiae Kansui), *Yuan Hua* (Flos Daphnes Genkwae), and *Yuan Zhi* (Radix Polygalae Tenuifoliae). If taken long-term, it may cause hypertension and/or edema. Contains glycyrrhetinic acid which could possibly cause a reduction in thyroid activity and basal metabolic rate.

The research on *Gan Cao* concurs that this medicinal is generally safe when used in small amounts as an envoy. It should not be taken long-term or as a single herb during pregnancy. When used as a single medicinal or in patients taking other potent Western pharmaceuticals, caution should be exercised to guard against potential toxicity and drug interaction.

COMMENTS

Unlike the preceding formula, this one is more useful in clinical practice. Besides wind heat asthma, it also treats heat pattern pneumonia and bronchitis.

MA ZI REN WAN

(Cannabis Seed Pills, a.k.a. Apricot Seed & Linum Formula)

Category: Draining and precipitating
Functions: Moistens the intestines and discharges heat, moves the qi and frees the flow of the stools
Chinese medical indications: Heat-induced fluid damage of the intestines and stomach with constipation, hard, dry stools, frequent urination, dry, yellow tongue fur, and a deep, rapid or floating, choppy pulse
Contraindications: Blood vacuity constipation, profound vacuity weakness, or pregnancy
Western medical indications: Constipation in the elderly or the weak, postpartum or postsurgical constipation, habitual constipation, chronic colitis, hemorrhoids
Potential formula toxicities & interactions:
FL/B&B: Prohibited during pregnancy
B&B: Use caution when treating weak or debilitated patients

POTENTIAL MEDICINAL TOXICITIES & INTERACTIONS:

Huo Ma Ren
(Semen Cannabis Sativae, cannabis seeds, marijuana seeds)

Standard daily dosage: 9-45g
B&G: Symptoms of overdose may include nausea, vomiting, diarrhea, numbness of the extremities, irritability, chorea, miosis, and in severe cases coma and death. Treatment is based on gastric lavage, fluids, and symptomatic therapy.
C&C: Contains alkaloids. Could possibly reduce the absorption and therapeutic effect of potassium and sodium iodides, sodium bicarbonate, aluminum hydroxide, and magnesium sulfate.
PDR: No health risks or side effects are known in conjunction with the proper administration of designated therapeutic dosages.

Bai Shao, Shao Yao
(Radix Albus Paeoniae Lactiflorae, white peony root)

Standard daily dosage: 6-30g
AH: Safe when used appropriately
B&G: Use with caution in debilitated patients with diarrhea. According

to some traditional sources, antagonizes *Shi Hu* (Herba Dendrobii) and *Mang Xiao* (Mirabilitum), counteracts *Bie Jia* (Carapax Amydae Sinensis) and *Xiao Ji* (Herba Cephalanopoloris Segeti), and is incompatible with *Li Lu* (Rhizoma Et Radix Veratri).

C&C: Contains calcium, tannic acid, potassium, and glycosides. Could possibly cause hyperkalemia when used with potassium-sparing diuretics. Could possibly reduce the effect of most antibiotics, cause digitalis intoxication and heart arrhythmias, and could possibly reduce the absorption and therapeutic effect of levadopa, isoniazid, chlorpromazine, calcium carbonate and gluconate, atropine, ephedrine, quinine, reserpine, vitamin B_1, trypsine, amylase, and pepsin. Vitamin C, nicotinic acid, glutamic acid, hydrochloric acid, and other highly acidic substances could possibly reduce the therapeutic effect of this medicinal.

Zhi Shi
(Fructus Immaturus Citri Aurantii, immature bitter orange)

Standard daily dosage: 3-9g

B&G: Use with caution during pregnancy or in debilitated patients.

C&C: Contains tannic acid. Highly acidic. Could possibly cause crystalluria and hematuria and reduce the absorption and biologic effect of most antibiotics, isoniazid, chlorpromazine, calcium carbonate and gluconate, atropine, ephedrine, quinine, reserpine, digitalis, vitamin B_1, trypsine, amylase, and pepsin, sodium bicarbonate, aluminum hydroxide, caffeine, opiates, scopolamine, and berbamin.

Da Huang, Dai Huang, Chuan Jun, Jun
(Radix Et Rhizoma Rhei, rhubarb root)

Standard daily dosage: 3-12g

AH: Do not use during pregnancy. Not to be used while nursing. Contraindicated in intestinal obstruction, abdominal pain of unknown origin, or any inflammatory condition of the intestines.

BR: Reduces absorption of oral drugs. Overuse may cause hypokalemia and increased toxicity of cardiac glycosides. May aggravate potassium loss from diuretics.

B&G: Use with extreme caution during pregnancy, menstruation, or postpartum. Contraindicated for nursing mothers since active ingredients enter the milk.

C&C: Contains alkaloids, tannic acid, potassium, and glycosides. Could possibly cause hyperkalemia when used with potassium-sparing diuretics. Vitamin C, nicotinic acid, glutamic acid, hydrochloric acid, and other highly acidic substances could possibly reduce the therapeutic effect of this medicinal.

PDR: Consult a physician before using this medicinal during pregnancy or while nursing. Contraindicated in cases of intestinal obstruction, acute inflammatory intestinal disease, appendicitis and abdominal pain of unknown origin.

Hou Po, Chuan Po
(Cortex Magnoliae Officinalis)

Standard daily dosage: 3-9g
AH: Not to be used during pregnancy (This medicinal is commonly used in China during pregnancy, especially for the treatment of nausea and vomiting.)
B&G: Use with caution during pregnancy. According to some traditional sources, antagonizes *Ze Xie* (Rhizoma Alismatis Orientalis) and *Han Shui Shi* (Calcitum).
C&C: Contains tannic acid and potassium. Could possibly cause hyperkalemia when used with potassium-sparing diuretics and reduce the absorption and biologic effect of most antibiotics, isoniazid, chlorpromazine, calcium carbonate and gluconate, atropine, ephedrine, quinine, reserpine, digitalis, vitamin B_1, trypsine, amylase, and pepsin.
PDR: No health risks or side effects are known in conjunction with the proper administration of designated therapeutic dosages.

Xing Ren, Ku Xing Ren
(Semen Pruni Armenicae, apricot kernel)

Standard daily dosage: 3-9g
AH: To be used only under the supervision of an expert qualified in the appropriate use of this substance.
B&G: Use with caution when treating infants or patients with diarrhea. Contains amygdalin and amygdalase which break down to hydrocyanic acid in the digestive tract. Lethal dosage in adults is 50-60 uncooked kernels; children 10 kernels. Eating this medicinal uncooked or in large quantities Could possibly cause dizziness, nausea, vomiting, and headache, which can progress to dyspnea, spasms, dilated pupils, arrhythmias, and coma. In the advent of overdosage activated charcoal and syrup of ipacec should be administered orally.
C&C: contains potassium and glycosides (including cyanophoric glycoside). If taken with codeine, morphine, or other opiates, hydrocyanic acid is produced which can lead to respiratory failure and death. Could possibly cause hyperkalemia when used with potassium-sparing diuretics. Vitamin C, nicotinic acid, glutamic acid, hydrochloric acid, and other highly acidic substances will reduce the therapeutic effect of this medicinal.

GLW: In case of poisoning, typically, 1-2 hours after ingestion there is a bitter taste and astringent feeling within the mouth, drooling, headache, dizziness, nausea, vomiting accompanied by watery diarrhea, heart palpitations, and lack of strength. In more serious cases, there is difficulty breathing. Sometimes one can smell cyanide on the person's breath. Eventually, breathing becomes weak, consciousness becomes unclear, and the pupils of the eye dilate widely with loss of reactivity to light. The teeth become clenched, blood pressure drops, there are generalized convulsions, and respiratory paralysis leads to death.

The maximum concentration of toxins in this medicinal are in the skin and the tip. When used in Chinese medicine, the kernels are blanched to remove the skin and the tips are broken off.

COMMENTS

Hu Ma Ren (Semen Lini Usitatissimi, flaxseed) can be substituted for *Huo Ma Ren*. Because *Da Huang* can cause melanosis coli, a precancerous condition of the bowel, it should not be used long-term. For chronic, recalcitrant constipation, *Run Chang Wan* (Moisten the Intestines Pills) or *Ji Chuan Jian* (Flow the River Brew) are safer choices.

MAI MEN DONG TANG
(Ophiopogon Decoction, a.k.a. Ophiopogon Combination)

Standard daily dosage: 6-15g
Category: Dryness-treating
Functions: Boosts the stomach and engenders fluids, downbears counterflow and stops coughing
Chinese medical indications: Lung wilting due to damaged lung yin manifesting in coughing, panting, wheezing, shortness of breath, a dry, uncomfortable sensation in the throat, a dry mouth, a dry, red tongue with scanty fur, and a vacuous, rapid pulse
Contraindications: Evils retained in the exterior and absence of qi and yin vacuity
Western medical indications: Gastritis, gastroesophageal reflux disorder (GERD), peptic ulcer, acute or chronic pharyngitis, chronic bronchitis, and pulmonary tuberculosis
Potential formula toxicities & interactions: None listed

POTENTIAL MEDICINAL TOXICITIES & INTERACTIONS:

Mai Men Dong, Mai Dong
(Tuber Ophiopogoni Japonici)

Standard daily dosage: 6-15g
AH: Safe when used appropriately
B&G: According to some traditional sources, antagonizes *Kuan Dong Hua* (Flos Tussilaginis Farfarae) and counteracts *Ku Shen* (Radix Sophorae Flavescentis) and *Bai Mu Er* (Fructificatio Tremellae Fuciformis).
C&C: Contains glycosides. Vitamin C, nicotinic acid, glutamic acid, hydrochloric acid, and other highly acidic substances could possibly reduce the therapeutic effect of this medicinal.

Ren Shen
(Radix Panacis Ginseng, ginseng)

Standard daily dosage: 1-30g
AH: Contraindicated in hypertension
BR: May cause manic episodes in patients on MAO-inhibitors. May cause hypertension if consumed with caffeine. Possible additive effects

to insulin. May reduce the anticoagulative effect of warfarin (Coumadin).
B&G: Contraindicated for hypertensive patients. Overdose can lead to
headache, insomnia, heart palpitations, and a rise in blood pressure. A
traditional antidote is mung bean soup.
C&C: Vitamin C, nicotinic acid, glutamic acid, hydrochloric acid, and
other highly acidic substances could possibly reduce the therapeutic
effect of this medicinal.
PDR: Contraindicated in patients with hypertension. Not recommended in
large doses during pregnancy or lactation due to potential neonatal androgenization. Enhances the effect of insulin and other antidiabetic agents.
Use with MAO-inhibitors may cause headaches, tremors, and manias.

Geng Mi
(Semen Oryzae Sativae, polished rice)

Standard daily dosage: 15-30g

No toxicity or interaction information listed in the sources

Da Zao, Hong Zao
(Fructus Zizyphi Jujubae, red dates)

Standard daily dosage: 10-30g (3-12 pieces)
AH: Safe when used appropriately
PDR: No health risks or side effects are known in conjunction with the
proper administration of designated therapeutic dosages.

Gan Cao
(Radix Glycyrrhizae Uralensis, licorice root)

Standard daily dosage: 2-12g
AH: Do not use during pregnancy. (This medicinal is routinely used in
Chinese medical gynecology during pregnancy as part of formulas
appropriately prescribed on the basis of pattern discrimination.) As a
single herb in high doses, it is contraindicated in diabetes, hypertension,
and liver disorders. Not for long-term use.
BR: May increase toxicity of cardiac glycosides. May increase potassium loss
due to diuretics and laxatives. Possible additive effect to corticosteroids. May
be synergistic with insulin in causing hypokalemia and sodium retention.
B&G: According to some traditional sources, incompatible with *Gan Sui*
(Radix Euphorbiae Kansui), *Yuan Hua* (Flos Daphnes Genkwae), and
Yuan Zhi (Radix Polygalae Tenuifoliae). If taken long-term, it may cause
hypertension and/or edema. Contains glycyrrhetinic acid which could
possibly cause a reduction in thyroid activity and basal metabolic rate.

The research on *Gan Cao* concurs that this medicinal is generally safe when used in small amounts as an envoy. It should not be taken long-term or as a single herb during pregnancy. When used as a single medicinal or in patients taking other potent Western pharmaceuticals, caution should be exercised to guard against potential toxicity and drug interaction.

Ban Xia
(Rhizoma Pinelliae Ternatae)

Standard daily dosage: 4.5-12g
AH: Do not use during pregnancy. (This medicinal is routinely used during pregnancy in China when indicated by disease and pattern discrimination.) Contraindicated in all hemorrhagic disorders.
B&G: Safe as long as it is properly prepared. Must be decocted with other herbs and not taken alone or uncooked. Toxic effects due to improper preparation or dosage include burning and numbness in throat and lips, nausea, and a feeling of pressure in the chest. Antidote is oral administration of raw ginger. Use with caution in patients with fever. According to some traditional sources, incompatible with *Wu Tou* (Radix Aconiti).
C&C: Contains alkaloids and glycosides. Could possibly reduce the absorption and therapeutic effect of potassium and sodium iodides, sodium bicarbonate, aluminum hydroxide, and magnesium sulfate. Vitamin C, nicotinic acid, glutamic acid, hydrochloric acid, and other highly acidic substances could possibly reduce the therapeutic effect of this medicinal.
GLW: Poisoning occurs within 15 minutes to three hours after ingestion of a suitable amount. Initially, there is burning pain in the mouth, tongue, and throat, and enlargement of the tongue. This is then followed by drooling, ulceration of the oral mucosa, unclear speech, difficulty swallowing, dizziness, low-grade fever, heart palpitations, numbness of the extremities, a somber white facial complexion, and a weak, forceless pulse. If severe, there may be convulsions and respiratory failure leading to death.

COMMENTS

Dang Shen (Radix Codonopsitis Pilosulae) or *Tai Zi Shen* (Radix Pseudostellariae Heterophyllae) is commonly substituted for *Ren Shen* in this formula, and usually, mix-fried *Gan Cao* is the form of that medicinal used. This formula may be used to treat yin damage nausea and vomiting due to chemo- or radiation therapy.

MU LI SAN
(Oyster Shell Powder)

Category: Securing and astringing
Functions: Secures the exterior and stops sweating
Chinese medical indications: Qi vacuity spontaneous sweating with heart palpitations, shortness of breath, fatigue, lack of strength, a pale red tongue with thin, white fur, and a faint pulse
Contraindications: Yin or yang desertion sweating
Western medical indications: Spontaneous sweating caused by weakness or debility
Potential formula toxicities & interactions: None listed

POTENTIAL MEDICINAL TOXICITIES & INTERACTIONS:

Mu Li
(Concha Ostreae, oyster shell)

Standard daily dosage: 15-30g
B&G: Contraindicated when the patient has high fever without sweating. Overdose may lead to indigestion or constipation. According to some traditional sources, works synergistically with *Bei Mu* (Bulbus Frittilariae), *Gan Cao* (Radix Glycyrrizae Uralensis), *Niu Xi* (Radix Achyranthis Bidentatae), and *Yuan Zhi* (Radix Polygalae Tenuifoliae) and has adverse effects when combined with *Ma Huang* (Herba Ephedrae), *Wu Zhu Yu* (Fructus Evodiae Rutecarpae), and *Xi Xin* (Herba Asari Cum Radice).
C&C: Contains calcium, iron, magnesium, and aluminum. Could possibly reduce the effects of most antibiotics, levadopa, and prednisolone, cause digitalis intoxication and heart arrhythmias, and hinder the absorption of isoniazid.

Huang Qi, Bei Qi
(Radix Astragali Membranacei, astragalus)

Standard daily dosage: 9-60g
AH: Safe when used appropriately
C&C: Contains alkaloids and potassium. Could possibly cause hyperkalemia when used with potassium-sparing diuretics. Could possibly reduce the absorption and therapeutic effect of potassium and sodium iodides, sodium bicarbonate, aluminum hydroxide, and magnesium sulfate.

PDR: Caution should be taken with patients receiving immunosuppressive therapy, such as transplant patients or patients with autoimmune disorders. May cause neurological dysfunction in high doses. May potentiate the risk of bleeding when used concomitantly with anticoagulants, antiplatelets, or antithrombotic agents.

Ma Huang Gen
(Radix Ephedrae, ephedra root)

Standard daily dosage: 3-9g

No toxicity or interaction information listed in the sources

The U.S. FDA has banned the inclusion of this medicinal in all dietary supplements.

Fu Xiao Mai
(Fructus Levis Tritici Aestivi)

Standard daily dosage: 9-15g
PDR: No health risks or side effects are known in conjunction with the proper administration of designated therapeutic dosages.

COMMENTS

These four ingredients may be added to other formulas or combined with other Chinese medicines for the treatment of the specific symptom of qi-vacuity spontaneous perspiration.

NUAN GAN JIAN
(Warm the Liver Brew)

Category: Qi-rectifying
Functions: Warms the liver and kidneys, moves the qi and stops pain
Chinese medical indications: Cold mounting due to a liver-kidney yang vacuity and qi stagnation with lower abdominal pain which is sharp, fixed, aggravated by cold, and accompanied by a pale tongue and a deep, tight or bowstring pulse
Contraindications: Heat or damp heat
Western medical indications: Inguinal hernia, varicocele, and hydrocele
Potential formula toxicities & interactions: None listed

POTENTIAL MEDICINAL TOXICITIES & INTERACTIONS:

Dang Gui
(Radix Angelicae Sinensis)

Standard daily dosage: 3-15g
AH: Do not use during pregnancy. (This medicinal is routinely used in Chinese medical gynecology during pregnancy as part of formulas appropriately prescribed on the basis of pattern discrimination.)
B&G: Use with caution in patients with diarrhea or abdominal distention.
C&C: Contains potassium. Could possibly cause hyperkalemia when used with potassium-sparing diuretics. May exaggerate the anticoagulative effect of warfarin (Coumadin).

Gou Qi Zi, Qi Zi
(Fructus Lycii Chinensis, lycium berries)

Standard daily dosage: 6-18g
AH: Not to be used during pregnancy. (No such prohibition exists in traditional Chinese medicine regarding this medicinal.)
C&C: Contains tannic acid and potassium. Could possibly cause hyperkalemia when used with potassium-sparing diuretics. Could possibly reduce the absorption and biologic effect of most antibiotics, isoniazid, chlorpromazine, calcium carbonate and gluconate, atropine, ephedrine, quinine, reserpine, digitalis, vitamin B_1, trypsine, amylase, and pepsin.
PDR: Not for use during pregnancy.

Xiao Hui Xiang
(Fructus Foeniculi Vulgaris, fennel)

Standard daily dosage: 3-9g
AH: Safe when used appropriately
PDR: Not for use during pregnancy or by small children.

Rou Gui, Gui Xin, Guan Gui
(Cortex Cinnamomi Cassiae, cinnamon bark)

Standard daily dosage: 1.5-4.5g
BR: Reduces absorption of tetracyclines.
B&G: Use with caution during pregnancy.
C&C: Contains tannic acid and potassium. Could possibly cause hyperkalemia when used with potassium-sparing diuretics. Could possibly reduce the absorption and biologic effect of most antibiotics, isoniazid, chlorpromazine, calcium carbonate and gluconate, atropine, ephedrine, quinine, reserpine, digitalis, vitamin B_1, trypsine, amylase, and pepsin.

Wu Yao, Tai Wu
(Radix Linderae Strychnifoliae)

Standard daily dosage: 3-9g

No toxicity or interaction information listed in the sources

Chen Xiang
(Lignum Aquilariae, aloeswood)

Standard daily dosage: 1.5-3g as a powder

No toxicity or interaction information listed in the sources

Fu Ling, Bai Fu Ling, Yun Ling
(Sclerotium Poriae Cocos)

Standard daily dosage: 9-15g
B&G: Large doses or long-term use is discouraged. Contraindicated in patients with frequent, copious urination. According to traditional sources, may counteract *Di Yu* (Radix Sanguisorbae Officinalis), *Qin Jiao* (Radix Gentianae Qinjiao), and *Bie Jia* (Carapax Amydae Sinensis).
C&C: Contains potassium. Could possibly cause hyperkalemia when used with potassium-sparing diuretics.

Sheng Jiang
(uncooked Rhizoma Zingiberis Officinalis, fresh ginger)

Standard daily dose: 3-9g
AH: Safe when used appropriately
BR: Reduces vomiting caused by chemotherapeutic drugs. Increases absorption of oral drugs.
PDR: Recommended safe dosage limit is six grams (6g). Avoid larger doses if being used to treat morning sickness or if used in patients taking anticoagulants.

COMMENTS

It is important for practitioners to rule out testicular cancer in patients complaining of cold-natured testicular pain. This formula is not capable of curing inguinal hernia but can reduce its discomfort and halt its progression.

PING WEI SAN
(Level the Stomach Powder,
a.k.a. Calm the Stomach Powder, Magnolia & Ginger Formula)

Category: Dampness-dispelling, turbidity-transforming
Functions: Dries dampness and transports the spleen, moves the qi and harmonizes the stomach
Chinese medical indications: Dampness and cold stagnating in the spleen and stomach with stomach duct and abdominal distention and fullness, loss of taste, torpid intake, heaviness of the limbs, loose stools or diarrhea, fatigue, somnolence, nausea and vomiting, belching/burping, acid regurgitation, a swollen, fat tongue with thick, white, slimy fur, and a moderate (*i.e.*, slightly slow) or soggy pulse
Contraindications: Yin-blood vacuity
Western medical indications: Acute and chronic gastritis, gastrectasis, gastric ulcer, peptic ulcer, indigestion (especially pediatric indigestion), gastric neurosis, obesity, chronic pancreatitis, and parasitic diseases
Potential formula toxicities & interactions:
FL/B&B: Use with caution during pregnancy

POTENTIAL MEDICINAL TOXICITIES & INTERACTIONS:

Cang Zhu
(Rhizoma Atractylodis)

Standard daily dosage: 4.5-9g
AH: Safe when used appropriately
B&G: Use with caution in patients with loose, watery stools.
PDR: No health risks or side effects are known in conjunction with the proper administration of designated therapeutic dosages.

Hou Po, Chuan Po
(Cortex Magnoliae Officinalis)

Standard daily dosage: 3-9g
AH: Not to be used during pregnancy. (This medicinal is commonly used in China during pregnancy, especially for the treatment of nausea and vomiting.)
B&G: Use with caution during pregnancy. According to some traditional sources, antagonizes *Ze Xie* (Rhizoma Alismatis Orientalis) and *Han Shui Shi* (Calcitum).
C&C: Contains tannic acid and potassium. Could possibly cause hyper-

kalemia when used with potassium-sparing diuretics and reduce the absorption and biologic effect of most antibiotics, isoniazid, chlorpromazine, calcium carbonate and gluconate, atropine, ephedrine, quinine, reserpine, digitalis, vitamin B_1, trypsine, amylase, and pepsin.
PDR: No health risks or side effects are known in conjunction with the proper administration of designated therapeutic dosages.

Chen Pi, Ju Pi, Ju Hong
(Pericarpium Citri Reticulatae, tangerine peel)

Standard daily dosage: 3-9g
AH: Safe when used appropriately
C&C: Contains potassium. Could possibly cause hyperkalemia when used with potassium-sparing diuretics.

Gan Cao
(Radix Glycyrrhizae Uralensis, licorice root)

Standard daily dosage: 2-12g
AH: Do not use during pregnancy. (This medicinal is routinely used in Chinese medical gynecology during pregnancy as part of formulas appropriately prescribed on the basis of pattern discrimination.) As a single herb in high doses, it is contraindicated in diabetes, hypertension, and liver disorders. Not for long-term use.
BR: May increase toxicity of cardiac glycosides. May increase potassium loss due to diuretics and laxatives. Possible additive effect to corticosteroids. May be synergistic with insulin in causing hypokalemia and sodium retention.
B&G: According to some traditional sources, incompatible with *Gan Sui* (Radix Euphorbiae Kansui), *Yuan Hua* (Flos Daphnes Genkwae), and *Yuan Zhi* (Radix Polygalae Tenuifoliae). If taken long-term, it may cause hypertension and/or edema. Contains glycyrrhetinic acid which could possibly cause a reduction in thyroid activity and basal metabolic rate.

The research on *Gan Cao* concurs that this medicinal is generally safe when used in small amounts as an envoy. It should not be taken long-term or as a single herb during pregnancy. When used as a single medicinal or in patients taking other potent Western pharmaceuticals, caution should be exercised to guard against potential toxicity and drug interaction.

Sheng Jiang
(uncooked Rhizoma Zingiberis Officinalis, fresh ginger)

Standard daily dose: 3-9g
AH: Safe when used appropriately

BR: Reduces vomiting caused by chemotherapeutic drugs. Increases absorption of oral drugs.

PDR: Recommended safe dosage limit is six grams (6g). Avoid larger doses if being used to treat morning sickness or if used in patients taking anticoagulants.

Da Zao, Hong Zao
(Fructus Zizyphi Jujubae, red dates)

Standard daily dosage: 10-30g (3-12 pieces)
AH: Safe when used appropriately
PDR: No health risks or side effects are known in conjunction with the proper administration of designated therapeutic dosages.

QING HAO BIE JIA TANG
(Artemisia Annua & Carapax Amydae Decoction)

Category: Vacuity heat-clearing
Functions: Nourishes yin and clears heat
Chinese medical indications: Yin vacuity heat in the later stages of a warm disease with night-time fever and morning coolness, no sweating as the fever recedes, emaciation but no loss of appetite, a red tongue with scanty fur, and a fine, rapid pulse
Contraindications: Early stage warm disease when evils are still in the qi aspect
Western medical indications: Advanced stages of various infectious diseases especially pulmonary and renal tuberculosis. Also useful for chronic nephritis, fevers of unknown etiology, typhoid fever convalescence, and postsurgical fever.
Potential formula toxicities & interactions:
FL/B&B: Not for fever from common cold or simple infections. Not for use in patients with spasms or convulsions.

POTENTIAL MEDICINAL TOXICITIES & INTERACTIONS:

Bie Jia
(Carapax Amydae Sinensis)

Standard daily dosage: 9-30g
B&G: Contraindicated in pregnancy and in patients who have not fully gotten over a cold. Use with caution in cases of impotence. According to some traditional sources, antagonizes *Ming Fan* (Alumen).

Qing Hao
(Herba Artemisiae Annuae Seu Apiaceae)

Standard daily dosage: 3-24g
AH: Not to be used during pregnancy.
B&G: Contraindicated in postpartum women with anemia. According to traditional sources, should not be used with *Sheng Di* (uncooked Radix Rehmanniae Glutinosae) or *Dang Gui* (Radix Angelicae Sinensis).
C&C: Contains tannic acid and potassium. Could possibly cause hyperkalemia when used with potassium-sparing diuretics. Could possibly reduce the absorption and biologic effect of most antibiotics, isoniazid, chlorpromazine, calcium carbonate and gluconate, atropine, ephedrine, quinine, reserpine, digitalis, vitamin B$_1$, trypsin, amylase, and pepsin.

Sheng Di, Sheng Di Huang
(uncooked Radix Rehmanniae Glutinosae)

Standard daily dosage: 9-30g
AH: Contraindicated in patients with diarrhea or lack of appetite
B&G: Contraindicated in pregnant women with anemias or digestive weakness
C&C: Contains potassium. Could possibly cause hyperkalemia when used with potassium-sparing diuretics.
PDR: No health risks or side effects are known in conjunction with the proper administration of designated therapeutic dosages.

Zhi Mu
(Rhizoma Anemarrhenae Aspheloidis)

Standard daily dosage: 6-12g
B&G: May cause diarrhea in some patients.
C&C: Contains potassium and glycosides. Could possibly cause hyperkalemia when used with potassium-sparing diuretics. Vitamin C, nicotinic acid, glutamic acid, hydrochloric acid, and other highly acidic substances could possibly reduce the therapeutic effect of this medicinal.
PDR: No health hazards are known in conjunction with the proper administration of designated therapeutic dosages.

Dan Pi, Mu Dan Pi
(Cortex Radicis Moutan, tree peony root bark)

Standard daily dosage: 6-12g
AH: Not to be used during pregnancy. (This ingredient is commonly used in China during pregnancy to treat heat in the blood and/or blood stasis.)
B&G: Should not be used during pregnancy or in patients with excessive sweating or profuse menstruation. Avoid using with garlic. According to some traditional sources, may counteract the effect of *Tu Si Zi* (Semen Cuscutae Chinensis), *Bei Mu* (Bulbus Fritillariae), and *Da Huang* (Radix Et Rhizoma Rhei).
C&C: Contains tannic acid, potassium, and glycosides. Could possibly cause hyperkalemia when used with potassium-sparing diuretics. Could possibly reduce the absorption and biologic effect of most antibiotics, isoniazid, chlorpromazine, calcium carbonate and gluconate, atropine, ephedrine, quinine, reserpine, digitalis, vitamin B_1, trypsine, amylase, and pepsin. Vitamin C, nicotinic acid, glutamic acid, hydrochloric acid, and other highly acidic substances could possibly reduce the therapeutic effect of this medicinal.

QING QI HUA TAN TANG
(Clear the Qi & Transform Phlegm Pills)

Category: Phlegm-transforming and heat-clearing
Functions: Clears heat and transforms phlegm, rectifies the qi and stops coughing
Chinese medical indications: Phlegm heat with cough and yellow, sticky phlegm which is difficult to expectorate, chest and diaphragmatic glomus and fullness, nausea, a red tongue with slimy, yellow fur, and a slippery, rapid pulse
Contraindications: None listed
Western medical indications: Acute and chronic bronchitis, bronchiectasis, chronic rhinitis, nasosinusitis, chronic tracheitis, and pneumonia
Potential formula toxicities & interactions: None listed

POTENTIAL MEDICINAL TOXICITIES & INTERACTIONS:

Dan Nan Xing
(bile-processed Rhizoma Arisaematis)

Standard daily dosage: 4.5-9g
B&G: Safe as long as it is properly prepared. Must be decocted properly with other medicinals and not taken alone or uncooked. Toxic effects due to improper preparation or dosage include irritation of the mouth and throat, edema and numbness of the lips, increase in saliva production, and voice problems. According to traditional sources, may counteract *Fu Zi* (Radix Lateralis Praeparatus Aconiti Carmichaeli), *Gan Jiang* (dry Rhizoma Zingiberis Officinalis), and *Sheng Jiang* (uncooked Rhizoma Zingiberis Officinalis).

Ban Xia
(Rhizoma Pinelliae Ternatae)

Standard daily dosage: 4.5-12g
AH: Do not use during pregnancy. (This medicinal is routinely used during pregnancy in China when indicated by disease and pattern discrimination.) Contraindicated in all hemorrhagic disorders.
B&G: Safe as long as it is properly prepared. Must be decocted with other herbs and not taken alone or uncooked. Toxic effects due to improper preparation or dosage include burning and numbness in throat and lips, nausea, and a feeling of pressure in the chest. Antidote is oral administration of raw ginger. Use with caution in patients with fever.

According to some traditional sources, incompatible with *Wu Tou* (Radix Aconiti).

C&C: Contains alkaloids and glycosides. Could possibly reduce the absorption and therapeutic effect of potassium and sodium iodides, sodium bicarbonate, aluminum hydroxide, and magnesium sulfate. Vitamin C, nicotinic acid, glutamic acid, hydrochloric acid, and other highly acidic substances could possibly reduce the therapeutic effect of this medicinal.

GLW: Poisoning occurs within 15 minutes to three hours after ingestion of a suitable amount. Initially, there is burning pain in the mouth, tongue, and throat, and enlargement of the tongue. This is then followed by drooling, ulceration of the oral mucosa, unclear speech, difficulty swallowing, dizziness, low-grade fever, heart palpitations, numbness of the extremities, a somber white facial complexion, and a weak, forceless pulse. If severe, there may be convulsions and respiratory failure leading to death.

Gua Lou Ren, Gua Lou Zi
(Semen Trichosanthis Kirlowii)

Standard daily dosage: 9-12g
AH: Safe when used appropriately
B&G: According to traditional sources, incompatible with *Wu Tou* (Radix Aconiti). Contains peimine which is fatal in animals at doses of 9mg/kg. Symptoms of toxicity include reduced breathing, mydriasis, tremors, and coma.
C&C: Contains alkaloids and glycosides. Could possibly reduce the absorption and therapeutic effect of potassium and sodium iodides, sodium bicarbonate, aluminum hydroxide, and magnesium sulfate. Vitamin C, nicotinic acid, glutamic acid, hydrochloric acid, and other highly acidic substances could possibly reduce the therapeutic effect of this medicinal.

Huang Qin, Tiao Qin
(Radix Scutellariae Baicalensis)

Standard daily dosage: 6-15g
AH: Safe when used appropriately
B&G: According to some traditional sources, counteracts *Dan Pi* (Cortex Radicis Moutan) and *Li Lu* (Rhizoma Et Radix Veratri).
C&C: Contains potassium and glycosides. Could possibly cause hyperkalemia when used with potassium-sparing diuretics. Vitamin C, nicotinic acid, glutamic acid, hydrochloric acid, and other highly acidic substances could possibly reduce the therapeutic effect of this medicinal.

Chen Pi, Ju Pi, Ju Hong
(Pericarpium Citri Reticulatae, tangerine peel)

Standard daily dosage: 3-9g
AH: Safe when used appropriately
C&C: Contains potassium. Could possibly cause hyperkalemia when used with potassium-sparing diuretics.

Xing Ren, Ku Xing Ren
(Semen Pruni Armenicae, apricot kernel)

Standard daily dosage: 3-12g
AH: To be used only under the supervision of an expert qualified in the appropriate use of this substance.
B&G: Use with caution when treating infants or patients with diarrhea. Contains amygdalin and amygdalase which break down to hydrocyanic acid in the digestive tract. Lethal dosage in adults is 50-60 uncooked kernels; children 10 kernels. Eating this medicinal uncooked or in large quantities could possibly cause dizziness, nausea, vomiting, and headache, which can progress to dyspnea, spasms, dilated pupils, arrhythmias, and coma. In the advent of overdose, activated charcoal and syrup of ipecac should be administered orally.
C&C: Contains potassium and glycosides (including cyanophoric glycoside). If taken with codeine, morphine, or other opiates, hydrocyanic acid is produced which can lead to respiratory failure and death. Could possibly cause hyperkalemia when used with potassium-sparing diuretics. Vitamin C, nicotinic acid, glutamic acid, hydrochloric acid, and other highly acidic substances will reduce the therapeutic effect of this medicinal.
GLW: In case of poisoning, typically, 1-2 hours after ingestion there is a bitter taste and astringent feeling within the mouth, drooling, headache, dizziness, nausea, vomiting accompanied by watery diarrhea, heart palpitations, and lack of strength. In more serious cases, there is difficulty breathing. Sometimes one can smell cyanide on the person's breath. Eventually, breathing becomes weak, consciousness becomes unclear, and the pupils of the eye dilate widely with loss of reactivity to light. The teeth become clenched, blood pressure drops, there are generalized convulsions, and respiratory paralysis leads to death.

The maximum concentration of toxins in this medicinal are in the skin and the tip. When used in Chinese medicine, the kernels are blanched to remove the skin and the tips are broken off.

Zhi Shi
(Fructus Immaturus Citri Aurantii, immature bitter orange)

Standard daily dosage: 3-9g

B&G: Use with caution during pregnancy or in debilitated patients.

C&C: Contains tannic acid. Highly acidic. Could possibly cause crystalluria and hematuria and reduce the absorption and biologic effect of most antibiotics, isoniazid, chlorpromazine, calcium carbonate and gluconate, atropine, ephedrine, quinine, reserpine, digitalis, vitamin B_1, trypsine, amylase, and pepsin, sodium bicarbonate, aluminum hydroxide, caffeine, opiates, scopolamine, and berbamin.

Fu Ling, Bai Fu Ling, Yun Ling
(Sclerotium Poriae Cocos)

Standard daily dosage: 9-15g

B&G: Large doses or long-term use is discouraged. Contraindicated in patients with frequent, copious urination. According to traditional sources, may counteract *Di Yu* (Radix Sanguisorbae Officinalis), *Qin Jiao* (Radix Gentianae Qinjiao), and *Bie Jia* (Carapax Amydae Sinensis).

C&C: Contains potassium. Could possibly cause hyperkalemia when used with potassium-sparing diuretics.

QING WEI SAN
(Clear the Stomach Powder, a.k.a. Coptis & Rehmannia Formula)

Category: Heat-clearing
Functions: Drains stomach fire, cools the blood, and nourishes yin
Chinese medical indications: Stomach heat manifesting as toothache, facial swelling, fever, bad breath, a dry mouth, a red tongue with scanty fur, and a surging, slippery, rapid pulse
Contraindications: Wind cold toothache or kidney vacuity tooth and gum disorders
Western medical indications: Stomatitis, trigeminal neuralgia, gingivitis, periodontal disease, glossitis, and idiopathic halitosis
Potential formula toxicities & interactions: None listed

POTENTIAL MEDICINAL TOXICITIES & INTERACTIONS:

Huang Lian, Chuan Lian
(Rhizoma Coptidis Chinensis)

Standard daily dosage: 1.5-9g
AH: Not to be used during pregnancy. (This medicinal is commonly used during pregnancy in China when indicated by disease and pattern discrimination.)
B&G: Contains berberine. Long-term use may damage the digestive system. According to some traditional sources, antagonizes *Ju Hua* (Flos Chrysanthemi Morifolii), *Xuan Shen* (Radix Scrophulariae Ningpoensis), *Bai Xian Pi* (Cortex Radicis Dictamni Dasycarpi), and *Jiang Can* (Bombyx Batryticatus). According to some traditional sources, counteracts *Kuan Dong Hua* (Flos Tussilaginis Farfarae) and *Niu Xi* (Radix Achyranthis Bidentatae), Some traditional sources say it should not be taken with pork.
C&C: Contains alkaloids, quercetin, and potassium. Could possibly cause hyperkalemia when used with potassium-sparing diuretics. Could possibly reduce the absorption and therapeutic effect of potassium and sodium iodides, sodium bicarbonate, calcium gluconate, carbonate, and lactate, aluminum hydroxide, magnesium and ferrous sulfates, and bismuth subcarbonate.

Sheng Ma
(Rhizoma Cimicifugae, black cohosh)

Standard daily dosage: 1.5-9g
AH: Not to be used during pregnancy. (This medicinal is commonly used during pregnancy in China.) Not to be used while nursing.
B&G: Contraindicated in cases of fully erupted measles and in patients

with breathing difficulties. Overdose causes headaches, dizziness, vomiting, tremors, gastroenteritis, and pathogenic erections.

C&C: Vitamin C, nicotinic acid, glutamic acid, hydrochloric acid, and other highly acidic substances could possibly reduce the therapeutic effect of this medicinal.

PDR: Not for use during pregnancy due to an increased risk of spontaneous abortion. Contains glycosides which may potentiate the effect of antihypertensive medications and result in hypotension.

Dan Pi, Mu Dan Pi
(Cortex Radicis Moutan, tree peony root bark)

Standard daily dosage: 6-12g
AH: Not to be used during pregnancy. (This ingredient is commonly used in China during pregnancy to treat heat in the blood and/or blood stasis.

B&G: Should not be used during pregnancy or in patients with excessive sweating or profuse menstruation. Avoid using with garlic.
According to some traditional sources, may counteract the effect of *Tu Si Zi* (Semen Cuscutae Chinensis), *Bei Mu* (Bulbus Fritillariae), and *Da Huang* (Radix Et Rhizoma Rhei).

C&C: Contains tannic acid, potassium, and glycosides. Could possibly cause hyperkalemia when used with potassium-sparing diuretics. Could possibly reduce the absorption and biologic effect of most antibiotics, isoniazid, chlorpromazine, calcium carbonate and gluconate, atropine, ephedrine, quinine, reserpine, digitalis, vitamin B_1, trypsine, amylase, and pepsin. Vitamin C, nicotinic acid, glutamic acid, hydrochloric acid, and other highly acidic substances could possibly reduce the therapeutic effect of this medicinal.

Sheng Di, Sheng Di Huang
(uncooked Radix Rehmanniae Glutinosae)

Standard daily dosage: 9-30g
AH: Contraindicated in patients with diarrhea or lack of appetite
B&G: Contraindicated in pregnant women with anemias or digestive weakness
C&C: Contains potassium. Could possibly cause hyperkalemia when used with potassium-sparing diuretics.
PDR: No health risks or side effects are known in conjunction with the proper administration of designated therapeutic dosages.

Dang Gui
(Radix Angelicae Sinensis)

Standard daily dosage: 3-15g

AH: Do not use during pregnancy. (This medicinal is routinely used in Chinese medical gynecology during pregnancy as part of formulas appropriately prescribed on the basis of pattern discrimination.)

B&G: Use with caution in patients with diarrhea or abdominal distention.

C&C: Contains potassium. Could possibly cause hyperkalemia when used with potassium-sparing diuretics. May exaggerate the anticoagulative effect of warfarin (Coumadin).

Comments

This formula is commonly used to treat dental caries and toothache due to stomach heat.

RUN CHANG WAN

(Moisten the Intestines Pills, a.k.a. Linum & Rhubarb Combination)

Category: Draining and precipitating
Functions: Moistens the intestines and frees the flow of the stools
Chinese medical indications: Intestinal dryness constipation with lusterless skin, dry mouth and unquenchable thirst, a dry tongue, and a fine pulse
Contraindications: None listed
Western medical indications: Constipation, especially in post-partum women and the elderly
Potential formula toxicities & interactions: None listed

POTENTIAL MEDICINAL TOXICITIES & INTERACTIONS:

Huo Ma Ren

(Semen Cannabis Sativae, cannabis seeds, marijuana seeds)

Standard daily dosage: 9-45g
B&G: Symptoms of overdose may include nausea, vomiting, diarrhea, numbness of the extremities, irritability, chorea, miosis, and, in severe cases, coma and death. Treatment is based on gastric lavage, fluids, and symptomatic therapy.
C&C: Contains alkaloids. Could possibly reduce the absorption and therapeutic effect of potassium and sodium iodides, sodium bicarbonate, aluminum hydroxide, and magnesium sulfate.
PDR: No health risks or side effects are known in conjunction with the proper administration of designated therapeutic dosages.

Tao Ren

(Semen Pruni Persicae, peach kernel)

Standard daily dosage: 4.5-9g
AH: Not to be used during pregnancy.
B&G: Contraindicated during pregnancy.
C&C: Contains potassium and glycosides (including cyanophoric gly-cosides). If taken with codeine, morphine, or other opiates, hydrocyanic acid is produced which can lead to respiratory failure and death. Could possibly cause hyperkalemia when used with potassium-sparing diuret-ics. Vitamin C, nicotinic acid, glutamic acid, hydrochloric acid, and

other highly acidic substances could possibly reduce the therapeutic effect of this medicinal.

GLW: In case of poisoning, typically, 1-2 hours after ingestion there is a bitter taste and astringent feeling within the mouth, drooling, headache, dizziness, nausea, vomiting accompanied by watery diarrhea, heart palpitations, and lack of strength. In more serious cases, there is difficulty breathing. Sometimes one can smell cyanide on the person's breath. Eventually, breathing becomes weak, consciousness becomes unclear, and the pupils of the eye dilate widely with loss of reactivity to light. The teeth become clenched, blood pressure drops, there are generalized convulsions, and respiratory paralysis leads to death.

Most of the toxins in this medicinal reside in the skin and tip. Therefore, this medicinal is blanched before using and its tip is broken off in order to make it less or non-toxic.

Dang Gui
(Radix Angelicae Sinensis)

Standard daily dosage: 3-15g

AH: Do not use during pregnancy. (This medicinal is routinely used in Chinese medical gynecology during pregnancy as part of formulas appropriately prescribed on the basis of pattern discrimination.)

B&G: Use with caution in patients with diarrhea or abdominal distention.

C&C: Contains potassium. Could possibly cause hyperkalemia when used with potassium-sparing diuretics. May exaggerate the anticoagulative effect of warfarin (Coumadin).

Sheng Di, Sheng Di Huang
(uncooked Radix Rehmanniae Glutinosae)

Standard daily dosage: 9-30g

AH: Contraindicated in patients with diarrhea or lack of appetite

B&G: Contraindicated in pregnant women with anemias or digestive weakness

C&C: Contains potassium. Could possibly cause hyperkalemia when used with potassium-sparing diuretics.

PDR: No health risks or side effects are known in conjunction with the proper administration of designated therapeutic dosages.

Zhi Ke, Zhi Qiao
(Fructus Citri Aurantii, bitter orange)

Standard daily dose: 3-9g

AH: Safe when used appropriately

B&G: Use with caution during pregnancy

C&C: Contains tannic acid. Highly acidic. Could possibly cause crystalluria and hematuria. Could possibly reduce the absorption and biologic effect of most antibiotics, isoniazid, chlorpromazine, calcium carbonate and gluconate, atropine, ephedrine, quinine, reserpine, digitalis, vitamin B_1, trypsine, amylase, and pepsin, sodium bicarbonate, aluminum hydroxide, caffeine, opiates, scopolamine, and berbamin.

PDR: May cause UV-sensitivity in light-skinned individuals. Otherwise, no health hazards are known in conjunction with the proper administration of designated therapeutic dosages.

COMMENTS

Huo Ma Ren can be substituted by *Hu Ma Ren* (Semen Lini Usitatissimi, flaxseed).

SANG JU YIN
(Mulberry Leaf & Chrysanthemum Beverage,
a.k.a. Morus & Chrysanthemum Combination)

Category: Exterior-resolving
Functions: Courses wind and clears heat, diffuses the lungs and stops cough
Chinese medical indications: Defensive aspect warm disease with slight fever, cough, slight thirst, thin, white tongue fur, and a floating, rapid pulse
Contraindications: Wind cold external contraction
Western medical indications: Common cold, flu, acute bronchitis, acute tonsillitis, epidemic conjunctivitis, headache, vertigo, and acute tracheitis
Potential formula toxicities & interactions: None listed

POTENTIAL MEDICINAL TOXICITIES & INTERACTIONS:

Sang Ye
(Folium Mori Albi, mulberry leaves)

Standard daily dose: 4.5-15g
AH: Safe when used appropriately
B&G: Long-term use in high dosages caused liver and kidney damage in mice.
C&C: Contains tannic acid and quercetin. Therefore, could conceivably reduce absorption and biologic effect of most antibiotics, isoniazid, chlorpromazine, calcium carbonate, gluconate, & lactate, atropine, ephedrine, quinine, reserpine, digitalis, vitamin B_1, trypsine, amylase, and pepsin, aluminum hydroxide, magnesium and ferrous sulfates, and bismuth subcarbonate.

Ju Hua, Gan Ju Hua, Hang Ju Hua
(Flos Chrysanthemi Morifolii, chrysanthemum flowers)

Standard daily dosage: 4.5-15g
B&G: Use with caution in patients with diarrhea and/or poor appetite.

Xing Ren, Ku Xing Ren
(Semen Pruni Armenicae, apricot kernel)

Standard daily dosage: 3-9g

AH: To be used only under the supervision of an expert qualified in the appropriate use of this substance.

B&G: Use with caution when treating infants or patients with diarrhea. Contains amygdalin and amygdalase which break down to hydrocyanic acid in the digestive tract. Lethal dosage in adults is 50-60 uncooked kernels; children 10 kernels. Eating this medicinal uncooked or in large quantities could possibly cause dizziness, nausea, vomiting, and headache which can progress to dyspnea, spasms, dilated pupils, arrhythmias, and coma. In the advent of overdose, activated charcoal and syrup of ipecac should be administered orally.

C&C: Contains potassium and glycosides (including cyanophoric glycoside). If taken with codeine, morphine, or other opiates, hydrocyanic acid is produced which can lead to respiratory failure and death. Could possibly cause hyperkalemia when used with potassium-sparing diuretics. Vitamin C, nicotinic acid, glutamic acid, hydrochloric acid, and other highly acidic substances may reduce the therapeutic effect of this medicinal.

GLW: In case of poisoning, typically, 1-2 hours after ingestion there is a bitter taste and astringent feeling within the mouth, drooling, headache, dizziness, nausea, vomiting accompanied by watery diarrhea, heart palpitations, and lack of strength. In more serious cases, there is difficulty breathing. Sometimes one can smell cyanide on the person's breath. Eventually, breathing becomes weak, consciousness becomes unclear, and the pupils of the eye dilate widely with loss of reactivity to light. The teeth become clenched, blood pressure drops, there are generalized convulsions, and respiratory paralysis leads to death.

The maximum concentration of toxins in this medicinal are in the skin and the tip. When used in Chinese medicine, the kernels are blanched to remove the skin and the tips are broken off.

Lian Qiao
(Fructus Forsythiae Suspensae, dried forsythia fruit pods)

Standard daily dosage: 6-15g
AH: Not to be used during pregnancy. (This medicinal is commonly used in China during pregnancy to treat wind heat external contractions and heat toxins.)
B&G: Contraindicated in patients with diarrhea, carbuncles that have already ulcerated, and skin ulcers.
C&C: Contains potassium and glycosides. Could possibly cause hyperkalemia when used with potassium-sparing diuretics. Vitamin C, nicotinic acid, glutamic acid, hydrochloric acid, and other highly acidic substances could possibly reduce the therapeutic effect of this medicinal.

Bo He
(Herba Menthae Haplocalycis, field mint)

Standard daily dose: 1.5-6g
AH: Safe when used appropriately
B&G: Not recommended for nursing mothers as it may inhibit lactation.

Jie Geng
(Radix Platycodi Grandiflori, bellflower root)

Standard daily dosage: 3-9g
AH: Contraindicated in hemoptysis, especially in cases of tuberculosis. Use with caution in bleeding peptic ulcer.
B&G: Contraindicated in patients with hemoptysis. According to some traditional sources, counteracts *Long Dan Cao* (Radix Gentiana Longdancao) and *Long Yan Rou* (Arillus Euphoriae Longanae).
C&C: Contains calcium and glycosides. Could possibly reduce the effect of most antibiotics, cause digitalis intoxication and heart arrhythmias, hinder the absorption of isoniazid, and reduce the biological effect of levadopa. Vitamin C, nicotinic acid, glutamic acid, hydrochloric acid, and other highly acidic substances could possibly reduce the therapeutic effect of this medicinal.

Gan Cao
(Radix Glycyrrhizae Uralensis, licorice root)

Standard daily dosage: 2-12g
AH: Do not use during pregnancy. (This medicinal is routinely used in Chinese medical gynecology during pregnancy as part of formulas appropriately prescribed on the basis of pattern discrimination.) As a single herb in high doses, it is contraindicated in diabetes, hypertension, and liver disorders. Not for long-term use.
BR: May increase toxicity of cardiac glycosides. May increase potassium loss due to diuretics and laxatives. Possible additive effect to corticosteroids. May be synergistic with insulin in causing hypokalemia and sodium retention.
B&G: According to some traditional sources, incompatible with *Gan Sui* (Radix Euphorbiae Kansui), *Yuan Hua* (Flos Daphnes Genkwae), and *Yuan Zhi* (Radix Polygalae Tenuifoliae). If taken long-term, it may cause hypertension and/or edema. Contains glycyrrhetinic acid which could possibly cause a reduction in thyroid activity and basal metabolic rate.

The research on *Gan Cao* concurs that this medicinal is generally safe when used in small amounts as an envoy. It should not be taken long-term or as a single herb during pregnancy. When used as a single medicinal or

in patients taking other potent Western pharmaceuticals, caution should be exercised to guard against potential toxicity and drug interaction.

Lu Gen, Wei Jing, Wei Gen
(Rhizoma Phragmitis Communis)

Standard daily dosage: 15-60g

PDR: No health risks or side effects are known in conjunction with the proper administration of designated therapeutic dosages.

SANG PIAO XIAO SAN
(Mantis Egg-case Powder)

Category: Securing and astringing
Functions: Regulates and supplements the heart and kidneys, astringes the essence and stops loss
Chinese medical indications: Polyuria and incontinence due to heart-kidney qi vacuity with turbid urine, impaired memory, a pale tongue with white fur, and a fine, slow, forceless pulse
Contraindications: Damp heat or vigorous fire in the lower burner
Western medical indications: Polyuria, spermatorrhea, nocturnal emissions, turbid urine, impaired memory due to nervous exhaustion, chronic nephritis, diabetes mellitus, tubular acidosis, primary aldosteronism, hyperparathyroidism, neurosis, prolapsed uterus, and autonomic dystonia
Potential formula toxicities & interactions: None listed

POTENTIAL MEDICINAL TOXICITIES & INTERACTIONS:

Sang Piao Xiao
(Ootheca Mantidis, mantis egg-case)

Standard daily dosage: 3-9g
B&G: According to some traditional sources, counteracts *Xuan Fu Hua* (Flos Inulae Racemosae).
C&C: Contains calcium, iron, and potassium. Could possibly cause hyperkalemia when used with potassium-sparing diuretics. Could possibly reduce the effect of most antibiotics, levadopa, and prednisolone, cause digitalis intoxication and heart arrhythmias, and hinder the absorption of isoniazid.

Long Gu
(Os Draconis, fossilized bone)

Standard daily dosage: 15-30g
B&G: According to some traditional sources, counteracts *Shi Gao* (Gypsum Fibrosum) and should not be mixed with fish.
C&C: Contains calcium, iron, magnesium, aluminum, and potassium. Could possibly cause hyperkalemia when used with potassium-sparing diuretics. Could possibly reduce the effect of most antibiotics, levadopa,

and prednisolone, cause digitalis intoxication and heart arrhythmias, and hinder the absorption of isoniazid.

Ren Shen
(Radix Panacis Ginseng, ginseng)

Standard daily dosage: 1-30g
AH: Contraindicated in hypertension
BR: May cause manic episodes in patients on MAO-inhibitors. May cause hypertension if consumed with caffeine. Possible additive effects to insulin. May reduce the anticoagulative effect of warfarin (Coumadin).
B&G: Contraindicated for hypertensive patients. Overdose can lead to headache, insomnia, heart palpitations, and a rise in blood pressure. A traditional antidote is mung bean soup.
C&C: Vitamin C, nicotinic acid, glutamic acid, hydrochloric acid, and other highly acidic substances could possibly reduce the therapeutic effect of this medicinal.
PDR: Contraindicated in patients with hypertension. Not recommended in large doses during pregnancy or lactation due to potential neonatal androgenization. Enhances the effect of insulin and other antidiabetic agents. Use with MAO-inhibitors may cause headaches, tremors, and manias.

Fu Shen
(Sclerotium Pararadicis Poriae Cocos)

Standard daily dosage: 9-60g
B&G: Large doses or long-term use is discouraged. Contraindicated in patients with frequent, copious urination. According to traditional sources, may counteract *Di Yu* (Radix Sanguisorbae Officinalis), *Qin Jiao* (Radix Gentianae Qinjiao), and *Bie Jia* (Carapax Amydae Sinensis).
C&C: Contains potassium. Could possibly cause hyperkalemia when used with potassium-sparing diuretics.

Yuan Zhi
(Radix Polygalae Tenuifoliae)

Standard daily dosage: 3-9g
AH: Contraindicated in gastritis or when gastric ulcers are present.
B&G: Contraindicated in gastritis or when gastric ulcers are present. According to some traditional sources, counteracts *Zhen Zhu* (Margarita) and *Li Lu* (Rhizoma Et Radix Veratri).

C&C: Contains glycosides. Vitamin C, nicotinic acid, glutamic acid, hydrochloric acid, and other highly acidic substances could possibly reduce the therapeutic effect of this medicinal.

Shi Chang Pu, Chang Pu
(Rhizoma Acori Graminei, sweetflag rhizome)

Standard daily dosage: 3-9g
AH: Do not use during pregnancy.
B&G: According to some traditional sources, antagonizes *Ma Huang* (Herba Ephedrae). Massive overdosage in mice led to convulsions, hypersensitivity to external stimuli, and death caused by stimulation of the spinal cord.
GLW: Symptoms of adverse reaction include headache, vomiting, vexation and agitation, sweating, stiffness of the neck, oral thirst, a rapid pulse, increased body temperature and blood pressure, slightly dilated pupils, a red flushed face, twitching muscles, generalized tension which may become convulsions, clenched teeth, arched-back rigidity, unclear thinking, cramping of the four limbs, dimming of consciousness, urinary block, and, eventually death due to respiratory paralysis.

Gui Ban
(Plastrum Testudinis, tortoise plastron)

Standard daily dosage: 9-30g
B&G: Contraindicated in pregnancy. According to some traditional sources, antagonizes *Sha Shen* (Radix Glehniae Littoralis) and *Ren Shen* (Radix Panacis Ginseng).

Dang Gui
(Radix Angelicae Sinensis)

Standard daily dosage: 3-15g
AH: Do not use during pregnancy. (This medicinal is routinely used in Chinese medical gynecology during pregnancy as part of formulas appropriately prescribed on the basis of pattern discrimination.)
B&G: Use with caution in patients with diarrhea or abdominal distention.
C&C: Contains potassium. Could possibly cause hyperkalemia when used with potassium-sparing diuretics. May exaggerate the anticoagulative effect of warfarin (Coumadin).

COMMENTS

Dang Shen (Radix Codonopsitis Pilosulae) may be substituted for *Ren Shen* in this formula.

SHEN FU TANG
(Ginseng & Aconite Decoction)

Category: Interior-warming
Functions: Rescues yang, strongly supplements source qi, and stems the desertion of qi due to yang detriment
Chinese medical indications: Yang qi desertion with cold extremities, sweating, weak breathing, shortness of breath, dizziness, an extremely pale facial complexion, a pale tongue, and a faint pulse on the verge of expiry
Contraindications: Not for long-term use; for emergency use only
Western medical indications: Cardiac failure, myocardial infarction, cardiogenic shock, postpartum hemorrhage, uterine bleeding, and other causes of hypovolemic shock
Potential formula toxicities & interactions:
B&B: A very strong formula that should only be administered in acute conditions. Extended use will damage the yin and consume blood.

POTENTIAL MEDICINAL TOXICITIES & INTERACTIONS:

Ren Shen
(Radix Panacis Ginseng, ginseng)

Standard daily dosage: 1-30g
AH: Contraindicated in hypertension
BR: May cause manic episodes in patients on MAO-inhibitors. May cause hypertension if consumed with caffeine. Possible additive effects to insulin. May reduce the anticoagulative effect of warfarin (Coumadin).
B&G: Contraindicated for hypertensive patients. Overdose can lead to headache, insomnia, heart palpitations, and a rise in blood pressure. A traditional antidote is mung bean soup.
C&C: Vitamin C, nicotinic acid, glutamic acid, hydrochloric acid, and other highly acidic substances could possibly reduce the therapeutic effect of this medicinal.
PDR: Contraindicated in patients with hypertension. Not recommended in large doses during pregnancy or lactation due to potential neonatal androgenization. Enhances the effect of insulin and other antidiabetic agents. Use with MAO-inhibitors may cause headaches, tremors, and manias.

Fu Zi, Shu Fu Zi, Fu Pian
(Radix Lateralis Praeparatus Aconiti Carmichaeli,
wolfsbane, monkshood)

Standard daily dosage: 1.5-15g
AH: To be used only under the supervision of an expert qualified in the appropriate use of this substance
B&G: Contraindicated during pregnancy. A very toxic medicinal which can be fatal if ingested in its uncooked form or in an inappropriate dose. It is generally combined with *Gan Cao* (Radix Glycyrhizae Uralensis) and *Gan Jiang* (dry Rhizoma Zingiberis Officinalis) in decoctions to reduce its toxicity. Symptoms of toxicity include drooling, gastric upset, light-headedness, blurred vision, and numbness and tingling of the extremities. More severe symptoms include premature atrial contractions, dyspnea, and reduced temperature and blood pressure. Emergency measures include the administration of atropine.
C&C: Contains alkaloids. Could possibly reduce the absorption and therapeutic effect of potassium and sodium iodides, sodium bicarbonate, aluminum hydroxide, and magnesium sulfate.
PDR: Contains nor-diterpene alkaloids, including aconitine. Highly toxic; small doses can be fatal.
GLW: If mild poisoning, there is a burning hot sensation in the mouth and on the tongue, numbness, and pain which gradually spreads to the four limbs and then to the whole body, nausea, vomiting, dizziness, heart palpitations, rapid breathing, vexation, agitation, restlessness, drooling. If more severe poisoning, there may be generalized sweating, paralysis, convulsions, urinary incontinence, dilated pupils, slowed reaction to light, slow heartbeat, arrhythmia, low blood pressure, a somber white facial complexion, reversal chilling of the four limbs, lowered body temperature, and circulatory collapse leading to death.

Sheng Jiang
(uncooked Rhizoma Zingiberis Officinalis, fresh ginger)

Standard daily dose: 3-9g
AH: Safe when used appropriately
BR: Reduces vomiting caused by chemotherapeutic drugs. Increases absorption of oral drugs.
PDR: Recommended safe dosage limit is six grams (6g). Avoid larger doses if being used to treat morning sickness or if used in patients taking anticoagulants.

Da Zao, Hong Zao
(Fructus Zizyphi Jujubae, red dates)

Standard daily dosage: 10-30g (3-12 pieces)
AH: Safe when used appropriately
PDR: No health risks or side effects are known in conjunction with the proper administration of designated therapeutic dosages.

COMMENTS

Because this formula is meant for emergency use, it is one where *Dang Shen* (Radix Codonopsitis Pilosulae) is not substituted for *Ren Shen*.

SHEN LING BAI ZHU SAN
(Ginseng, Poria & Atractylodes Powder, a.k.a.
Ginseng & Atractylodes Formula)

Category: Qi-supplementing
Functions: Fortifies the spleen and supplements the qi, eliminates dampness and stops diarrhea
Chinese medical indications: Spleen vacuity with internally engendered dampness resulting in loose stools, diarrhea, torpid intake, fatigue, lack of strength, chest and stomach duct oppression and distention, a pale white or sallow yellow facial complexion, a pale tongue with white fur, and a fine, moderate (*i.e.*, slightly slow) or forceless, moderate pulse
Contraindications: Yin vacuity heat
Western medical indications: Diarrhea from chronic gastritis, chronic hepatitis, chronic bronchitis, chronic nephritis, diabetes mellitus, malabsorption symdromes, and malnutrition in children
Potential formula toxicities & interactions: None listed

POTENTIAL MEDICINAL TOXICITIES & INTERACTIONS:

Ren Shen
(Radix Panacis Ginseng, ginseng)

Standard daily dosage: 1-30g
AH: Contraindicated in hypertension.
BR: May cause manic episodes in patients on MAO-inhibitors. May cause hypertension if consumed with caffeine. Possible additive effects to insulin. May reduce the anticoagulative effect of warfarin (Coumadin).
B&G: Contraindicated for hypertensive patients. Overdose can lead to headache, insomnia, heart palpitations, and a rise in blood pressure. A traditional antidote is mung bean soup.
C&C: Vitamin C, nicotinic acid, glutamic acid, hydrochloric acid, and other highly acidic substances could possibly reduce the therapeutic effect of this medicinal.
PDR: Contraindicated in patients with hypertension. Not recommended in large doses during pregnancy or lactation due to potential neonatal androgenization. Enhances the effect of insulin and other antidiabetic agents. Use with MAO-inhibitors may cause headaches, tremors, and manias.

Bai Zhu
(Rhizoma Atractylodis Macrocephalae)

Standard daily dosage: 4.5-9g
AH: Safe when used appropriately
B&G: When rats were fed 0.5g/kg of this medicinal for two months, they developed a mild lymphopenia and anemia but suffered no damage to the brain, heart, or liver.

Fu Ling, Bai Fu Ling, Yun Ling
(Sclerotium Poriae Cocos)

Standard daily dosage: 9-15g
B&G: Large doses or long-term use is discouraged. Contraindicated in patients with frequent, copious urination. According to traditional sources, may counteract *Di Yu* (Radix Sanguisorbae Officinalis), *Qin Jiao* (Radix Gentianae Qinjiao), and *Bie Jia* (Carapax Amydae Sinensis). **C&C:** Contains potassium. Could possibly cause hyperkalemia when used with potassium-sparing diuretics.

Gan Cao
(Radix Glycyrrhizae Uralensis, licorice root)

Standard daily dosage: 2-12g
AH: Do not use during pregnancy. (This medicinal is routinely used in Chinese medical gynecology during pregnancy as part of formulas appropriately prescribed on the basis of pattern discrimination.) As a single herb in high doses, it is contraindicated in diabetes, hypertension, and liver disorders. Not for long-term use.
BR: May increase toxicity of cardiac glycosides. May increase potassium loss due to diuretics and laxatives. Possible additive effect to corticosteroids. May be synergistic with insulin in causing hypokalemia and sodium retention.
B&G: According to some traditional sources, incompatible with *Gan Sui* (Radix Euphorbiae Kansui), *Yuan Hua* (Flos Daphnes Genkwae), and *Yuan Zhi* (Radix Polygalae Tenuifoliae). If taken long-term, it may cause hypertension and/or edema. Contains glycyrrhetinic acid which could possibly cause a reduction in thyroid activity and basal metabolic rate.

The research on *Gan Cao* concurs that this medicinal is generally safe when used in small amounts as an envoy. It should not be taken long-term or as a single herb during pregnancy. When used as a single medicinal or in patients taking other potent Western pharmaceuticals, caution should be exercised to guard against potential toxicity and drug interaction.

Shan Yao
(Radix Dioscoreae Oppositae)

Standard daily dosage: 9-30g
AH: Safe when used appropriately
B&G: According to some traditional sources, antagonizes *Gan Sui* (Radix Euphorbiae Kansui).
C&C: Contains alkaloids, potassium, amylase, and glycosides. Could possibly cause hyperkalemia when used with potassium-sparing diuretics. Could possibly reduce the absorption and therapeutic effect of potassium and sodium iodides, sodium bicarbonate, aluminum hydroxide, magnesium sulfate, tetracyclines, sulphanomides, and aspirin. Vitamin C, nicotinic acid, glutamic acid, hydrochloric acid, and other highly acidic substances could possibly reduce the therapeutic effect of this medicinal.
PDR: Use of this medicinal may reduce the antiinflammatory effect of indomethacin. May have an additive estrogenic effect when administered with estrogen-containing drugs. Poisoning in overdoses may occur from the picrotoxin-like effect of dioscorin.

Bai Bian Dou, Bian Dou
(Semen Dolichoris Lablab, hyacinth bean)

Standard daily dosage: 9-21g
B&G: Contraindicated in patients with intermittent chills and fevers.
C&C: Contains alkaloids. Could possibly reduce the absorption and therapeutic effect of potassium and sodium iodides, sodium bicarbonate, aluminum hydroxide, and magnesium sulfate.

Lian Zi, Lian Zi Rou, Lian Rou, Lian Ren
(Semen Nelumbinis Nuciferae)

Standard daily dosage: 6-15g
AH: Contraindicated in constipation and stomach distention.
B&G: Contraindicated in constipation and stomach distention.
PDR: No health risks or side effects are known in conjunction with the proper administration of designated therapeutic dosages.

Yi Yi Ren, Yi Ren, Yi Mi, Yi Mi Ren, Yi Ren Mi
(Semen Coicis Lachryma-jobi, Job's tears barley)

Standard daily dosage: 9-30g
AH: Not to be used during pregnancy.

B&G: Use with caution during pregnancy.
C&C: Contains potassium. Could possibly cause hyperkalemia when used with potassium-sparing diuretics.

Sha Ren
(Fructus Amomi)

Standard daily dosage: 1.5-6g
AH: Safe when used appropriately
PDR: Use with caution in patients with gallstones since it can trigger colic due to its motility-enhancing effect.

Jie Geng
(Radix Platycodi Grandiflori, bellflower root)

Standard daily dosage: 3-9g
AH: Contraindicated in hemoptysis, especially in cases of tuberculosis. Use with caution in bleeding peptic ulcer.
B&G: Contraindicated in patients with hemoptysis. According to some traditional sources, counteracts *Long Dan Cao* (Radix Gentiana Longdancao) and *Long Yan Rou* (Arillus Euphoriae Longanae).
C&C: Contains calcium and glycosides. Could possibly reduce the effect of most antibiotics, cause digitalis intoxication and heart arrhythmias, hinder the absorption of isoniazid, and reduce the biological effect of levadopa. Vitamin C, nicotinic acid, glutamic acid, hydrochloric acid, and other highly acidic substances could possibly reduce the therapeutic effect of this medicinal.

COMMENTS

Dang Shen (Radix Codonopsitis Pilosulae) is commonly substituted for *Ren Shen* in this formula.

SHENG HUA TANG
(Engendering & Transforming Decoction)

Category: Blood-quickening
Functions: Quickens the blood, transforms stasis, and warms the channels
Chinese medical indications: Uterine cold as a result of qi and blood vacuity postpartum manifesting as nonprecipitation of the lochia, chilly pain in the lower abdomen, a pale but purplish tongue or possible static macules or speckles, and a fine, deep, choppy pulse
Contraindications: Heat stasis or postpartum bleeding due to heat causing the blood to move frenetically outside its vessels
Western medical indications: Retention of lochia, retention of placental fragments and other postpartum complaints associated with stale blood retained in the lower abdomen, chronic endometritis, puerperal infection, and trichomonas vaginitis
Potential formula toxicities & interactions:
FL/B&B: Contraindicated during pregnancy and with most hemorrhagic disorders. Use with care in postpartum disorders since this formula may be too harsh.

POTENTIAL MEDICINAL TOXICITIES & INTERACTIONS:

Dang Gui
(Radix Angelicae Sinensis)

Standard daily dosage: 3-15g
AH: Do not use during pregnancy. (This medicinal is routinely used in Chinese medical gynecology during pregnancy as part of formulas appropriately prescribed on the basis of pattern discrimination.)
B&G: Use with caution in patients with diarrhea or abdominal distention.
C&C: Contains potassium. Could possibly cause hyperkalemia when used with potassium-sparing diuretics. May exaggerate the anticoagulative effect of warfarin (Coumadin).

Chuan Xiong
(Radix Ligustici Wallichii)

Standard daily dosage: 3-9g (In China today, it is not uncommon for this medicinal to be prescribed up to 15 grams per day in decoction.)
AH: Do not use during pregnancy. (This medicinal is routinely used in Chinese medical gynecology during pregnancy as part of formulas appropriately prescribed on the basis of pattern discrimination.)
B&G: Not for patients with migraine headache or excessive menstrual bleeding. Overdosage causes vomiting and dizziness. According to some

traditional texts, antagonizes *Shan Zhu Yu* (Fructus Corni Officinalis) and *Huang Qi* (Radix Astragali Membranacei), counteracts *Hua Shi* (Talcum) and *Huang Lian* (Rhizoma Coptidis Chinensis), and is incompatible with *Li Lu* (Rhizoma Et Radix Veratri).

C&C: Contains alkaloids and potassium. Could possibly cause hyperkalemia when used with potassium-sparing diuretics. Could possibly reduce the absorption and therapeutic effect of potassium and sodium iodides, sodium bicarbonate, aluminum hydroxide, and magnesium sulfate.

Pao Jiang

(blast-fried Rhizoma Zingiberis Officinalis) (Toxicity and usage information not specific to *Pao Jiang* or blast-fried Rhizoma Zingiberis Officinalis. Assumedly, blast-frying does change the chemotherapeutic actions of this medicinal.)

Standard daily dosage: 3-12g

AH: Not to be used during pregnancy. Patients with gallstones must consult a practitioner prior to use.

BR: Reduces vomiting caused by chemotherapeutic drugs. Increases absorption of oral drugs.

B&G: Use with caution during pregnancy.

PDR: Recommended safe dosage limit is six grams (6g). Avoid larger doses if being used to treat morning sickness or if used in patients taking anticoagulants.

Gan Cao

(Radix Glycyrrhizae Uralensis, licorice root)

Standard daily dosage: 2-12g

AH: Do not use during pregnancy. (This medicinal is routinely used in Chinese medical gynecology during pregnancy as part of formulas appropriately prescribed on the basis of pattern discrimination.) As a single herb in high doses, it is contraindicated in diabetes, hypertension, and liver disorders. Not for long-term use.

BR: May increase toxicity of cardiac glycosides. May increase potassium loss due to diuretics and laxatives. Possible additive effect to corticosteroids. May be synergistic with insulin in causing hypokalemia and sodium retention.

B&G: According to some traditional sources, incompatible with *Gan Sui* (Radix Euphorbiae Kansui), *Yuan Hua* (Flos Daphnes Genkwae), and *Yuan Zhi* (Radix Polygalae Tenuifoliae). If taken long-term, it may cause hypertension and/or edema. Contains glycyrrhetinic acid which could possibly cause a reduction in thyroid activity and basal metabolic rate.

The research on *Gan Cao* concurs that this medicinal is generally safe when used in small amounts as an envoy. It should not be taken long-term or as a single herb during pregnancy. When used as a single medicinal or in patients taking other potent Western pharmaceuticals, caution should be exercised to guard against potential toxicity and drug interaction.

Tao Ren
(Semen Pruni Persicae, peach kernel)

Standard daily dosage: 4.5-9g
AH: Not to be used during pregnancy.
B&G: Contraindicated during pregnancy.
C&C: Contains potassium and glycosides (including cyanophoric glycosides). If taken with codeine, morphine, or other opiates, hydrocyanic acid is produced which can lead to respiratory failure and death. Could possibly cause hyperkalemia when used with potassium-sparing diuretics. Vitamin C, nicotinic acid, glutamic acid, hydrochloric acid, and other highly acidic substances could possibly reduce the therapeutic effect of this medicinal.
GLW: In case of poisoning, typically, 1-2 hours after ingestion there is a bitter taste and astringent feeling within the mouth, drooling, headache, dizziness, nausea, vomiting accompanied by watery diarrhea, heart palpitations, and lack of strength. In more serious cases, there is difficulty breathing. Sometimes one can smell cyanide on the person's breath. Eventually, breathing becomes weak, consciousness becomes unclear, and the pupils of the eye dilate widely with loss of reactivity to light. The teeth become clenched, blood pressure drops, there are generalized convulsions, and respiratory paralysis leads to death.

Most of the toxins in this medicinal reside in the skin and tip. Therefore, this medicinal is blanched before using and its tip is broken off in order to make it less or non-toxic.

COMMENTS

Some Chinese doctors administer this formula prophylactically postpartum and postabortion, whether spontaneous or artificial.

SHENG MAI SAN
(Engender the Pulse Powder)

Category: Qi-supplementing
Functions: Supplements the qi and engenders fluids, preserves the yin and stops excessive sweating
Chinese medical indications: Lung qi and yin dual vacuity with chronic cough and scanty phlegm which is difficult to expectorate, shortness of breath, spontaneous perspiration, a dry mouth and tongue, a pale red tongue with scanty fur, and a vacuous, rapid or fine, rapid pulse
Contraindications: Unresolved evils and/or undamaged fluids
Western medical indications: Superventricular arrhythmias, rheumatic heart disease, coronary artery disease, post-bypass debility, chronic bronchitis, and pulmonary tuberculosis
Potential formula toxicities & interactions:
B&B: Using this formula in patients with an externally contracted illness, such as a cold or flu, may prolong the infection.

POTENTIAL MEDICINAL TOXICITIES & INTERACTIONS:

Ren Shen
(Radix Panacis Ginseng, ginseng)

Standard daily dosage: 1-30g
AH: Contraindicated in hypertension.
BR: May cause manic episodes in patients on MAO-inhibitors. May cause hypertension if consumed with caffeine. Possible additive effects to insulin. May reduce the anticoagulative effect of warfarin (Coumadin).
B&G: Contraindicated for hypertensive patients. Overdose can lead to headache, insomnia, heart palpitations, and a rise in blood pressure. A traditional antidote is mung bean soup.
C&C: Vitamin C, nicotinic acid, glutamic acid, hydrochloric acid, and other highly acidic substances could possibly reduce the therapeutic effect of this medicinal.
PDR: Contraindicated in patients with hypertension. Not recommended in large doses during pregnancy or lactation due to potential neonatal androgenization. Enhances the effect of insulin and other antidiabetic agents. Use with MAO-inhibitors may cause headaches, tremors, and manias.

Mai Men Dong, Mai Dong
(Tuber Ophiopogoni Japonici)

Standard daily dosage: 6-15g
AH: Safe when used appropriately
B&G: According to some traditional sources, antagonizes *Kuan Dong Hua* (Flos Tussilaginis Farfarae) and counteracts *Ku Shen* (Radix Sophorae Flavescentis) and *Bai Mu Er* (Fructificatio Tremellae Fuciformis).
C&C: Contains glycosides. Vitamin C, nicotinic acid, glutamic acid, hydrochloric acid, and other highly acidic substances could possibly reduce the therapeutic effect of this medicinal.

Wu Wei Zi
(Fructus Schisandrae Chinensis, schisandra)

Standard daily dosage: 1.5-9g
AH: Safe when used appropriately
B&G: Occasionally causes heartburn. In mice, toxic doses were 10-15g/kg. Symptoms of overdose included restlessness, insomnia, or dyspnea.
C&C: Contains potassium. Highly acidic. Could possibly cause crystalluria and hematuria. Could possibly cause hyperkalemia when used in large doses with potassium-sparing diuretics. Could possibly reduce the therapeutic effect of sodium bicarbonate, aluminum hydroxide, many antibiotics (especially aminoglycosides and sulfas), reserpine, caffeine, opiates, scopolamine, and berbamin.
PDR: No health risks or side effects are known in conjunction with the proper administration of designated therapeutic dosages.

COMMENTS

Dang Shen (Radix Codonopsitis Pilosulae) or *Tai Zi Shen* (Radix Pseudostellariae Heterophyllae) are commonly substituted for *Ren Shen* in this formula, especially when this formula is combined with another formula or heavily modified.

SHI HUI SAN
(Ten Ashes Powder, a.k.a. Ten Partially Charred
Substances Powder)

Category: Bleeding-stopping
Functions: Cools the blood and stops bleeding
Chinese medical indications: Fire blazing in the upper and
middle burners damaging the blood vessels and resulting in
hematemesis or hemoptysis
Contraindications: Qi, yin, and/or yang vacuity bleeding
Western medical indications: Hematemesis, hemoptysis, epistaxis, acute hemorrhagic esophagitis or gastritis, bleeding peptic ulcer, hemorrhagic febrile diseases, functional uterine bleeding, and pulmonary tuberculosis
Potential formula toxicities & interactions: None listed

POTENTIAL MEDICINAL TOXICITIES & INTERACTIONS:

Da Ji
(Herba Seu Radix Cirsii Japonici)

Standard daily dosage: 4.5-60g

No toxicity or interaction information listed in sources

Xiao Ji
(Herba Cephalanoploris Segeti)

Standard daily dosage: 4.5-60g
C&C: Contains alkaloids, potassium, and glycosides. Could possibly
cause hyperkalemia when used with potassium-sparing diuretics and
reduce the absorption and therapeutic effect of potassium and sodium
iodides, sodium bicarbonate, aluminum hydroxide, and magnesium sulfate. Vitamin C, nicotinic acid, glutamic acid, hydrochloric acid, and
other highly acidic substances could possibly reduce the therapeutic
effect of this medicinal.

He Ye
(Folium Nelumbinis Nuciferae, lotus leaves)

Standard daily dosage: 9-30g
AH: Safe when used appropriately

B&G: According to traditional sources, may counteract *Fu Ling* (Sclerotium Poria Cocos).
PDR: No health risks or side effects are known in conjunction with the proper administration of designated therapeutic dosages.

Ce Bai Ye
(Cacumen Biotae Orientalis)

Standard daily dosage: 6-15g
B&G: Long-term use or a large dose may cause dizziness and gastric upset.

Bai Mao Gen, Mao Gen
(Rhizoma Imperatae Cylindricae)

Standard daily dosage: 9-60g
AH: Safe when used appropriately
C&C: Contains potassium. Highly acidic. Could possibly cause crystal-luria and hematuria. Could possibly cause hyperkalemia when used with potassium-sparing diuretics and could possibly reduce the therapeutic effect of sodium bicarbonate, aluminum hydroxide, many antibiotics (especially aminoglycosides and sulfas), reserpine, caffeine, opiates, scopolamine, and berbamin.

Qian Cao Gen, Qian Cao
(Radix Rubiae Cordifoliae)

Standard daily dosage: 6-9g

No toxicity or interaction information listed in the sources

Zhi Zi, Shan Zhi, Shan Zhi Zi
(Fructus Gardeniae Jasminoidis, dried gardenia fruit pod)

Standard daily dosage: 3-12g
AH: Safe when used appropriately
B&G: Contains geniposide which caused diarrhea in mice.
C&C: Contains potassium and glycosides. Could possibly cause hyper-kalemia when used with potassium-sparing diuretics. Vitamin C, nico-tinic acid, glutamic acid, hydrochloric acid, and other highly acidic sub-stances could possibly reduce the therapeutic effect of this medicinal.

Da Huang, Dai Huang, Chuan Jun, Jun
(Radix Et Rhizoma Rhei, rhubarb root)

Standard daily dosage: 3-12g
AH: Do not use during pregnancy. Not to be used while nursing. Contraindicated in intestinal obstruction, abdominal pain of unknown origin, or any inflammatory condition of the intestines.
BR: Reduces absorption of oral drugs. Overuse may cause hypokalemia and increased toxicity of cardiac glycosides. May aggravate potassium loss from diuretics.
B&G: Use with extreme caution during pregnancy, menstruation, or postpartum. Contraindicated for nursing mothers since active ingredients enter the milk.
C&C: Contains alkaloids, tannic acid, potassium, and glycosides. Could possibly cause hyperkalemia when used with potassium-sparing diuretics. Vitamin C, nicotinic acid, glutamic acid, hydrochloric acid, and other highly acidic substances could possibly reduce the therapeutic effect of this medicinal.
PDR: Consult a physician before using this medicinal during pregnancy or while nursing. Contraindicated in cases of intestinal obstruction, acute inflammatory intestinal disease, appendicitis and abdominal pain of unknown origin.

Dan Pi, Mu Dan Pi
(Cortex Radicis Moutan, tree peony root bark)

Standard daily dosage: 6-12g
AH: Not to be used during pregnancy. (This ingredient is commonly used in China during pregnancy to treat heat in the blood and/or blood stasis.)
B&G: Should not be used during pregnancy or in patients with excessive sweating or profuse menstruation. Avoid using with garlic. According to some traditional sources, may counteract the effect of *Tu Si Zi* (Semen Cuscutae Chinensis), *Bei Mu* (Bulbus Fritillariae), and *Da Huang* (Radix Et Rhizoma Rhei).
C&C: Contains tannic acid, potassium, and glycosides. Could possibly cause hyperkalemia when used with potassium-sparing diuretics. Could possibly reduce the absorption and biologic effect of most antibiotics, isoniazid, chlorpromazine, calcium carbonate and gluconate, atropine, ephedrine, quinine, reserpine, digitalis, vitamin B_1, trypsine, amylase, and pepsin. Vitamin C, nicotinic acid, glutamic acid, hydrochloric acid, and other highly acidic substances could possibly reduce the therapeutic effect of this medicinal.

Zong Lu Tan
(carbonized Fibra Stipulae Trachycarpi)

Standard daily dosage: 9-15g

No toxicity or interaction information listed in the sources

COMMENTS

Although specifically for blood heat bleeding, some Chinese doctors use this formula in ready-made form as an all-purpose first aid styptic. This is based on Ye Tian-shi's three principles of treating bleeding: 1) First stop the bleeding, 2) treat the cause, and 3) treat the root. In that case, this formula is employed to first stop the bleeding by any means possible.

SHI XIAO SAN
(Loose a Smile Powder, a.k.a. Sudden Smile Powder)

Category: Blood-quickening
Functions: Quickens the blood and dispels stasis, dissipates binding and stops pain
Chinese medical indications: Static blood resulting in menstrual irregularities, painful menstruation, nonprecipitation of the lochia, and postpartum abdominal pain
Contraindications: Spleen-stomach qi vacuity and pregnancy
Western medical indications: Retention of lochia, dysmenorrhea, amenorrhea, irregular menstruation, postpartum abdominal pain, endometriosis, and angina pectoris
Potential formula toxicities & interactions:
FL/B&B: Contraindicated during pregnancy because *Pu Huang* (Pollen Typhae) may cause uterine contractions

POTENTIAL MEDICINAL TOXICITIES & INTERACTIONS:

Wu Ling Zhi
(Excrementum Trogopterori Seu Pteromi, flying squirrel feces)

Standard daily dosage: 3-9g
B&G: Use with caution during pregnancy. Traditionally considered to be antagonized by *Ren Shen* (Radix Panacis Ginseng).

Pu Huang
(Pollen Typhae, cat-tail pollen)

Standard daily dosage: 4.5-12g
B&G: Use with caution during pregnancy.
C&C: Contains potassium. Could possibly cause hyperkalemia when used with potassium-sparing diuretics.

COMMENTS

This formula is seldom used in this simple, discrete form. Instead, more commonly, the ingredients in this formula are added to other formulas when the ability to stop pain is wanted.

Si Jun Zi Tang
(Four Gentlemen Decoction, a.k.a. Four Major Herb Combination)

Category: Qi-supplementing
Functions: Fortifies the spleen and supplements the qi
Chinese medical indications: Spleen qi vacuity with a pale facial complexion, a faint, low voice and/or disinclination to speak due to fatigue, fatigue, lack of strength, loose stools, a pale tongue, and a fine, forceless pulse
Contraindications: Vacuity heat, constipation, high fever
Western medical indications: Chronic gastritis, gastric and duodenal ulcer, gastrointestinal weakness and dysfunction, gastroptysis, irritable bowel syndrome, diabetes mellitus, uterine fibroids, anemia, vomiting, and diarrhea
Potential formula toxicities & interactions:
FL/B&B: Prolonged use may result in a dry mouth, extreme thirst, agitation, irritability, or constipation.

POTENTIAL MEDICINAL TOXICITIES & INTERACTIONS:

Ren Shen
(Radix Panacis Ginseng, ginseng)

Standard daily dosage: 1-30g
AH: Contraindicated in hypertension
BR: May cause manic episodes in patients on MAO-inhibitors. May cause hypertension if consumed with caffeine. Possible additive effects to insulin. May reduce the anticoagulative effect of warfarin (Coumadin).
B&G: Contraindicated for hypertensive patients. Overdose can lead to headache, insomnia, heart palpitations, and a rise in blood pressure. A traditional antidote is mung bean soup.
C&C: Vitamin C, nicotinic acid, glutamic acid, hydrochloric acid, and other highly acidic substances could possibly reduce the therapeutic effect of this medicinal.
PDR: Contraindicated in patients with hypertension. Not recommended in large doses during pregnancy or lactation due to potential neonatal androgenization. Enhances the effect of insulin and other antidiabetic agents. Use with MAO-inhibitors may cause headaches, tremors, and manias.

Bai Zhu
(Rhizoma Atractylodis Macrocephalae)

Standard daily dosage: 4.5-9g
AH: Safe when used appropriately
B&G: When rats were fed 0.5g/kg of this medicinal for two months, they developed a mild lymphopenia and anemia but suffered no damage to the brain, heart, or liver.

Fu Ling, Bai Fu Ling, Yun Ling
(Sclerotium Poriae Cocos)

Standard daily dosage: 9-15g
B&G: Large doses or long-term use is discouraged. Contraindicated in patients with frequent, copious urination. According to traditional sources, may counteract *Di Yu* (Radix Sanguisorbae Officinalis), *Qin Jiao* (Radix Gentianae Qinjiao), and *Bie Jia* (Carapax Amydae Sinensis).
C&C: Contains potassium. Could possibly cause hyperkalemia when used with potassium-sparing diuretics.

Gan Cao
(Radix Glycyrrhizae Uralensis, licorice root)

Standard daily dosage: 2-12g
AH: Do not use during pregnancy. (This medicinal is routinely used in Chinese medical gynecology during pregnancy as part of formulas appropriately prescribed on the basis of pattern discrimination.) As a single herb in high doses, it is contraindicated in diabetes, hypertension, and liver disorders. Not for long-term use.
BR: May increase toxicity of cardiac glycosides. May increase potassium loss due to diuretics and laxatives. Possible additive effect to corticosteroids. May be synergistic with insulin in causing hypokalemia and sodium retention.
B&G: According to some traditional sources, incompatible with *Gan Sui* (Radix Euphorbiae Kansui), *Yuan Hua* (Flos Daphnes Genkwae), and *Yuan Zhi* (Radix Polygalae Tenuifoliae). If taken long-term, it may cause hypertension and/or edema. Contains glycyrrhetinic acid which could possibly cause a reduction in thyroid activity and basal metabolic rate.

The research on *Gan Cao* concurs that this medicinal is generally safe when used in small amounts as an envoy. It should not be taken long-term or as a single herb during pregnancy. When used as a single medicinal or in patients taking other potent Western pharmaceuticals, caution should be exercised to guard against potential toxicity and drug interaction.

COMMENTS

Although this formula is one of the most famous in Chinese medicine, it is rarely prescribed in this simple form since real-life patients rarely present simple spleen qi vacuity. However, either some or all of the ingredients in this formula are often added to other formulas to fortify the spleen and supplement the qi, especially if the symptom of spleen qi vacuity is loose stools. Typically, *Dang Shen* (Radix Codonopsitis Pilosulae) is substituted for *Ren Shen* in this formula.

SI NI SAN
(Four Counterflows Powder, a.k.a.
Bupleurum & Chih-shih Formula)

Category: Harmonizing
Functions: Out-thrusts the exterior and resolves depression,
courses the liver and fortifies the spleen
Chinese medical indications: Yang reversal due to a combination of
liver depression and spleen vacuity with cold hands and feet caused
primarily by psychoemotional stress, easy anger, possible chest
oppression, a red tongue with yellow fur, and a bowstring pulse
Contraindications: None listed
Western medical indications: Gastritis, Raynaud's phenome-
non or disease, peptic ulcer, cholecystitis, gallstones, hepatitis,
intercostal neuralgia, biliary acariasis, hernia, acute appendicitis,
pancreatitis, intestinal obstruction, allergic colitis, psychogenic
diarrhea, mastitis, and fibrocystic breast disease
Potential formula toxicities & interactions:
FL: May cause abdominal distention in some patients. If so,
reduce the amount of *Gan Cao* (Radix Glycyrrhizae Uralensis).

POTENTIAL MEDICINAL TOXICITIES & INTERACTIONS:

Gan Cao
(Radix Glycyrrhizae Uralensis, licorice root)

Standard daily dosage: 2-12g
AH: Do not use during pregnancy. (This medicinal is routinely used in
Chinese medical gynecology during pregnancy as part of formulas
appropriately prescribed on the basis of pattern discrimination.) As a single herb in high doses, it is contraindicated in diabetes, hypertension,
and liver disorders. Not for long-term use.
BR: May increase toxicity of cardiac glycosides. May increase potassium loss due to diuretics and laxatives. Possible additive effect to corticosteroids. May be synergistic with insulin in causing hypokalemia and
sodium retention.
B&G: According to some traditional sources, incompatible with *Gan Sui*
(Radix Euphorbiae Kansui), *Yuan Hua* (Flos Daphnes Genkwae), and
Yuan Zhi (Radix Polygalae Tenuifoliae). If taken long-term, it may cause
hypertension and/or edema. Contains glycyrrhetinic acid which could
possibly cause a reduction in thyroid activity and basal metabolic rate.

The research on *Gan Cao* concurs that this medicinal is generally safe when used in small amounts as an envoy. It should not be taken long-term or as a single herb during pregnancy. When used as a single medicinal or in patients taking other potent Western pharmaceuticals, caution should be exercised to guard against potential toxicity and drug interaction.

Zhi Shi
(Fructus Immaturus Citri Aurantii, immature bitter orange)

Standard daily dosage: 3-9g
B&G: Use with caution during pregnancy or in debilitated patients.
C&C: Contains tannic acid. Highly acidic. Could possibly cause crystalluria and hematuria and reduce the absorption and biologic effect of most antibiotics, isoniazid, chlorpromazine, calcium carbonate and gluconate, atropine, ephedrine, quinine, reserpine, digitalis, vitamin B_1, trypsine, amylase, and pepsin, sodium bicarbonate, aluminum hydroxide, caffeine, opiates, scopolamine, and berbamin.

Chai Hu
(Radix Bupleuri)

Standard daily dosage: 3-12g
AH: Safe when used appropriately
B&G: May occasionally cause nausea and vomiting, in which case the dose should then be reduced significantly.
C&C: Vitamin C, nicotinic acid, glutamic acid, hydrochloric acid, and other highly acidic substances could possibly reduce the therapeutic effect of this medicinal.
PDR: Not to be administered during pregnancy. (This medicinal is routinely used in Chinese medical gynecology during pregnancy as part of formulas appropriately prescribed on the basis of pattern discrimination.) Overdose may lead to gastroenteritis, intestinal colic, and diarrhea due to saponin content.

Bai Shao, Shao Yao
(Radix Albus Paeoniae Lactiflorae, white peony root)

Standard daily dosage: 6-30g
AH: Safe when used appropriately
B&G: Use with caution in debilitated patients with diarrhea. According to some traditional sources, antagonizes *Shi Hu* (Herba Dendrobii) and *Mang Xiao* (Mirabilitum), counteracts *Bie Jia* (Carapax Amydae Sinensis) and *Xiao Ji* (Herba Cephalanopoloris Segeti), and is incompatible with *Li Lu* (Rhizoma Et Radix Veratri).
C&C: Contains calcium, tannic acid, potassium, and glycosides. Could possibly cause hyperkalemia when used with potassium-sparing diuret-

ics. Could possibly reduce the effect of most antibiotics, cause digitalis intoxication and heart arrhythmias, and could possibly reduce the absorption and therapeutic effect of levadopa, isoniazid, chlorpromazine, calcium carbonate and gluconate, atropine, ephedrine, quinine, reserpine, vitamin B_1, trypsine, amylase, and pepsin. Vitamin C, nicotinic acid, glutamic acid, hydrochloric acid, and other highly acidic substances could possibly reduce the therapeutic effect of this medicinal.

COMMENTS

Although this formula is rarely prescribed in this simple, discrete form, this formula is considered the model for all qi and blood harmonizing formulas.

SI NI TANG

(Four Counterflows Decoction, a.k.a.
Aconite & G.L. Combination)

Category: Interior-warming
Functions: Returns or rescues yang and stems counterflow
Chinese medical indications: Kidney yang vacuity/vacuity cold
resulting in extremely cold extremities, aversion to cold, sleeping
with the knees drawn up, fatigue, somnolence, vomiting, diarrhea
with undigested food, chilly abdominal pain, a pale tongue with
slimy, white fur, and a deep, fine or deep, forceless pulse
Contraindications: True heat and false cold
Western medical indications: Influenza, intestinal fever,
cholera, diarrhea, neurotic vomiting, indigestion, edema, jaundice, hypopituitarism, hypothyroidism, adrenal insufficiency,
intractable arthritis, prostration, heart failure, cardiac insufficiency, and coma
Potential formula toxicities & interactions: None listed

POTENTIAL MEDICINAL TOXICITIES & INTERACTIONS:

Fu Zi, Shu Fu Zi, Fu Pian

(Radix Lateralis Praeparatus Aconiti Carmichaeli, wolfsbane, monkshood)

Standard daily dosage: 1.5-15g
AH: To be used only under the supervision of an expert qualified in the
appropriate use of this substance.
B&G: Contraindicated during pregnancy. A very toxic medicinal which can be
fatal if ingested in its uncooked form or in an inappropriate dose. It is generally
combined with *Gan Cao* (Radix Glycyrhizae Uralensis) and *Gan Jiang* (dry
Rhizoma Zingiberis Officinalis) in decoctions to reduce its toxicity. Symptoms
of toxicity include drooling, gastric upset, light-headedness, blurred vision, and
numbness and tingling of the extremities. More severe symptoms include premature atrial contractions, dyspnea, and reduced temperature and blood pressure. Emergency measures include the administration of atropine.
C&C: Contains alkaloids. Could possibly reduce the absorption and
therapeutic effect of potassium and sodium iodides, sodium bicarbonate,
aluminum hydroxide, and magnesium sulfate.
PDR: Contains nor-diterpene alkaloids, including aconitine. Highly
toxic. Small doses can be fatal.
GLW: If mild poisoning, there is a burning hot sensation in the mouth and on

the tongue, numbness, and pain which gradually spreads to the four limbs and then to the whole body, nausea, vomiting, dizziness, heart palpitations, rapid breathing, vexation, agitation, restlessness, drooling. If more severe, there may be generalized sweating, paralysis, convulsions, urinary incontinence, dilated pupils, slowed reaction to light, slow heartbeat, arrhythmia, low blood pressure, a somber white facial complexion, reversal chilling of the four limbs, lowered body temperature and circulatory collapse leading to death.

Gan Jiang
(dry Rhizoma Zingiberis Officinalis, dry ginger)

Standard daily dosage: 3-12g
AH: Not to be used during pregnancy. Patients with gallstones should consult a practitioner prior to use.
B&G: Use with caution during pregnancy.

Gan Cao
(Radix Glycyrrhizae Uralensis, licorice root)

Standard daily dosage: 2-12g
AH: Do not use during pregnancy. (This medicinal is routinely used in Chinese medical gynecology during pregnancy as part of formulas appropriately prescribed on the basis of pattern discrimination.) As a single herb in high doses, it is contraindicated in diabetes, hypertension, and liver disorders. Not for long-term use.
BR: May increase toxicity of cardiac glycosides. May increase potassium loss due to diuretics and laxatives. Possible additive effect to corticosteroids. May be synergistic with insulin in causing hypokalemia and sodium retention.
B&G: According to some traditional sources, incompatible with *Gan Sui* (Radix Euphorbiae Kansui), *Yuan Hua* (Flos Daphnes Genkwae), and *Yuan Zhi* (Radix Polygalae Tenuifoliae). If taken long-term, it may cause hypertension and/or edema. Contains glycyrrhetinic acid which could possibly cause a reduction in thyroid activity and basal metabolic rate.

The research on *Gan Cao* concurs that this medicinal is generally safe when used in small amounts as an envoy. It should not be taken long-term or as a single herb during pregnancy. When used as a single medicinal or in patients taking other potent Western pharmaceuticals, caution should be exercised to guard against potential toxicity and drug interaction.

COMMENTS

It is extremely important to differentiate this formula from the preceding one. In the case of this formula, there is true internal cold. In the case of *Si Ni San* (Four Counterflows Powder), there is only seeming cold, while, in actuality, there may be even depressive heat internally.

Si Shen Wan
(Four Spirits Pills, a.k.a. Dioscorea Combination)

Category: Securing and astringing
Functions: Warms and supplements the kidneys, astringes the intestines and stops diarrhea
Chinese medical indications: Daybreak or cockcrow diarrhea due to spleen-kidney yang vacuity with torpid intake, indigestion, fatigue, somnolence, low back soreness and cold lower limbs, a pale tongue with thin, white fur, and a deep, slow, forceless pulse
Contraindications: Intestinal and stomach accumulation and stagnation
Western medical indications: Chronic colitis, chronic dysentery, autonomic dystonia of the intestinal tract, intestinal tuberculosis, allergic colitis, tabes dorsalis, and pancreatic dysfunction
Potential formula toxicities & interactions: None listed

POTENTIAL MEDICINAL TOXICITIES & INTERACTIONS:

Bu Gu Zhi, Po Gu Zhi
(Fructus Psoraleae Corylifoliae)

Standard daily dosage: 3-9g
B&G: Contraindicated in patients with fever or constipation. Can be hard to digest. According to some traditional sources, antagonizes *Gan Cao* (Radix Glycyrrhizae Uralensis). Extremely large doses have had some teratogenic effects when given to rats and guinea pigs.

Wu Zhu Yu
(Fructus Evodiae Rutecarpae)

Standard daily dosage: 3-9g
AH: Do not exceed recommended dose.
B&G: Very drying. Should not be used long-term. According to some traditional sources, antagonizes *Dan Shen* (Radix Salviae Miltiorrhizae) and counteracts *Zi Shi Ying* (Flouritum). Overdose may cause the throat to become extremely dry. Large doses stimulate the central nervous system and can lead to visual disturbances and hallucinations.
C&C: Contains alkaloids and quercetin. Could possibly reduce the absorption and therapeutic effect of potassium and sodium iodides, sodi-

um bicarbonate, calcium gluconate, carbonate, and lactate, aluminum hydroxide, magnesium and ferrous sulfates, and bismuth subcarbonate.
GLW: Symptoms of adverse reaction include vomiting, abdominal pain, diarrhea, increased body temperature, visual disturbances, visual hallucinations, and falling hair. In pregnant women, toxicity may cause abortion.

Rou Dou Kou, Rou Guo, Rou Kou
(Semen Myristicae Fragantis, nutmeg)

Standard daily dosage: 1.5-9g
AH: Not to be used during pregnancy.
BR: May potentiate psychoactive drugs, especially MAO-inhibitors.
B&G: Contains myristicin, a hallucinogen. Doses of 1.9g/kg were fatal in cats with liver damage found on autopsy. In humans, ingestion of 7.5g of the powdered herb can lead to dizziness or stupor. Deaths from large overdoses have been reported in humans.

Wu Wei Zi
(Fructus Schisandrae Chinensis, schisandra)

Standard daily dosage: 1.5-9g
B&G: Occasionally causes heartburn. In mice, toxic doses were 10-15g/kg. Symptoms of overdose included restlessness, insomnia, or dyspnea.
C&C: Contains potassium. Highly acidic. Could possibly cause crystalluria and hematuria. Could possibly cause hyperkalemia when used in large doses with potassium-sparing diuretics. Could possibly reduce the therapeutic effect of sodium bicarbonate, aluminum hydroxide, many antibiotics (especially aminoglycosides and sulfas), reserpine, caffeine, opiates, scopolamine, and berbamin.
PDR: No health risks or side effects are known in conjunction with the proper administration of designated therapeutic dosages.

COMMENTS

A couple or all four ingredients in this formula are often added to other formulas when diarrhea or dysentery is complicated by kidney qi not securing.

SI WU TANG
(Four Materials Decoction, a.k.a. Tang-kuei Four Combination)

Category: Blood-supplementing
Functions: Supplements and harmonizes the blood
Chinese medical indications: Blood vacuity resulting in dizziness, blurred vision, a lusterless facial complexion, pale lips and nails, generalized muscle tension and cramps, menstrual irregularities, scanty menstruation, blocked menstruation, a pale tongue, and a fine, bowstring or fine, choppy pulse
Contraindications: Severe blood loss leading to qi desertion or spleen vacuity with poor appetite and loose stools
Western medical indications: Dysmenorrhea, irregular menstruation, uterine bleeding, anemia due to various causes, threatened miscarriage, abdominal pain during pregnancy, postpartum weakness, scanty lactation, hemafecia, dry skin, constipation, and neurgenic headache
Potential formula toxicities & interactions: None listed

POTENTIAL MEDICINAL TOXICITIES & INTERACTIONS:

Shu Di, Shu Di Huang
(cooked Radix Rehmanniae Glutinosae)

Standard daily dosage: 9-30g
AH: Contraindicated in patients with diarrhea or indigestion
B&G: Overuse can lead to abdominal distention and loose stools. Side effects include diarrhea, abdominal pain, dizziness, lethargy, and heart palpitations which often disappear upon continued administration of the herb.
PDR: No health risks or side effects are known in conjunction with the proper administration of designated therapeutic dosages.

Bai Shao, Shao Yao
(Radix Albus Paeoniae Lactiflorae, white peony root)

Standard daily dosage: 6-30g
AH: Safe when used appropriately
B&G: Use with caution in debilitated patients with diarrhea. According to some traditional sources, antagonizes *Shi Hu* (Herba Dendrobii) and *Mang Xiao* (Mirabilitum), counteracts *Bie Jia* (Carapax Amydae Sinensis) and *Xiao Ji* (Herba Cephalanopoloris Segeti), and is incompatible with *Li Lu* (Rhizoma Et Radix Veratri).

C&C: Contains calcium, tannic acid, potassium, and glycosides. Could possibly cause hyperkalemia when used with potassium-sparing diuretics, could possibly reduce the effect of most antibiotics, could possibly cause digitalis intoxication and heart arrhythmias, and could possibly reduce the absorption and therapeutic effect of levadopa, isoniazid, chlorpromazine, calcium carbonate and gluconate, atropine, ephedrine, quinine, reserpine, vitamin B$_1$, trypsine, amylase, and pepsin. Vitamin C, nicotinic acid, glutamic acid, hydrochloric acid, and other highly acidic substances could possibly reduce the therapeutic effect of this medicinal.

Dang Gui
(Radix Angelicae Sinensis)

Standard daily dosage: 3-15g
AH: Do not use during pregnancy. (This medicinal is routinely used in Chinese medical gynecology during pregnancy as part of formulas appropriately prescribed on the basis of pattern discrimination.)
B&G: Use with caution in patients with diarrhea or abdominal distention.
C&C: Contains potassium. Could possibly cause hyperkalemia when used with potassium-sparing diuretics. May exaggerate the anticoagulative effect of warfarin (Coumadin).

Chuan Xiong
(Radix Ligustici Wallichii)

Standard daily dosage: 3-9g (In China today, it is not uncommon for this medicinal to be prescribed up to 15 grams per day in decoction.)
AH: Do not use during pregnancy. (This medicinal is routinely used in Chinese medical gynecology during pregnancy as part of formulas appropriately prescribed on the basis of pattern discrimination.)
B&G: Not for patients with migraine headache or excessive menstrual bleeding. Overdosage causes vomiting and dizziness. According to some traditional texts, antagonizes *Shan Zhu Yu* (Fructus Corni Officinalis) and *Huang Qi* (Radix Astragali Membranacei), counteracts *Hua Shi* (Talcum) and *Huang Lian* (Rhizoma Coptidis Chinensis), and is incompatible with *Li Lu* (Rhizoma Et Radix Veratri).
C&C: Contains alkaloids and potassium. Could possibly cause hyperkalemia when used with potassium-sparing diuretics. Could possibly reduce the absorption and therapeutic effect of potassium and sodium iodides, sodium bicarbonate, aluminum hydroxide, and magnesium sulfate.

COMMENTS

Since blood vacuity rarely manifests as a single, discrete pattern, this formula is hardly ever indicated in its pure form. Nevertheless, this formula is an important teaching model, if not such a clinically useful one.

SU HE XIANG WAN
(Liquid Styrax Pills)

Category: Orifice-opening
Functions: Aromatically opens the orifices, moves the qi, and stops pain
Chinese medical indications: Acute damp cold and phlegm turbidity obstruction disorders with sudden collapse, loss of consciousness, clenched jaw, chest and abdominal fullness, pain, and cold, am urge to vomit or defecate without doing either, a pale facial complexion, purple lips, profuse phlegm and saliva, cold extremities, a pale tongue with slimy, glossy fur, and a deep, slippery pulse
Contraindications: Pregnancy
Western medical indications: Partial or total loss of consciousness due to cerebralvascular accident, uremic or hepatic coma, encephalitis, hysteria, seizure disorder, psychosis, schizophrenia, postconcussion syndrome, cholera-like illness, angina pectoris, and coronary artery disease
Potential formula toxicities & interactions:
FL/B&B: Do not use in high doses or long-term due to the possibility of mercury toxicity from *Zhu Sha* (Cinnabaris). To help prevent mercury poisoning, the formula should not be heated.

POTENTIAL MEDICINAL TOXICITIES & INTERACTIONS:

Su He Xiang
(Styrax Liquidis)

Standard daily dosage: 0.3-1g in pills and powders
B&G: Use with caution during pregnancy. Contraindicated in patients with high fever, coma, spontaneous sweating, and collapse.
PDR: No health risks or side effects are known in conjunction with the proper administration of designated therapeutic dosages.

She Xiang
(Secretio Moschi Moschiferi, musk)

Standard daily dosage: 0.016-0.15g in pills and powders
B&G: Contraindicated during pregnancy. Use with caution in cases of hypertension.

Bing Pian
(Borneol)

Standard daily dosage: 0.3-0.9g in pills and powders
B&G: Use with caution during pregnancy. Do not expose to heat.

An Xi Xiang
(Benzoinum)

Standard daily dosage: 0.3-1.5g in pills and powders
PDR: No health risks or side effects are known in conjunction with the proper administration of designated therapeutic dosages.

Mu Xiang
(Radix Aucklandiae Lappae)

Standard daily dosage: 1.5-9g
AH: Safe when used appropriately
PDR: No health risks or side effects are known in conjunction with the proper administration of designated therapeutic dosages.

Tan Xiang, Bai Tan Xiang
(Lignum Santali Albi, sandlewood)

Standard daily dosage: 3-9g
AH: Contraindicated in kidney diseases involving the parenchyma of the kidney. Not for use beyond six weeks without consultation with a physician.
PDR: Contraindicated in patients with kidney disease.

Chen Xiang
(Lignum Aquilariae, aloeswood)

Standard daily dosage: 1.5-3g as a powder

No toxicity or interaction information listed in the sources

Ru Xiang
(Resina Olibani, frankincense)

Standard daily dosage: 3-9g
B&G: Contraindicated during pregnancy

Ding Xiang
(Flos Caryophylli, cloves)

Standard daily dosage: 0.5-1g as a powder; 1.5-4.5g in decoction
AH: Safe when used appropriately
B&G: Contraindicated in the presence of fever. Do not combine with *Yu Jin* (Tuber Curcumae). LD50 of oral preparations varied from 1.6-5g/kg in animals.
C&C: Contains quercetin. Could possibly reduce the absorption of calcium gluconate, carbonate, and lactate, aluminum hydroxide, magnesium and ferrous sulfates, and bismuth subcarbonate.

Xiang Fu
(Rhizoma Cyperi Rotundi)

Standard daily dosage: 4.5-12g
AH: Safe when used appropriately

Bi Ba
(Fructus Piperis Longi)

Standard daily dosage: 1.5-4.5g
B&G: Contraindicated in patients with fever.

Xi Jiao
(Cornu Rhinocerotis, rhinoceros horn)

Standard daily dosage: 1-2g as a powder
B&G: Use with great caution during pregnancy. Should only be used in the presence of high fever. According to traditional sources, may antagonize *Chuan Wu* (Radix Aconiti Carmichaeli), *Cao Wu* (Radix Aconiti Kusnezoffii), and *Lei Wan* (Sclerotium Omphaliae Lapidescentis).

Because *Xi Jiao* is from an endangered species, it is now commonly substituted by *Shui Niu Jiao* (Cornu Bubali, water buffalo horn. Standard daily dosage of this ingredient in decoction is 4.5-9g.

Zhu Sha
(Cinnabaris, cinnabar)

Standard daily dosage: 0.2-2.7g in pills and powders
B&G: Contains mercuric sulfide which is highly toxic. Should not be used in large amounts or long-term. To prevent mercury poisoning, do not heat.

GLW: Symptoms of adverse reaction include burning pain in the oral cavity and throat, swelling and distention of the mucosa, bleeding, ulceration, and a metallic taste in the mouth, nausea, vomiting, abdominal pain, diarrhea, mucus in the stools or hemafecia. If severe, there is hemorrhagic enteritis, clenched teeth, fright reversal, and trembling. If the kidneys are poisoned, there is edema, scanty urination, albuminuria, and acute kidney failure, syncope, convulsions, low blood pressure, shock, and eventual respiratory failure.

He Zi
(Fructus Terminaliae Chebulae)

Standard daily dosage: 3-9g
AH: Contraindicated in acute cough, acute diarrhea, and early stage dysentery.
B&G: May inhibit digestive function in some patients.
C&C: Contains tannic acid and alkalis. May hinder the absorption and reduce the therapeutic effect of most antibiotics. When combined with isoniazid, tetracyclines, rifampin, chlorpromazine, or erythromycin may cause hepatoxicity.
PDR: Contains large amounts of tannin. Large doses may lead to constipation. Overdosages could possibly cause liver and kidney damage.

Bai Zhu
(Rhizoma Atractylodis Macrocephalae)

Standard daily dosage: 4.5-9g
AH: Safe when used appropriately
B&G: When rats were fed 0.5g/kg of this medicinal for two months, they developed a mild lymphopenia and anemia but suffered no damage to the brain, heart, or liver.

COMMENTS

This formula is given as a ready-made medicinal. In China, it is sold in little vials meant to be carried around by the patient the same way one might carry nitroglycerine tablets.

Suan Zao Ren Tang
(Zizyphus Spinosa Decoction, a.k.a.
Sour Jujube Decoction, Zizyphus Combination)

Category: Spirit-quieting
Functions: Nourishes the blood and quiets the spirit, clears heat and eliminates vexation
Chinese medical indications: Liver-heart blood vacuity with vacuity heat and easy anger, insomnia, heart palpitations, night sweats, dizziness, a dry mouth and parched throat, a dry, red tongue, and bowstring, fine, rapid pulse
Contraindications: None listed
Western medical indications: Insomnia, nervous exhaustion, night sweats, impaired memory, nightmares, fearful crying and irritability in teething infants, neurasthenia, and schizophrenia
Potential formula toxicities & interactions: None listed

POTENTIAL MEDICINAL TOXICITIES & INTERACTIONS:

Suan Zao Ren
(Semen Zizyphi Spinosae)

Standard daily dosage: 9-18g
AH: Not to be used during pregnancy. (No such prohibition exists for this medicinal in traditional Chinese medicine.)

Fu Ling, Bai Fu Ling, Yun Ling
(Sclerotium Poriae Cocos)

Standard daily dosage: 9-15g
B&G: Large doses or long-term use is discouraged. Contraindicated in patients with frequent, copious urination. According to traditional sources, may counteract *Di Yu* (Radix Sanguisorbae Officinalis), *Qin Jiao* (Radix Gentianae Qinjiao), and *Bie Jia* (Carapax Amydae Sinensis).
C&C: Contains potassium. Could possibly cause hyperkalemia when used with potassium-sparing diuretics.

Zhi Mu
(Rhizoma Anemarrhenae Aspheloidis)

Standard daily dosage: 6-12g
AH: Safe when used appropriately
B&G: May cause diarrhea in some patients.
C&C: Contains potassium and glycosides. Could possibly cause hyper-kalemia when used with potassium-sparing diuretics. Vitamin C, nico-

tinic acid, glutamic acid, hydrochloric acid, and other highly acidic substances could possibly reduce the therapeutic effect of this medicinal.
PDR: No health hazards are known in conjunction with the proper administration of designated therapeutic dosages.

Chuan Xiong
(Radix Ligustici Wallichii)

Standard daily dosage: 3-9g (In China today, it is not uncommon for this medicinal to be prescribed up to 15 grams per day in decoction.)
AH: Do not use during pregnancy. (This medicinal is routinely used in Chinese medical gynecology during pregnancy as part of formulas appropriately prescribed on the basis of pattern discrimination.)
B&G: Not for patients with migraine headache or excessive menstrual bleeding. Overdosage causes vomiting and dizziness. According to some traditional texts, antagonizes *Shan Zhu Yu* (Fructus Corni Officinalis) and *Huang Qi* (Radix Astragali Membranacei), counteracts *Hua Shi* (Talcum) and *Huang Lian* (Rhizoma Coptidis Chinensis), and is incompatible with *Li Lu* (Rhizoma Et Radix Veratri).
C&C: Contains alkaloids and potassium. Could possibly cause hyperkalemia when used with potassium-sparing diuretics. Could possibly reduce the absorption and therapeutic effect of potassium and sodium iodides, sodium bicarbonate, aluminum hydroxide, and magnesium sulfate.

Gan Cao
(Radix Glycyrrhizae Uralensis, licorice root)

Standard daily dosage: 2-12g
AH: Do not use during pregnancy. (This medicinal is routinely used in Chinese medical gynecology during pregnancy as part of formulas appropriately prescribed on the basis of pattern discrimination.) As a single herb in high doses, it is contraindicated in diabetes, hypertension, and liver disorders. Not for long-term use.
BR: May increase toxicity of cardiac glycosides. May increase potassium loss due to diuretics and laxatives. Possible additive effect to corticosteroids. May be synergistic with insulin in causing hypokalemia and sodium retention.
B&G: According to some traditional sources, incompatible with *Gan Sui* (Radix Euphorbiae Kansui), *Yuan Hua* (Flos Daphnes Genkwae), and *Yuan Zhi* (Radix Polygalae Tenuifoliae). If taken long-term, it may cause hypertension and/or edema. Contains glycyrrhetinic acid which could possibly cause a reduction in thyroid activity and basal metabolic rate.

The research on *Gan Cao* concurs that this medicinal is generally safe when used in small amounts as an envoy. It should not be taken long-term or as a single herb during pregnancy. When used as a single medicinal or in patients taking other potent Western pharmaceuticals, caution should be exercised to guard against potential toxicity and drug interaction.

TIAN MA GOU TENG YIN
(Gastrodia & Uncaria Beverage)

Category: Wind-treating
Functions: Levels the liver and extinguishes wind, clears heat and quickens the blood, supplements and boosts the liver and kidneys
Chinese medical indications: Ascendant liver yang hyperactivity with internal stirring of the liver wind resulting in headache, dizziness, tinnitus, blurred vision, a sensation of heat rushing up to the head, insomnia, profuse dreams, a red tongue, and a bowstring, rapid pulse
Contraindications: None listed
Western medical indications: Cerebrovascular disease, transitory ischemic attacks, hemiplegia, essential hypertension, renal hypertension, hypertensive encephalopathy, aphasia, apraxia, epilepsy, puerperal eclampsia, trigeminal neuralgia, and neurosis
Potential formula toxicities & interactions: None listed

POTENTIAL MEDICINAL TOXICITIES & INTERACTIONS:

Tian Ma
(Rhizoma Gastrodiae Elatae)

Standard daily dosage: 3-9g
AH: Safe when used appropriately.
B&G: LD50 in mice via intraperitoneal injection is 51g/kg; in rabbits 12g/kg. Signs of toxicity in rabbits included lethargy, reduced deep tendon reflexes, loss of appetite, tachycardia, and slow waves on the EEG. Many of the rabbits died within 48 hours.
C&C: Contains glycosides. Vitamin C, nicotinic acid, glutamic acid, hydrochloric acid, and other highly acidic substances could possibly reduce the therapeutic effect of this medicinal.

Gou Teng
(Ramulus Uncariae Cum Uncis)

Standard daily dosage: 6-15g
AH: Safe when used appropriately
B&G: LD50 in mice for one dose in a decoction is 29g/kg.
C&C: Contains alkaloids and potassium. Could possibly cause hyper-

kalemia when used with potassium-sparing diuretics. Could possibly reduce the absorption and therapeutic effect of potassium and sodium iodides, sodium bicarbonate, aluminum hydroxide, and magnesium sulfate.
PDR: No health risks or side effects are known in conjunction with the proper administration of designated therapeutic dosages.

Shi Jue Ming
(Concha Haliotidis, abalone shell)

Standard daily dosage: 9-30g
B&G: According to some traditional sources, counteracts *Xuan Fu Hua* (Flos Inulae Racemosae).
C&C: Highly alkaline. Contains calcium. Toxic when taken with some antibiotics (aminoglycosides) and quinidine. Could possibly cause hyperkalemia when taken with potassium-sparing diuretics. Could possibly cause digitalis intoxication and heart arrhythmias. Could possibly reduce the therapeutic effect of most antibiotics, isoniazid, levadopa.

Zhi Zi, Shan Zhi, Shan Zhi Zi
(Fructus Gardeniae Jasminoidis)

Standard daily dosage: 3-12g
B&G: Contains geniposide which caused diarrhea in mice.
C&C: Contains potassium and glycosides. Could possibly cause hyperkalemia when used with potassium-sparing diuretics. Vitamin C, nicotinic acid, glutamic acid, hydrochloric acid, and other highly acidic substances could possibly reduce the therapeutic effect of this medicinal.

Huang Qin, Tiao Qin
(Radix Scutellariae Baicalensis)

Standard daily dosage: 6-15g
AH: Safe when used appropriately
B&G: According to some traditional sources, counteracts *Dan Pi* (Cortex Radicis Moutan) and *Li Lu* (Rhizoma Et Radix Veratri).
C&C: Contains potassium and glycosides. Could possibly cause hyperkalemia when used with potassium-sparing diuretics. Vitamin C, nicotinic acid, glutamic acid, hydrochloric acid, and other highly acidic substances could possibly reduce the therapeutic effect of this medicinal.

Yi Mu Cao, Kun Cao
(Herba Leonuri Heterophylli, motherwort)

Standard daily dosage: 9-60g
AH: Not to be used during pregnancy
B&G: Contraindicated during pregnancy. Oral administration in pregnant rabbits resulted in miscarriages. LD50 for intravenous injection in mice was 572mg/kg.
C&C: Contains alkaloids and potassium. Could possibly cause hyperkalemia when used with potassium-sparing diuretics. Could possibly reduce the absorption and therapeutic effect of potassium and sodium iodides, sodium bicarbonate, aluminum hydroxide, and magnesium sulfate.
PDR: Not for use during pregnancy.
GLW: Symptoms of adverse reaction include generalized lack of strength, inability to move the lower limbs, paralysis, generalized soreness, numbness, and pain, chest oppression, sweating, low blood pressure, and weak respiration. However, the mind and speech remain clear.

Chuan Niu Xi
(Radix Cyathulae)

Standard daily dosage: 9-15g
AH: Not to be used during pregnancy
B&G: Contraindicated during pregnancy or in patients with excessive menstruation.

Du Zhong
(Cortex Eucommiae Ulmoidis)

Standard daily dosage: 6-15g
AH: Safe when used appropriately
B&G: Has a mild sedative effect in large doses. According to some traditional sources, antagonizes *Xuan Shen* (Radix Scrophulariae Ningpoensis).
C&C: Contains tannic acid. Could possibly reduce the absorption and biologic effect of most antibiotics, isoniazid, chlorpromazine, calcium carbonate and gluconate, atropine, ephedrine, quinine, reserpine, digitalis, vitamin B_1, trypsine, amylase, and pepsin.

This medicinal contains latex. Therefore, some patients taking this medicinal may have an allergic reaction if they are allergic to latex.

Sang Ji Sheng, Sang Ji
(Ramulus Loranthi Seu Visci, mulberry mistletoe)

Standard daily dosage: 9-30g
B&G: Contains avicularin. Overdose has been shown to cause vomiting, diarrhea, and death in experimental animals.
C&C: Contains quercetin, potassium, and glycosides. Could possibly cause hyperkalemia when used with potassium-sparing diuretics. Could possibly reduce the absorption of calcium gluconate, carbonate, and lactate, aluminum hydroxide, magnesium and ferrous sulfates, and bismuth subcarbonate. Vitamin C, nicotinic acid, glutamic acid, hydrochloric acid, and other highly acidic substances could possibly reduce the therapeutic effect of this medicinal.

Ye Jiao Teng
(Caulis Polygoni Multiflori)

Standard daily dosage: 9-30g

No toxicity or interaction information listed in the sources

Fu Ling, Bai Fu Ling, Yun Ling
(Sclerotium Poriae Cocos)

Standard daily dosage: 9-15g
B&G: Large doses or long-term use is discouraged. Contraindicated in patients with frequent, copious urination. According to traditional sources, may counteract *Di Yu* (Radix Sanguisorbae Officinalis), *Qin Jiao* (Radix Gentianae Qinjiao), and *Bie Jia* (Carapax Amydae Sinensis).
C&C: Contains potassium. Could possibly cause hyperkalemia when used with potassium-sparing diuretics.

TIAN WANG BU XIN DAN
(Heavenly Emperor Supplement the Heart Elixir, a.k.a.
Ginseng & Zizyphus Formula)

Category: Spirit-quieting
Functions: Enriches the yin and nourishes the blood, supplements the heart and quiets the spirit
Chinese medical indications: Heart-kidney qi and yin vacuity with easy anger, heart palpitations, fatigue, anxiety, insomnia, inability to concentrate, impaired memory, possible night sweats, a red tongue with scanty fur, and a fine, rapid pulse
Contraindications: Not for long-term use
Western medical indications: Drug dependency (especially tranquillizers or sleeping pills), neurasthenia, heart disease, menopausal syndrome, chronic urticaria, and apthous ulcers
Potential formula toxicities & interactions:
FL/B&B*Zhu Sha* (Cinnabaris) is a toxic substance that should not be taken long-term.

POTENTIAL MEDICINAL TOXICITIES & INTERACTIONS:

Sheng Di, Sheng Di Huang
(uncooked Radix Rehmanniae Glutinosae)

Standard daily dosage: 9-30g
AH: Contraindicated in patients with diarrhea or lack of appetite
B&G: Contraindicated in pregnant women with anemias or digestive weakness
C&C: Contains potassium. Could possibly cause hyperkalemia when used with potassium-sparing diuretics.
PDR: No health risks or side effects are known in conjunction with the proper administration of designated therapeutic dosages.

Ren Shen
(Radix Panacis Ginseng, ginseng)

Standard daily dosage: 1-30g
AH: Contraindicated in hypertension
BR: May cause manic episodes in patients on MAO-inhibitors. May cause hypertension if consumed with caffeine. Possible additive effects to insulin. May reduce the anticoagulative effect of warfarin (Coumadin).

B&G: Contraindicated for hypertensive patients. Overdose can lead to headache, insomnia, heart palpitations, and a rise in blood pressure. A traditional antidote is mung bean soup.

C&C: Vitamin C, nicotinic acid, glutamic acid, hydrochloric acid, and other highly acidic substances could possibly reduce the therapeutic effect of this medicinal.

PDR: Contraindicated in patients with hypertension. Not recommended in large doses during pregnancy or lactation due to potential neonatal androgenization. Enhances the effect of insulin and other antidiabetic agents. Use with MAO-inhibitors may cause headaches, tremors, and manias.

Tian Men Dong, Tian Dong
(Tuber Asparagi Cochinensis)

AH: Safe when used appropriately

B&G: Contraindicated in patients with loss of appetite and diarrhea or cough from the common cold.

PDR: Contains steroid saponins and flavinoids. Should not be administered in the presence of kidney diseases due to the irritating effect of the saponins. Otherwise considered safe with the proper administration of designated therapeutic dosages.

Mai Men Dong, Mai Dong
(Tuber Ophiopogoni Japonici)

Standard daily dosage: 6-15g

AH: Safe when used appropriately

B&G: According to some traditional sources, antagonizes *Kuan Dong Hua* (Flos Tussilaginis Farfarae) and counteracts *Ku Shen* (Radix Sophorae Flavescentis) and *Bai Mu Er* (Fructificatio Tremellae Fuciformis).

C&C: Contains glycosides. Vitamin C, nicotinic acid, glutamic acid, hydrochloric acid, and other highly acidic substances could possibly reduce the therapeutic effect of this medicinal.

Xuan Shen, Yuan Shen
(Radix Scrophulariae Ningpoensis)

Standard daily dosage: 9-30g

C&C: Contains alkaloids, potassium, and glycosides. Could possibly cause hyperkalemia when used with potassium-sparing diuretics. Could possibly reduce the absorption and therapeutic effect of potassium and sodium iodides, sodium bicarbonate, aluminum hydroxide, and magnesium sulfate. Vitamin C, nicotinic acid, glutamic acid, hydrochloric acid, and other highly acidic substances Could possibly reduce the therapeutic effect of this medicinal.

Dan Shen
(Radix Salviae Miltiorrhizae)

Standard daily dosage: 6-60g
AH: Safe when used appropriately
BR: Possible additive effect to warfarin (Coumadin)
B&G: According to traditional texts, incompatible with *Li Lu* (Rhizoma Et Radix Veratri). Administration of tinctures of this herb can lead to pruritus, stomach ache, or reduced appetite.
C&C: Contains potassium. Could possibly cause hyperkalemia when used with potassium-sparing diuretics. Increases the absorption and decreases the clearance of warfarin (Coumadin) which can adversely affect prothrombin time. Should not be used in cancer patients taking antineoplastic drugs since this medicinal can hinder their therapeutic effect and promote tumor metastasis. Hinders the absorption of magnesium oxide, calcium carbonate, and aluminum hydroxide.
PDR: No health risks or side effects are known in conjunction with the proper administration of designated therapeutic dosages.

Fu Ling, Bai Fu Ling, Yun Ling
(Sclerotium Poriae Cocos)

Standard daily dosage: 9-15g
B&G: Large doses or long-term use is discouraged. Contraindicated in patients with frequent, copious urination. According to traditional sources, may counteract *Di Yu* (Radix Sanguisorbae Officinalis), *Qin Jiao* (Radix Gentianae Qinjiao), and *Bie Jia* (Carapax Amydae Sinensis).
C&C: Contains potassium. Could possibly cause hyperkalemia when used with potassium-sparing diuretics.

Yuan Zhi
(Radix Polygalae Tenuifoliae)

Standard daily dosage: 3-9g
AH: Contraindicated in gastritis or when gastric ulcers are present.
B&G: Contraindicated in gastritis or when gastric ulcers are present. According to some traditional sources, counteracts *Zhen Zhu* (Margarita) and *Li Lu* (Rhizoma Et Radix Veratri).
C&C: Contains glycosides. Vitamin C, nicotinic acid, glutamic acid,

hydrochloric acid, and other highly acidic substances could possibly reduce the therapeutic effect of this medicinal.

Dang Gui
(Radix Angelicae Sinensis)

Standard daily dosage: 3-15g
AH: Do not use during pregnancy. (This medicinal is routinely used in Chinese medical gynecology during pregnancy as part of formulas appropriately prescribed on the basis of pattern discrimination.)
B&G: Use with caution in patients with diarrhea or abdominal distention.
C&C: Contains potassium. Could possibly cause hyperkalemia when used with potassium-sparing diuretics. May exaggerate the anticoagulative effect of warfarin (Coumadin).

Wu Wei Zi
(Fructus Schisandrae Chinensis, schisandra)

Standard daily dosage: 1.5-9g
AH: Safe when used appropriately
B&G: Occasionally causes heartburn. In mice, toxic doses were 10-15g/kg. Symptoms of overdose include restlessness, insomnia, or dyspnea.
C&C: Contains potassium. Highly acidic. Could possibly cause crystalluria and hematuria. Could possibly cause hyperkalemia when used in large doses with potassium-sparing diuretics. Could possibly reduce the therapeutic effect of sodium bicarbonate, aluminum hydroxide, many antibiotics (especially aminoglycosides and sulfas), reserpine, caffeine, opiates, scopolamine, and berbamin.
PDR: No health risks or side effects are known in conjunction with the proper administration of designated therapeutic dosages.

Bai Zi Ren
(Semen Biotae Orientalis)

Standard daily dosage: 6-18g
B&G: Contraindicated in patients with loose stools or phlegm disorders. According to some traditional sources, antagonizes *Ju Hua* (Flos Chrysanthemum Morifolii).
C&C: Contains glycosides. Vitamin C, nicotinic acid, glutamic acid, hydrochloric acid, and other highly acidic substances could possibly reduce the therapeutic effect of this medicinal.

Suan Zao Ren
(Semen Zizyphi Spinosae)

Standard daily dosage: 9-18g

AH: Not to be used during pregnancy. (No such prohibition exists for this medicinal in traditional Chinese medicine.)

Jie Geng
(Radix Platycodi Grandiflori, bellflower root)

Standard daily dosage: 3-9g
AH: Contraindicated in hemoptysis, especially in cases of tuberculosis. Use with caution in bleeding peptic ulcer.
B&G: Contraindicated in patients with hemoptysis. According to some traditional sources, counteracts *Long Dan Cao* (Gentiana Longdancao) and *Long Yan Rou* (Arillus Euphoriae Longanae).
C&C: Contains calcium and glycosides. Could possibly reduce the effect of most antibiotics, cause digitalis intoxication and heart arrhythmias, hinder the absorption of isoniazid, and reduce the biological effect of levadopa. Vitamin C, nicotinic acid, glutamic acid, hydrochloric acid, and other highly acidic substances could possibly reduce the therapeutic effect of this medicinal.

Zhu Sha
(Cinnabaris, cinnabar)

Standard daily dosage: 0.2-2.7g in pills and powders
B&G: Contains mercuric sulfide which is highly toxic. Should not be used in large amounts or long-term. To prevent mercury poisoning, do not heat.
GLW: Symptoms of adverse reaction include burning pain in the oral cavity and throat, swelling and distention of the mucosa, bleeding, ulceration, and a metallic taste in the mouth, nausea, vomiting, abdominal pain, diarrhea, mucus in the stools or hemafecia. If severe, there is hemorrhagic enteritis, clenched teeth, fright reversal, and trembling. If the kidneys are poisoned, there is edema, scanty urination, albuminuria, and acute kidney failure, syncope, convulsions, low blood pressure, shock, and eventual respiratory failure.

Long Yan Rou, Yuan Rou
(Arillus Euphoriae Longanae, longan fruit)

Standard daily dosage: 6-30g

No toxicity or interaction information listed in the sources

COMMENTS

Dang Shen (Radix Codonopsitis Pilosulae) is commonly substituted for *Ren Shen* in this formula. *Hu Po* (Succinum) or *Long Gu* (Os Draconis) is commonly substituted for *Zhu Sha*.

TONG XIE YAO FANG
(Painful Diarrhea Essential Formula)

Category: Harmonizing
Functions: Courses the liver and rectifies the qi, fortifies the spleen and supplements the qi
Chinese medical indications: Liver-spleen disharmony resulting in colicky abdominal and diarrhea associated with psycho-emotional stress, borborygmus, thin, white tongue fur, and a bowstring pulse
Contraindications: None listed
Western medical indications: Irritable bowel syndrome, colitis, acute gastroenteritis, bacillary dysentery, and hyperthyroidism
Potential formula toxicities & interactions: None listed

POTENTIAL MEDICINAL TOXICITIES & INTERACTIONS:

Bai Zhu
(Rhizoma Atractylodis Macrocephalae)

Standard daily dosage: 4.5-9g
AH: Safe when used appropriately
B&G: When rats were fed 0.5g/kg of this medicinal for two months, they developed a mild lymphopenia and anemia but suffered no damage to the brain, heart, or liver.

Bai Shao, Shao Yao
(Radix Albus Paeoniae Lactiflorae, white peony root)

Standard daily dosage: 6-30g
AH: Safe when used appropriately
B&G: Use with caution in debilitated patients with diarrhea. According to some traditional sources, antagonizes *Shi Hu* (Herba Dendrobii) and *Mang Xiao* (Mirabilitum), counteracts *Bie Jia* (Carapax Amydae Sinensis) and *Xiao Ji* (Herba Cephalanopoloris Segeti), and is incompatible with *Li Lu* (Rhizoma Et Radix Veratri).
C&C: Contains calcium, tannic acid, potassium, and glycosides. Could possibly cause hyperkalemia when used with potassium-sparing diuretics. Could possibly reduce the effect of most antibiotics, cause digitalis intoxication and heart arrhythmias, and could possibly reduce the absorption and therapeutic effect of levadopa, isoniazid, chlorpromazine, calcium carbonate and gluconate, atropine, ephedrine, quinine, reser-

pine, vitamin B_1, trypsine, amylase, and pepsin. Vitamin C, nicotinic acid, glutamic acid, hydrochloric acid, and other highly acidic substances could possibly reduce the therapeutic effect of this medicinal.

Chen Pi, Ju Pi, Ju Hong
(Pericarpium Citri Reticulatae, tangerine peel)

Standard daily dosage: 3-9g
AH: Safe when used appropriately
C&C: Contains potassium. Could possibly cause hyperkalemia when used with potassium-sparing diuretics.

Fang Feng
(Radix Ledebouriellae Divaricatae)

Standard daily dosage: 3-9g
AH: Safe when used appropriately
B&G: According to some traditional sources, may antagonize *Gan Jiang* (dry Rhizoma Zingiberis Officinalis), *Li Lu* (Rhizoma Et Radix Veratri) and counteracts *Bei Xie* (Rhizoma Dioscoreae Hypoglaucae).
C&C: Contains glycosides. Vitamin C, nicotinic acid, glutamic acid, hydrochloric acid, and other highly acidic substances could possibly reduce the therapeutic effect of this medicinal.

COMMENTS

The ingredients in this formula commonly form the basis of prescriptions for the treatment of all types of diarrhea manifesting as a liver-spleen disharmony.

WAN DAI TANG
(End [Abnormal] Vaginal Discharge Decoction)

Category: Securing and astringing, uterus-stabilizing
Functions: Fortifies the spleen and supplements the center, transforms dampness and stops vaginal discharge
Chinese medical indications: Liver-spleen disharmony resulting in profuse, white or pale yellow, abnormal vaginal discharge which is thin in consistency, continuous, and not foul-smelling, fatigue, a pale facial complexion, loose stools, a pale tongue with white fur, and a soggy, bowstring, possibly moderate (*i.e.*, slightly slow) pulse
Contraindications: Depressive or damp heat
Western medical indications: Abnormal vaginal discharge, hemophilus vaginitis, vulvitis, cervical inflammation, diarrhea, edema during pregnancy, edema during menstruation, and headache
Potential formula toxicities & interactions:
FL/B&B: Should not be used if discharge is dark yellow, contains blood, and is thick, sticky, and foul-smelling. Use of this formula under these conditions will exacerbate the condition.

POTENTIAL MEDICINAL TOXICITIES & INTERACTIONS:

Bai Zhu
(Rhizoma Atractylodis Macrocephalae)

Standard daily dosage: 4.5-9g
AH: Safe when used appropriately
B&G: When rats were fed 0.5g/kg of this medicinal for two months, they developed a mild lymphopenia and anemia but suffered no damage to the brain, heart, or liver.

Shan Yao
(Radix Dioscoreae Oppositae)

Standard daily dosage: 9-30g
AH: Safe when used appropriately
B&G: According to some traditional sources, antagonizes *Gan Sui* (Radix Euphorbiae Kansui).
C&C: Contains alkaloids, potassium, amylase, and glycosides. Could possibly cause hyperkalemia when used with potassium-sparing diuretics.

Could possibly reduce the absorption and therapeutic effect of potassium and sodium iodides, sodium bicarbonate, aluminum hydroxide, magnesium sulfate, tetracyclines, sulphanomides, and aspirin. Vitamin C, nicotinic acid, glutamic acid, hydrochloric acid, and other highly acidic substances could possibly reduce the therapeutic effect of this medicinal.
PDR: Use of this medicinal may reduce the antiinflammatory effect of indomethacin. May have an additive estrogenic effect when administered with estrogen-containing drugs. Poisoning in overdoses may occur from the picrotoxin-like effect of dioscorin.

Ren Shen
(Radix Panacis Ginseng, ginseng)

Standard daily dosage: 1-30g
AH: Contraindicated in hypertension
BR: May cause manic episodes in patients on MAO-inhibitors. May cause hypertension if consumed with caffeine. Possible additive effects to insulin. May reduce the anticoagulative effect of warfarin (Coumadin).
B&G: Contraindicated for hypertensive patients. Overdose can lead to headache, insomnia, heart palpitations, and a rise in blood pressure. A traditional antidote is mung bean soup.
C&C: Vitamin C, nicotinic acid, glutamic acid, hydrochloric acid, and other highly acidic substances could possibly reduce the therapeutic effect of this medicinal.
PDR: Contraindicated in patients with hypertension. Not recommended in large doses during pregnancy or lactation due to potential neonatal androgenization. Enhances the effect of insulin and other antidiabetic agents. Use with MAO-inhibitors may cause headaches, tremors, and manias.

Cang Zhu
(Rhizoma Atractylodis)

Standard daily dosage: 4.5-9g
B&G: Use with caution in patients with loose, watery stools.
PDR: No health risks or side effects are known in conjunction with the proper administration of designated therapeutic dosages.

Chen Pi, Ju Pi, Ju Hong
(Pericarpium Citri Reticulatae, tangerine peel)

Standard daily dosage: 3-9g
AH: Safe when used appropriately
C&C: Contains potassium. Could possibly cause hyperkalemia when used with potassium-sparing diuretics.

Che Qian Zi, Che Qian Ren
(Semen Plantaginis, plantain seeds)

Standard daily dosage: 4.5-9g
B&G: Contraindicated during pregnancy.
C&C: Contains glycosides. Highly acidic. Could possibly cause crystalluria and hematuria and reduce the therapeutic effect of sodium bicarbonate, aluminum hydroxide, many antibiotics (especially aminoglycosides and sulfas), reserpine, caffeine, opiates, scopolamine, and berbamin. Vitamin C, nicotinic acid, glutamic acid, hydrochloric acid, and other highly acidic substances could possibly reduce the therapeutic effect of this medicinal.

Chai Hu
(Radix Bupleuri)

Standard daily dosage: 3-12g
AH: Safe when used appropriately
B&G: May occasionally cause nausea and vomiting, in which case the dose should then be reduced significantly.
C&C: Vitamin C, nicotinic acid, glutamic acid, hydrochloric acid, and other highly acidic substances could possibly reduce the therapeutic effect of this medicinal.
PDR: Not to be administered during pregnancy. (This medicinal is routinely used in Chinese medical gynecology during pregnancy as part of formulas appropriately prescribed on the basis of pattern discrimination.) Overdose may lead to gastroenteritis, intestinal colic, and diarrhea due to saponin content.

Jing Jie Sui, Jing Jie
(Herba Seu Flos Schizonepetae Tenuifoliae)

Standard daily dosage: 3-9g

No toxicity or interaction information listed in the sources

Gan Cao
(Radix Glycyrrhizae Uralensis, licorice root)

Standard daily dosage: 2-12g
AH: Do not use during pregnancy. (This medicinal is routinely used in Chinese medical gynecology during pregnancy as part of formulas appropriately prescribed on the basis of pattern discrimination.) As a single herb in high doses, it is contraindicated in diabetes, hypertension, and liver disorders. Not for long-term use.
BR: May increase toxicity of cardiac glycosides. May increase potassium loss due to diuretics and laxatives. Possible additive effect to corticosteroids. May be synergistic with insulin in causing hypokalemia and sodium retention.

B&G: According to some traditional sources, incompatible with *Gan Sui* (Radix Euphorbiae Kansui), *Yuan Hua* (Flos Daphnes Genkwae), and *Yuan Zhi* (Radix Polygalae Tenuifoliae). If taken long-term, it may cause hypertension and/or edema. Contains glycyrrhetinic acid which could possibly cause a reduction in thyroid activity and basal metabolic rate.

The research on *Gan Cao* concurs that this medicinal is generally safe when used in small amounts as an envoy. It should not be taken long-term or as a single herb during pregnancy. When used as a single medicinal or in patients taking other potent Western pharmaceuticals, caution should be exercised to guard against potential toxicity and drug interaction.

COMMENTS

Dang Shen (Radix Codonopsitis Pilosulae) is commonly substituted for *Ren Shen* in this formula.

WEN DAN TANG
(Warm the Gallbladder Decoction, a.k.a.
Bamboo & Hoelen Combination)

Category: Phlegm-transforming
Functions: Rectifies the qi and transforms phlegm, clears the gallbladder and harmonizes the stomach
Chinese medical indications: Gallbladder-stomach disharmony (a.k.a. liver-stomach disharmony) with phlegm heat resulting in dizziness, nausea and vomiting, insomnia, heart palpitations, easy fright, chest oppression, a bitter taste in the mouth, slight thirst, slimy, yellow tongue fur, and a slippery, bowstring pulse
Contraindications: None listed
Western medical indications: Mood disorders, such as depression and anxiety, obsessive compulsive disorder, early stages of schizophrenia, chronic gastritis, peptic ulcer, chronic hepatitis, Meniere's disease, and chronic bronchitis
Potential formula toxicities & interactions: None listed

POTENTIAL MEDICINAL TOXICITIES & INTERACTIONS:

Zhu Rhu
(Caulis Bambusae In Taeniis, bamboo shavings)

Standard daily dosage: 4.5-9g
C&C: Contains potassium. Could possibly cause hyperkalemia when used with potassium-sparing diuretics.

Zhi Shi
(Fructus Immaturus Citri Aurantii, immature bitter orange)

Standard daily dosage: 3-9g
B&G: Use with caution during pregnancy or in debilitated patients.
C&C: Contains tannic acid. Highly acidic. Could possibly cause crystalluria and hematuria and reduce the absorption and biologic effect of most antibiotics, isoniazid, chlorpromazine, calcium carbonate and gluconate, atropine, ephedrine, quinine, reserpine, digitalis, vitamin B_1, trypsine, amylase, and pepsin, sodium bicarbonate, aluminum hydroxide, caffeine, opiates, scopolamine, and berbamin.

Ban Xia
(Rhizoma Pinelliae Ternatae)

Standard daily dosage: 4.5-12g

AH: Do not use during pregnancy. (This medicinal is routinely used during pregnancy in China when indicated by disease and pattern discrimination.) Contraindicated in all hemorrhagic disorders.

B&G: Safe as long as it is properly prepared. Must be decocted with other herbs and not taken alone or uncooked. Toxic effects due to improper preparation or dosage include burning and numbness in throat and lips, nausea, and a feeling of pressure in the chest. Antidote is oral administration of raw ginger. Use with caution in patients with fever. According to some traditional sources, incompatible with *Wu Tou* (Radix Aconiti).

C&C: Contains alkaloids and glycosides. Could possibly reduce the absorption and therapeutic effect of potassium and sodium iodides, sodium bicarbonate, aluminum hydroxide, and magnesium sulfate. Vitamin C, nicotinic acid, glutamic acid, hydrochloric acid, and other highly acidic substances could possibly reduce the therapeutic effect of this medicinal.

GLW: Poisoning occurs within 15 minutes to three hours after ingestion of a suitable amount. Initially, there is burning pain in the mouth, tongue, and throat, and enlargement of the tongue. This is then followed by drooling, ulceration of the oral mucosa, unclear speech, difficulty swallowing, dizziness, low-grade fever, heart palpitations, numbness of the extremities, a somber white facial complexion, and a weak, forceless pulse. If severe, there may be convulsions and respiratory failure leading to death.

Chen Pi, Ju Pi, Ju Hong
(Pericarpium Citri Reticulatae, tangerine peel)

Standard daily dosage: 3-9g

AH: Safe when used appropriately

C&C: Contains potassium. Could possibly cause hyperkalemia when used with potassium-sparing diuretics.

Fu Ling, Bai Fu Ling, Yun Ling
(Sclerotium Poriae Cocos)

Standard daily dosage: 9-15g

B&G: Large doses or long-term use is discouraged. Contraindicated in patients with frequent, copious urination. According to traditional sources, may counteract *Di Yu* (Radix Sanguisorbae Officinalis), *Qin Jiao* (Radix Gentianae Qinjiao), and *Bie Jia* (Carapax Amydae Sinensis).

C&C: Contains potassium. Could possibly cause hyperkalemia when used with potassium-sparing diuretics.

Gan Cao
(Radix Glycyrrhizae Uralensis, licorice root)

Standard daily dosage: 2-12g
AH: Do not use during pregnancy. (This medicinal is routinely used in Chinese medical gynecology during pregnancy as part of formulas appropriately prescribed on the basis of pattern discrimination.) As a single herb in high doses, it is contraindicated in diabetes, hypertension, and liver disorders. Not for long-term use.
BR: May increase toxicity of cardiac glycosides. May increase potassium loss due to diuretics and laxatives. Possible additive effect to corticosteroids. May be synergistic with insulin in causing hypokalemia and sodium retention.
B&G: According to some traditional sources, incompatible with *Gan Sui* (Radix Euphorbiae Kansui), *Yuan Hua* (Flos Daphnes Genkwae), and *Yuan Zhi* (Radix Polygalae Tenuifoliae). If taken long-term, it may cause hypertension and/or edema. Contains glycyrrhetinic acid which could possibly cause a reduction in thyroid activity and basal metabolic rate.

The research on *Gan Cao* concurs that this medicinal is generally safe when used in small amounts as an envoy. It should not be taken long-term or as a single herb during pregnancy. When used as a single medicinal or in patients taking other potent Western pharmaceuticals, caution should be exercised to guard against potential toxicity and drug interaction.

Sheng Jiang
(uncooked Rhizoma Zingiberis Officinalis, fresh ginger)

Standard daily dose: 3-9g
AH: Safe when used appropriately
BR: Reduces vomiting caused by chemotherapeutic drugs. Increases absorption of oral drugs.
PDR: Recommended safe dosage limit is six grams (6g). Avoid larger doses if being used to treat morning sickness or if used in patients taking anticoagulants.

Da Zao, Hong Zao
(Fructus Zizyphi Jujubae, red dates)

Standard daily dosage: 10-30g (3-12 pieces)
AH: Safe when used appropriately
PDR: No health risks or side effects are known in conjunction with the proper administration of designated therapeutic dosages.

COMMENTS

This formula forms the base for a whole family of related formulas. The most famous of these is *Huang Lian Wen Dan Tang* (Coptis Warm the Gallbladder Decoction) and *Shi Wei Wen Dan Tang* (Ten Flavors Warm the Gallbladder Decoction).

AH= AHPA, B&B= BENSKY & BAROLET, B&G= BENSKY & GAMBLE, BR= BRINKER,
C&C= CHAN & CHEUNG, FL= FLAWS, GLW= GAO LU WEN, PDR= PHYSICIAN'S DESK REFERENCE

WEN JING TANG
(Warm the Menses Decoction, a.k.a. Tang-kuei & Evodia Combination)

Category: Blood-quickening
Functions: Warms the menses and dispels cold, nourishes the blood and dispels stasis
Chinese medical indications: Vacuity cold of the chong and ren with blood stasis resulting in mild, enduring uterine bleeding, menstrual irregularity, continuous leaking, midcycle bleeding, chilly pain and distention in the lower abdomen, infertility, dry lips and mouth, low-grade fever at dusk, warm palms and soles, a pale, purple tongue or possible static macules or speckles, and a fine, deep, slow, and bowstring pulse
Contraindications: Concretions and conglomerations due to blood stasis and replete evils
Western medical indications: Functional uterine bleeding, irregular menstruation, primary dysmenorrhea, infertility, polycystic ovarian syndrome, chronic pelvic inflammatory disease, and perimenopausal syndrome
Potential formula toxicities & interactions: None listed

POTENTIAL MEDICINAL TOXICITIES & INTERACTIONS:

Wu Zhu Yu
(Fructus Evodiae Rutecarpae)

Standard daily dosage: 3-9g
AH: Do not exceed recommended dose.
B&G: Very drying. Should not be used long-term. According to some traditional sources, antagonizes *Dan Shen* (Radix Salviae Miltiorrhizae) and counteracts *Zi Shi Ying* (Fluoritum). Overdose may cause the throat to become extremely dry. Large doses stimulate the central nervous system and can lead to visual disturbances and hallucinations.
C&C: Contains alkaloids and quercetin. Could possibly reduce the absorption and therapeutic effect of potassium and sodium iodides, sodium bicarbonate, calcium gluconate, carbonate, and lactate, aluminum hydroxide, magnesium and ferrous sulfates, and bismuth subcarbonate.
GLW: Symptoms of adverse reaction include vomiting, abdominal pain, diarrhea, increased body temperature, visual disturbances, visual hallucinations, and falling hair. In pregnant women, toxicity may cause abortion.

Gui Zhi
(Ramulus Cinnamomi Cassiae, cinnamon twigs)

Standard daily dosage: 3-15g
AH: Safe when used appropriately
B&G: Use with caution in the presence of fever, during pregnancy, or during excessive menstruation.
PDR: Contraindicated during pregnancy.

Dang Gui
(Radix Angelicae Sinensis)

Standard daily dosage: 3-15g
AH: Do not use during pregnancy. (This medicinal is routinely used in Chinese medical gynecology during pregnancy as part of formulas appropriately prescribed on the basis of pattern discrimination.)
B&G: Use with caution in patients with diarrhea or abdominal distention.
C&C: Contains potassium. Could possibly cause hyperkalemia when used with potassium-sparing diuretics. May exaggerate the anticoagulative effect of warfarin (Coumadin).

Chuan Xiong
(Radix Ligustici Wallichii)

Standard daily dosage: 3-9g (In China today, it is not uncommon for this medicinal to be prescribed up to 15 grams per day in decoction.)
AH: Do not use during pregnancy. (This medicinal is routinely used in Chinese medical gynecology during pregnancy as part of formulas appropriately prescribed on the basis of pattern discrimination.)
B&G: Not for patients with migraine headache or excessive menstrual bleeding. Overdosage causes vomiting and dizziness. According to some traditional texts, antagonizes *Shan Zhu Yu* (Fructus Corni Officinalis) and *Huang Qi* (Radix Astragali Membranacei), counteracts *Hua Shi* (Talcum) and *Huang Lian* (Rhizoma Coptidis Chinensis), and is incompatible with *Li Lu* (Rhizoma Et Radix Veratri).
C&C: Contains alkaloids and potassium. Could possibly cause hyperkalemia when used with potassium-sparing diuretics. Could possibly reduce the absorption and therapeutic effect of potassium and sodium iodides, sodium bicarbonate, aluminum hydroxide, and magnesium sulfate.

Bai Shao, Shao Yao
(Radix Albus Paeoniae Lactiflorae, white peony root)

Standard daily dosage: 6-30g
AH: Safe when used appropriately
B&G: Use with caution in debilitated patients with diarrhea. According to some traditional sources, antagonizes *Shi Hu* (Herba Dendrobii) and

Mang Xiao (Mirabilitum), counteracts *Bie Jia* (Carapax Amydae Sinensis) and *Xiao Ji* (Herba Cephalanopoloris Segeti), and is incompatible with *Li Lu* (Rhizoma Et Radix Veratri).

C&C: Contains calcium, tannic acid, potassium, and glycosides. Could possibly cause hyperkalemia when used with potassium-sparing diuretics. Could possibly reduce the effect of most antibiotics, cause digitalis intoxication and heart arrhythmias, and could possibly reduce the absorption and therapeutic effect of levadopa, isoniazid, chlorpromazine, calcium carbonate and gluconate, atropine, ephedrine, quinine, reserpine, vitamin B_1, trypsine, amylase, and pepsin. Vitamin C, nicotinic acid, glutamic acid, hydrochloric acid, and other highly acidic substances could possibly reduce the therapeutic effect of this medicinal.

E Jiao
(Gelatinum Corii Asini, donkey skin glue)

Standard daily dosage: 3-15g
B&G: According to some traditional sources, counteracts *Da Huang* (Radix Et Rhizoma Rhei).

Mai Men Dong, Mai Dong
(Tuber Ophiopogoni Japonici)

Standard daily dosage: 6-15g
AH: Safe when used appropriately
B&G: According to some traditional sources, antagonizes *Kuan Dong Hua* (Flos Tussilaginis Farfarae) and counteracts *Ku Shen* (Radix Sophorae Flavescentis) and *Bai Mu Er* (Fructificatio Tremellae Fuciformis).
C&C: Contains glycosides. Vitamin C, nicotinic acid, glutamic acid, hydrochloric acid, and other highly acidic substances could possibly reduce the therapeutic effect of this medicinal.

Dan Pi, Mu Dan Pi
(Cortex Radicis Moutan, tree peony root bark)

Standard daily dosage: 6-12g
AH: Not to be used during pregnancy. (This ingredient is commonly used in China during pregnancy to treat heat in the blood and/or blood stasis.)
B&G: Should not be used during pregnancy or in patients with excessive sweating or profuse menstruation. Avoid using with garlic. According to some traditional sources, may counteract the effect of *Tu Si Zi* (Semen Cuscutae Chinensis), *Bei Mu* (Bulbus Fritillariae), and *Da Huang* (Radix Et Rhizoma Rhei).
C&C: Contains tannic acid, potassium, and glycosides. Could possibly cause hyperkalemia when used with potassium-sparing diuretics. Could possibly reduce the absorption and biologic effect of most antibiotics, isoniazid,

chlorpromazine, calcium carbonate and gluconate, atropine, ephedrine, quinine, reserpine, digitalis, vitamin B$_1$, trypsin, amylase, and pepsin. Vitamin C, nicotinic acid, glutamic acid, hydrochloric acid, and other highly acidic substances could possibly reduce the therapeutic effect of this medicinal.

Ren Shen
(Radix Panacis Ginseng, ginseng)

Standard daily dosage: 1-30g

AH: Contraindicated in hypertension

BR: May cause manic episodes in patients on MAO-inhibitors. May cause hypertension if consumed with caffeine. Possible additive effects to insulin. May reduce the anticoagulative effect of warfarin (Coumadin).

B&G: Contraindicated for hypertensive patients. Overdose can lead to headache, insomnia, heart palpitations, and a rise in blood pressure. A traditional antidote is mung bean soup.

C&C: Vitamin C, nicotinic acid, glutamic acid, hydrochloric acid, and other highly acidic substances could possibly reduce the therapeutic effect of this medicinal.

PDR: Contraindicated in patients with hypertension. Not recommended in large doses during pregnancy or lactation due to potential neonatal androgenization. Enhances the effect of insulin and other antidiabetic agents. Use with MAO-inhibitors may cause headaches, tremors, and manias.

Gan Cao
(Radix Glycyrrhizae Uralensis, licorice root)

Standard daily dosage: 2-12g

AH: Do not use during pregnancy. (This medicinal is routinely used in Chinese medical gynecology during pregnancy as part of formulas appropriately prescribed on the basis of pattern discrimination.) As a single herb in high doses, it is contraindicated in diabetes, hypertension, and liver disorders. Not for long-term use.

BR: May increase toxicity of cardiac glycosides. May increase potassium loss due to diuretics and laxatives. Possible additive effect to corticosteroids. May be synergistic with insulin in causing hypokalemia and sodium retention.

B&G: According to some traditional sources, incompatible with *Gan Sui* (Radix Euphorbiae Kansui), *Yuan Hua* (Flos Daphnes Genkwae), and *Yuan Zhi* (Radix Polygalae Tenuifoliae). If taken long-term, it may cause hypertension and/or edema. Contains glycyrrhetinic acid which could possibly cause a reduction in thyroid activity and basal metabolic rate.

The research on *Gan Cao* concurs that this medicinal is generally safe when used in small amounts as an envoy. It should not be taken long-term or as a single herb during pregnancy. When used as a single medicinal or

in patients taking other potent Western pharmaceuticals, caution should be exercised to guard against potential toxicity and drug interaction.

Sheng Jiang
(uncooked Rhizoma Zingiberis Officinalis, fresh ginger)

Standard daily dose: 3-9g
AH: Safe when used appropriately
BR: Reduces vomiting caused by chemotherapeutic drugs. Increases absorption of oral drugs.
PDR: Recommended safe dosage limit is six grams (6g). Avoid larger doses if being used to treat morning sickness or if used in patients taking anticoagulants.

Ban Xia
(Rhizoma Pinelliae Ternatae)

Standard daily dosage: 4.5-12g
AH: Do not use during pregnancy. (This medicinal is routinely used during pregnancy in China when indicated by disease and pattern discrimination.) Contraindicated in all hemorrhagic disorders.
B&G: Safe as long as it is properly prepared. Must be decocted with other herbs and not taken alone or uncooked. Toxic effects due to improper preparation or dosage include burning and numbness in throat and lips, nausea, and a feeling of pressure in the chest. Antidote is oral administration of raw ginger. Use with caution in patients with fever. According to some traditional sources, incompatible with *Wu Tou* (Radix Aconiti).
C&C: Contains alkaloids and glycosides. Could possibly reduce the absorption and therapeutic effect of potassium and sodium iodides, sodium bicarbonate, aluminum hydroxide, and magnesium sulfate. Vitamin C, nicotinic acid, glutamic acid, hydrochloric acid, and other highly acidic substances could possibly reduce the therapeutic effect of this medicinal.
GLW: Poisoning occurs within 15 minutes to three hours after ingestion of a suitable amount. Initially, there is burning pain in the mouth, tongue, and throat, and enlargement of the tongue. This is then followed by drooling, ulceration of the oral mucosa, unclear speech, difficulty swallowing, dizziness, low-grade fever, heart palpitations, numbness of the extremities, a somber white facial complexion, and a weak, forceless pulse. If severe, there may be convulsions and respiratory failure leading to death.

COMMENTS

Dang Shen (Radix Codonopsitis Pilosulae) is commonly substituted for *Ren Shen* in this formula.

WU LING SAN
(Five [Ingredients] Poria Powder, a.k.a.
Hoelen Five Herb Formula)

Category: Dampness-dispelling
Functions: Disinhibits water and seeps dampness, warms yang
and transforms the qi
Chinese medical indications: Spleen vacuity failing to trans-
port water with edema, generalized bodily heaviness, diarrhea,
strangury
Contraindications: Long-term use in cases of spleen and/or kidney vacuity
Western medical indications: Chronic nephritis edema, acute
and chronic nephritis, chronic renal failure, acute gastritis, cardiac edema from congestive heart failure, gastroptosis, gastrectasis, ascites due to liver cirrhosis, infectious hepatitis, urinary
retention, scrotal hydrocele, acute gastroenteritis with diarrhea,
Meniere's disease, genitourinary infections, neurogenic bladder
syndrome
Potential formula toxicities & interactions:
FL: Do not use for prolonged period of time
B&B: Symptoms of overdose may include dizziness, vertigo, a
bland taste in the mouth, and reduced appetite

POTENTIAL MEDICINAL TOXICITIES & INTERACTIONS:

Ze Xie
(Rhizoma Alismatis Orientalis)

Standard daily dosage: 6-15g
AH: Prolonged use may cause gastrointestinal irritation.
B&G: Although considered safe, prolonged usage may irritate the intestinal tract and could possibly cause gastroenteritis.
C&C: Contains alkaloids and potassium. Could possibly cause hyperkalemia when used with potassium-sparing diuretics and reduce the
absorption and therapeutic effect of potassium and sodium iodides, sodium bicarbonate, aluminum hydroxide, magnesium sulfate.
PDR: Contains triterpenes, sesquiterpenes, flavone sulfate, and caffeic
acid derivatives. No health hazards or side effects with proper administration of designated therapeutic dosages.

Fu Ling, Bai Fu Ling, Yun Ling
(Sclerotium Poriae Cocos)

Standard daily dosage: 9-15g
B&G: Large doses or long-term use is discouraged. Contraindicated in patients with frequent, copious urination. According to traditional sources, may counteract *Di Yu* (Radix Sanguisorbae Officinalis), *Qin Jiao* (Radix Gentianae Qinjiao), and *Bie Jia* (Carapax Amydae Sinensis).

Zhu Ling
(Sclerotium Polypori Umbellati)

Standard daily dosage: 6-15g
AH: Safe when used appropriately

Bai Zhu
(Rhizoma Atractylodis Macrocephalae)

Standard daily dosage: 4.5-9g
B&G: When rats were fed 0.5g/kg of this medicinal for two months, they developed a mild lymphopenia and anemia but suffered no damage to the brain, heart, or liver.

Gui Zhi
(Ramulus Cinnamomi Cassiae, cinnamon twigs)

Standard daily dosage: 3-15g
AH: Safe when used appropriately
B&G: Use with caution in the presence of fever, during pregnancy, or during excessive menstruation.
PDR: Contraindicated during pregnancy.

WU MEI WAN

(Mume Pills, a.k.a. Mume Formula)

Category: Worm-killing
Functions: Warms the viscera and quiets roundworms
Chinese medical indications: Roundworm reversal with heat in the stomach and cold in the intestines. However, can also be used to treat complex combinations of qi and blood vacuity due to spleen vacuity, qi and blood stagnation and stasis, and damp heat. Classic symptamology includes intermittent attacks of abdominal pain, chest oppression, easy anger, vexatious heat in the chest and stomach duct region accompanied by vomiting after eating, and cold hands and feet. Commonly, there is a red tongue with geographically peeled fur.
Contraindications: Damp heat dysentery
Western medical indications: Ascariasis (including biliary), chronic dysentery, chronic gastritis, gastric ulcer, postgastrectomy syndrome, neurosis, insomnia, and uterine complaints associated with candidiasis
Potential formula toxicities & interactions: None listed

POTENTIAL MEDICINAL TOXICITIES & INTERACTIONS:

Wu Mei

(Fructus Pruni Mume)

Standard daily dosage: 3-9g
AH: Safe when used appropriately
C&C: Highly acidic. Could possibly cause crystalluria and hematuria. Could possibly reduce the therapeutic effect of sodium bicarbonate, aluminum hydroxide, many antibiotics (especially aminoglycosides and sulfas), reserpine, caffeine, opiates, scopolamine, and berbamin.

Chuan Jiao

(Pericarpium Zanthoxyli Bungeani, Sichuan peppercorn husk)

Standard daily dosage: 1.5-6g
AH: Not to be used during pregnancy.
B&G: Use with caution during pregnancy. According to some traditional sources, counteracts *Kuan Dong Hua* (Flos Tussilaginis Farfarae), *Fu Zi* (Radix Lateralis Praeparatus Aconiti Carmichaeli), and *Fang Feng*

(Radix Ledebouriellae Divaricatae) and antagonizes *Gua Lou* (Fructus Trichosanthis Kirlowii). Can inhibit lactation.

Xi Xin
(Herba Asari Cum Radice)

Standard daily dosage: 1-3g
AH: Do not use during pregnancy. Contains aristolochic acid (AA). Do not exceed recommended dose.
B&G: Nephrotoxic. Use with caution in patients with renal problems. According to some traditional sources, may antagonize *Shan Zhu Yu* (Fructus Corni Officinalis) and *Huang Qi* (Radix Astragali Membranacei).
PDR: Not to be used during pregnancy.
GLW: Symptoms of adverse reaction include headache, vomiting, vexation and agitation, sweating, stiffness of the neck, oral thirst, a rapid pulse, increased body temperature and blood pressure, slightly dilated pupils, a red flushed face, twitching muscles, generalized tension which may become convulsions, clenched teeth, arched-back rigidity, unclear thinking, cramping of the four limbs, dimming of consciousness, urinary block, and, eventually, death due to respiratory paralysis.

Xi Xin is on the FDA's "B List" of herbs which may potentially contain aristolochic acid (AA). *Xi Xin* is harvested in China mostly from *Asarum sieboldi* and *Asarum heteropoides*, neither of which have conclusively been shown to contain AA. However, other species of *Asarum* are sometimes substituted, and these may contain AA. As of this writing, the FDA has set no acceptable limit to AA consumption by humans.

Huang Lian
(Rhizoma Coptidis Chinensis)

Standard daily dosage: 1.5-9g
AH: Do not use during pregnancy. (This medicinal is commonly used during pregnancy in China when indicated by disease and pattern discrimination.)
B&G: Contains berberine. Long-term use may damage the digestive system, According to some traditional sources, antagonizes *Ju Hua* (Flos Chrysanthemi Morifolii), *Xuan Shen* (Radix Scrophulariae Ningpoensis), *Bai Xian Pi* (Cortex Radicis Dictamni Dasycarpi), *Jiang Can* (Bombyx Batryticatus). According to some traditional sources, counteracts *Kuan Dong Hua* (Flos Tussilaginis Farfarae) and *Niu Xi* (Radix Achyranthis Bidentatae). Some traditional sources say it should not be taken with pork.

C&C: Contains alkaloids, quercetin, and potassium. Could possibly cause hyperkalemia when used with potassium-sparing diuretics. Could possibly reduce the absorption and therapeutic effect of potassium and sodium iodides, sodium bicarbonate, calcium gluconate, carbonate, and lactate, aluminum hydroxide, magnesium and ferrous sulfates, and bismuth subcarbonate.

Gan Jiang
(dry Rhizoma Zingiberis Officinalis, dry ginger)

Standard daily dosage: 3-12g
AH: Not to be used during pregnancy. Patients with gallstones should consult a practitioner prior to use.
B&G: Use with caution during pregnancy.

Huang Bai, Huang Bo
(Cortex Phellodendri)

Standard daily dosage: 3-12g
AH: Not to be used during pregnancy. (This medicinal is commonly used during pregnancy in China.)
B&G: Chinese literature reports one case of a patient who developed a skin rash after ingestion.
C&C: Contains alkaloids & quercetin. Could possibly reduce the absorption and therapeutic effect of potassium and sodium iodides, sodium bicarbonate, calcium gluconate, carbonate, and lactate, aluminum hydroxide, magnesium and ferrous sulfates, and bismuth subcarbonate.

Fu Zi, Shu Fu Zi, Fu Pian
(Radix Lateralis Praeparatus Aconiti Carmichaeli, wolfsbane, monkshood)

Standard daily dosage: 1.5-15g
AH: To be used only under the supervision of an expert qualified in the appropriate use of this substance
B&G: Contraindicated during pregnancy. A very toxic medicinal which can be fatal if ingested in its uncooked form or in an inappropriate dose. It is generally combined with *Gan Cao* (Radix Glycyrhizae Uralensis) and *Gan Jiang* (dry Rhizoma Zingiberis Officinalis) in decoctions to reduce its toxicity. Symptoms of toxicity include drooling, gastric upset, light-headedness, blurred vision, and numbness and tingling of the extremities. More severe symptoms include premature atrial contractions, dyspnea, and reduced temperature and blood pressure. Emergency measures include the administration of atropine.
C&C: Contains alkaloids. Could possibly reduce the absorption and

therapeutic effect of potassium and sodium iodides, sodium bicarbonate, aluminum hydroxide, and magnesium sulfate.

PDR: Contains nor-diterpene alkaloids, including aconitine. Highly toxic; small doses can be fatal.

GLW: If mild poisoning, there is a burning hot sensation in the mouth and on the tongue, numbness, and pain which gradually spreads to the four limbs and then to the whole body, nausea, vomiting, dizziness, heart palpitations, rapid breathing, vexation, agitation, restlessness, drooling. If more severe poisoning, there may be generalized sweating, paralysis, convulsions, urinary incontinence, dilated pupils, slowed reaction to light, slow heartbeat, arrhythmia, low blood pressure, a somber white facial complexion, reversal chilling of the four limbs, lowered body temperature, and circulatory collapse leading to death.

Gui Zhi
(Ramulus Cinnamomi Cassiae, cinnamon twigs)

Standard daily dosage: 3-15g

AH: Safe when used appropriately

B&G: Use with caution in the presence of fever, during pregnancy, or during excessive menstruation.

PDR: Contraindicated during pregnancy.

Ren Shen
(Radix Panacis Ginseng, ginseng)

Standard daily dosage: 1-30g

AH: Contraindicated in hypertension

BR: May cause manic episodes in patients on MAO-inhibitors. May cause hypertension if consumed with caffeine. Possible additive effects to insulin. May reduce the anticoagulative effect of warfarin (Coumadin).

B&G: Contraindicated for hypertensive patients. Overdose can lead to headache, insomnia, heart palpitations, and a rise in blood pressure. A traditional antidote is mung bean soup.

C&C: Vitamin C, nicotinic acid, glutamic acid, hydrochloric acid, and other highly acidic substances could possibly reduce the therapeutic effect of this medicinal.

PDR: Contraindicated in patients with hypertension. Not recommended in large doses during pregnancy or lactation due to potential neonatal androgenization. Enhances the effect of insulin and other antidiabetic agents. Use with MAO-inhibitors may cause headaches, tremors, and manias.

Dang Gui
(Radix Angelicae Sinensis)

Standard daily dosage: 3-15g
AH: Do not use during pregnancy. (This medicinal is routinely used in Chinese medical gynecology during pregnancy as part of formulas appropriately prescribed on the basis of pattern discrimination.)
B&G: Use with caution in patients with diarrhea or abdominal distention.
C&C: Contains potassium. Could possibly cause hyperkalemia when used with potassium-sparing diuretics. May exaggerate the anticoagulative effect of warfarin (Coumadin).

COMMENTS

While this formula is the main one for killing or dispelling worms in Chinese medicine, it actually has a rather broad scope of indications. It can be used whenever there is a complex combination of spleen qi and/or yang vacuity, blood vacuity, qi stagnation, blood stasis, and damp heat. In that case, Chinese doctors speak of a vacuity and repletion, hot and cold condition. *Dang Shen* (Radix Codonopsitis Pilosulae) is commonly substituted for *Ren Shen* in this formula.

WU ZHU YU TANG
(Evodia Decoction, a.k.a. Evodia Combination)

Category: Interior-warming
Functions: Warms and supplements the liver and stomach, downbears counterflow and stops vomiting
Chinese medical indications: Vacuity cold of the stomach and/or liver with vomiting immediately after eating, clamoring stomach, acid regurgitation, dry heaves, spitting of clear fluids, headache at the vertex, diarrhea, cold hands and feet, slimy, white tongue fur, and a fine, bowstring, or fine, slow pulse
Contraindications: Vomiting and acid regurgitation due to heat
Western medical indications: Chronic gastritis, acute gastroenteritis, cholecystitis, morning sickness, neurogenic headache, migraine headache, abdominal migraine, hypertension, trigeminal neuralgia, and Meniere's disease
Potential formula toxicities & interactions:
B&B: For severe nausea, the decoction should be taken cool to insure that it will not be regurgitated. Occasional side effects include chest discomfort, dizziness, and a worsening of headache. These symptoms generally resolve within 30 minutes of taking the decoction.

POTENTIAL MEDICINAL TOXICITIES & INTERACTIONS:

Wu Zhu Yu
(Fructus Evodiae Rutecarpae)

Standard daily dosage: 3-9g
AH: Do not exceed recommended dose.
B&G: Very drying. Should not be used long-term. According to some traditional sources, antagonizes *Dan Shen* (Radix Salviae Miltiorrhizae) and counteracts *Zi Shi Ying* (Fluoritum). Overdose may cause the throat to become extremely dry. Large doses stimulate the central nervous system and can lead to visual disturbances and hallucinations.
C&C: Contains alkaloids and quercetin. Could possibly reduce the absorption and therapeutic effect of potassium and sodium iodides, sodium bicarbonate, calcium gluconate, carbonate, and lactate, aluminum hydroxide, magnesium and ferrous sulfates, and bismuth subcarbonate.
GLW: Symptoms of adverse reaction include vomiting, abdominal pain, diarrhea, increased body temperature, visual disturbances, visual hallucinations, and falling hair. In pregnant women, toxicity may cause abortion.

Sheng Jiang
(uncooked Rhizoma Zingiberis Officinalis, fresh ginger)

Standard daily dose: 3-9g
AH: Safe when used appropriately
BR: Reduces vomiting caused by chemotherapeutic drugs. Increases absorption of oral drugs.
PDR: Recommended safe dosage limit is six grams (6g). Avoid larger doses if being used to treat morning sickness or if used in patients taking anticoagulants.

Ren Shen
(Radix Panacis Ginseng, ginseng)

Standard daily dosage: 1-30g
AH: Contraindicated in hypertension
BR: May cause manic episodes in patients on MAO-inhibitors. May cause hypertension if consumed with caffeine. Possible additive effects to insulin. May reduce the anticoagulative effect of warfarin (Coumadin).
B&G: Contraindicated for hypertensive patients. Overdose can lead to headache, insomnia, heart palpitations, and a rise in blood pressure. A traditional antidote is mung bean soup.
C&C: Vitamin C, nicotinic acid, glutamic acid, hydrochloric acid, and other highly acidic substances could possibly reduce the therapeutic effect of this medicinal.
PDR: Contraindicated in patients with hypertension. Not recommended in large doses during pregnancy or lactation due to potential neonatal androgenization. Enhances the effect of insulin and other antidiabetic agents. Use with MAO-inhibitors may cause headaches, tremors, and manias.

Da Zao, Hong Zao
(Fructus Zizyphi Jujubae, red dates)

Standard daily dosage: 10-30g (3-12 pieces)
AH: Safe when used appropriately
PDR: No health risks or side effects are known in conjunction with the proper administration of designated therapeutic dosages.

COMMENTS

When used for the first aid treatment of migraine headache with nausea, this formula may actually provoke vomiting. However, if it does, the migraine pain will abate after the vomiting as will the nausea.

XI JIAO DI HUANG TANG
(Rhinoceros Horn & Rehmannia Decoction)

Category: Heat-clearing, blood-cooling
Functions: Drains fire and resolves toxins
Chinese medical indications: Heat evils in the blood aspect with fever, various types of hemorrhagic conditions, red skin macules, black, tarry stools, abdominal distention and fullness, thirst with an inability to swallow, a crimson tongue with thorn-like papillae, and a fine, rapid pulse
Contraindications: Bleeding due to yang vacuity or spleen-stomach vacuity
Western medical indications: Various sorts of hemorrhage including infectious febrile diseases with hemorrhage, measles, septicemia, encephalitis, meningitis, toxemia, uremia, hepatic coma, thrombocytopenic purpura, bleeding and pus in the anterior chamber of the eye, iridocyclitis, glaucoma, acute leukemia, mental illness, and burns
Potential formula toxicities & interactions: None listed

POTENTIAL MEDICINAL TOXICITIES & INTERACTIONS:

Xi Jiao
(Cornu Rhinocerotis, rhinoceros horn)

Standard daily dosage: 1-2g as a powder
B&G: Use with great caution during pregnancy. Should only be used in the presence of high fever. According to traditional sources, may antagonize *Chuan Wu* (Radix Aconiti Carmichaeli), *Cao Wu* (Radix Aconiti Kusnezoffii), and *Lei Wan* (Sclerotium Omphaliae Lapidescentis).

Because *Xi Jiao* is from an endangered species, it is now commonly substituted by *Shui Niu Jiao* (Cornu Bubali, water buffalo horn). Standard daily dosage of this ingredient in decoction is 4.5-9g.

Sheng Di, Sheng Di Huang
(uncooked Radix Rehmanniae Glutinosae)

Standard daily dosage: 9-30g
AH: Contraindicated in patients with diarrhea or lack of appetite
B&G: Contraindicated in pregnant women with anemias or digestive weakness
C&C: Contains potassium. Could possibly cause hyperkalemia when used with potassium-sparing diuretics.

PDR: No health risks or side effects are known in conjunction with the proper administration of designated therapeutic dosages.

Bai Shao, Shao Yao
(Radix Albus Paeoniae Lactiflorae, white peony root)

Standard daily dosage: 6-30g
AH: Safe when used appropriately
B&G: Use with caution in debilitated patients with diarrhea. According to some traditional sources, antagonizes *Shi Hu* (Herba Dendrobii) and *Mang Xiao* (Mirabilitum), counteracts *Bie Jia* (Carapax Amydae Sinensis) and *Xiao Ji* (Herba Cephalanopoloris Segeti), and is incompatible with *Li Lu* (Rhizoma Et Radix Veratri).
C&C: Contains calcium, tannic acid, potassium, and glycosides. Could possibly cause hyperkalemia when used with potassium-sparing diuretics. Could possibly reduce the effect of most antibiotics, cause digitalis intoxication and heart arrhythmias, and could possibly reduce the absorption and therapeutic effect of levadopa, isoniazid, chlorpromazine, calcium carbonate and gluconate, atropine, ephedrine, quinine, reserpine, vitamin B$_1$, trypsine, amylase, and pepsin. Vitamin C, nicotinic acid, glutamic acid, hydrochloric acid, and other highly acidic substances could possibly reduce the therapeutic effect of this medicinal.

Dan Pi, Mu Dan Pi
(Cortex Radicis Moutan, tree peony root bark)

Standard daily dosage: 6-12g
AH: Not to be used during pregnancy. (This ingredient is commonly used in China during pregnancy to treat heat in the blood and/or blood stasis.)
B&G: Should not be used during pregnancy or in patients with excessive sweating or profuse menstruation. Avoid using with garlic. According to some traditional sources, may counteract the effect of *Tu Si Zi* (Semen Cuscutae Chinensis), *Bei Mu* (Bulbus Fritillariae), and *Da Huang* (Radix Et Rhizoma Rhei).
C&C: Contains tannic acid, potassium, and glycosides. Could possibly cause hyperkalemia when used with potassium-sparing diuretics. Could possibly reduce the absorption and biologic effect of most antibiotics, isoniazid, chlorpromazine, calcium carbonate and gluconate, atropine, ephedrine, quinine, reserpine, digitalis, vitamin B$_1$, trypsine, amylase, and pepsin. Vitamin C, nicotinic acid, glutamic acid, hydrochloric acid, and other highly acidic substances could possibly reduce the therapeutic effect of this medicinal.

COMMENTS

Shui Niu Jiao (Cornu Bubali) and *Chi Shao* (Radix Rubrus Paeoniae Lactiflorae) are commonly substituted for *Xi Jiao* and *Bai Shao* respectively.

Xiang Ru San

(Elsholtzia Powder, a.k.a. Elsholtzia Combination)

Category: Exterior-resolving
Functions: Resolves the exterior and dissipates cold, transforms dampness and harmonizes the middle
Chinese medical indications: Exterior cold with interior dampness contracted in the summer manifesting as aversion to cold with skin that is warm to the touch, no sweating, heaviness of the head, headache, abdominal pain, vomiting, diarrhea, chest oppression, fatigue, slimy, white tongue fur, and a floating pulse
Contraindications: Summerheat conditions
Western medical indications: Upper respiratory infection (especially in the summertime), gastroenteritis, bacillary dysentery, and cholera
Potential formula toxicities & interactions: None listed

POTENTIAL MEDICINAL TOXICITIES & INTERACTIONS:

Xiang Ru
(Herba Elsholtziae Seu Moslae)

Standard daily dosage: 3-9g
AH: Safe when used appropriately
B&G: May cause vomiting if taken in a hot decoction. Adding *Huang Qin* (Radix Scutellariae Baicalensis) and *Huang Lian* (Rhizoma Coptidis Chinensis) reduces this effect.

Bai Bian Dou, Bian Dou
(Semen Dolichoris Lablab, hyacinth beans)

Standard daily dosage: 9-21g
B&G: Contraindicated in patients with intermittent chills and fevers.
C&C: Contains alkaloids. Could possibly reduce the absorption and therapeutic effect of potassium and sodium iodides, sodium bicarbonate, aluminum hydroxide, and magnesium sulfate.

Hou Po, Chuan Po
(Cortex Magnoliae Officinalis)

Standard daily dosage: 3-9g
AH: Do not use during pregnancy. (This medicinal is commonly used in China during pregnancy, especially for the treatment of nausea and vomiting.)

B&G: Use with caution during pregnancy. According to some traditional sources, antagonizes *Ze Xie* (Rhizoma Alismatis Orientalis) and *Han Shui Shi* (Calcitum).

C&C: Contains tannic acid and potassium. Could possibly cause hyperkalemia when used with potassium-sparing diuretics. Could possibly reduce the absorption and biologic effect of most antibiotics, isoniazid, chlorpromazine, calcium carbonate and gluconate, atropine, ephedrine, quinine, reserpine, digitalis, vitamin B_1, trypsine, amylase, and pepsin.

PDR: No health risks or side effects are known in conjunction with the proper administration of designated therapeutic dosages.

XIAO CHAI HU TANG
(Minor Bupleurum Decoction)

Category: Harmonizing

Functions: 1) Harmonizes and resolves the *shao yang* aspect; 2) harmonizes the liver, spleen, stomach, and intestines, clears heat and transforms phlegm

Chinese medical indications: 1) Intermittent fever and chills, dry throat, a bitter or sour taste in the mouth, dizziness, easy anger, chest and rib-side oppression and fullness, possible cough with yellow phlegm, heartburn, nausea and vomiting, reduced appetite, half white and half yellow tongue fur, and a bowstring, possibly rapid and/or slippery pulse; 2) fatigue, easy anger, burping/belching, nausea and vomiting, diarrhea, heartburn, a possible bitter taste in the mouth, white or yellow tongue fur, and a bowstring, possibly slippery and/or rapid pulse

Contraindications: Repletion above and vacuity below, ascendant liver yang hyperactivity, and liver fire flaming upward

Western medical indications: Common cold with lingering fever, acute and chronic bronchitis, pleuritis, pneumonia, pulmonary tuberculosis, sinusitis, malaria, acute or chronic viral hepatitis, cholecystitis, jaundice, otitis media, mumps, mastitis, puerperal fever, gastric ulcer, stomach ache, lymphadenitis, and tonsillitis

Potential formula toxicities & interactions:

B&B: If taken long-term, could possibly cause headache, dizziness, and bleeding of the gums in some patients. Use with caution in patients with hypertension. Some patients may experience fever and chills due to the out-thrusting action of this formula.

POTENTIAL MEDICINAL TOXICITIES & INTERACTIONS:

Chai Hu
(Radix Bupleuri)

Standard daily dosage: 3-12g

AH: Safe when used appropriately

B&G: May occasionally cause nausea and vomiting, in which case the dose should then be reduced significantly.

C&C: Vitamin C, nicotinic acid, glutamic acid, hydrochloric acid, and other highly acidic substances could possibly reduce the therapeutic effect of this medicinal.

PDR: Not to be administered during pregnancy. (This medicinal is routinely used in Chinese medical gynecology during pregnancy as part of formulas appropriately prescribed on the basis of pattern discrimination.) Overdose may lead to gastroenteritis, intestinal colic, and diarrhea due to saponin content.

Huang Qin, Tiao Qin
(Radix Scutellariae Baicalensis)

Standard daily dosage: 6-15g
AH: Safe when used appropriately
B&G: According to some traditional sources, counteracts *Dan Pi* (Cortex Radicis Moutan) and *Li Lu* (Rhizoma Et Radix Veratri).
C&C: Contains potassium and glycosides. Could possibly cause hyperkalemia when used with potassium-sparing diuretics. Vitamin C, nicotinic acid, glutamic acid, hydrochloric acid, and other highly acidic substances could possibly reduce the therapeutic effect of this medicinal.

Ren Shen
(Radix Panacis Ginseng, ginseng)

Standard daily dosage: 1-30g
AH: Contraindicated in hypertension
BR: May cause manic episodes in patients on MAO-inhibitors. May cause hypertension if consumed with caffeine. Possible additive effects to insulin. May reduce the anticoagulative effect of warfarin (Coumadin).
B&G: Contraindicated for hypertensive patients. Overdose can lead to headache, insomnia, heart palpitations, and a rise in blood pressure. A traditional antidote is mung bean soup.
C&C: Vitamin C, nicotinic acid, glutamic acid, hydrochloric acid, and other highly acidic substances could possibly reduce the therapeutic effect of this medicinal.
PDR: Contraindicated in patients with hypertension. Not recommended in large doses during pregnancy or lactation due to potential neonatal androgenization. Enhances the effect of insulin and other antidiabetic agents. Use with MAO-inhibitors may cause headaches, tremors, and manias.

Ban Xia
(Rhizoma Pinelliae Ternatae)

Standard daily dosage: 4.5-12g
AH: Do not use during pregnancy. (This medicinal is routinely used during pregnancy in China when indicated by disease and pattern discrimination.) Contraindicated in all hemorrhagic disorders.
B&G: Safe as long as it is properly prepared. Must be decocted with other herbs and not taken alone or uncooked. Toxic effects due to improper preparation or dosage include burning and numbness in throat and lips,

nausea, and a feeling of pressure in the chest. Antidote is oral administration of raw ginger. Use with caution in patients with fever. According to some traditional sources, incompatible with *Wu Tou* (Radix Aconiti).
C&C: Contains alkaloids and glycosides. Could possibly reduce the absorption and therapeutic effect of potassium and sodium iodides, sodium bicarbonate, aluminum hydroxide, and magnesium sulfate. Vitamin C, nicotinic acid, glutamic acid, hydrochloric acid, and other highly acidic substances could possibly reduce the therapeutic effect of this medicinal.
GLW: Poisoning occurs within 15 minutes to three hours after ingestion of a suitable amount. Initially, there is burning pain in the mouth, tongue, and throat, and enlargement of the tongue. This is then followed by drooling, ulceration of the oral mucosa, unclear speech, difficulty swallowing, dizziness, low-grade fever, heart palpitations, numbness of the extremities, a somber white facial complexion, and a weak, forceless pulse. If severe, there may be convulsions and respiratory failure leading to death.

Gan Cao
(Radix Glycyrrhizae Uralensis, licorice root)

Standard daily dosage: 2-12g
AH: Do not use during pregnancy. (This medicinal is routinely used in Chinese medical gynecology during pregnancy as part of formulas appropriately prescribed on the basis of pattern discrimination.) As a single herb in high doses, it is contraindicated in diabetes, hypertension, and liver disorders. Not for long-term use.
BR: May increase toxicity of cardiac glycosides. May increase potassium loss due to diuretics and laxatives. Possible additive effect to corticosteroids. May be synergistic with insulin in causing hypokalemia and sodium retention.
B&G: According to some traditional sources, incompatible with *Gan Sui* (Radix Euphorbiae Kansui), *Yuan Hua* (Flos Daphnes Genkwae), and *Yuan Zhi* (Radix Polygalae Tenuifoliae). If taken long-term, it may cause hypertension and/or edema. Contains glycyrrhetinic acid which could possibly cause a reduction in thyroid activity and basal metabolic rate.

The research on *Gan Cao* concurs that this medicinal is generally safe when used in small amounts as an envoy. It should not be taken long-term or as a single herb during pregnancy. When used as a single medicinal or in patients taking other potent Western pharmaceuticals, caution should be exercised to guard against potential toxicity and drug interaction.

Sheng Jiang
(uncooked Rhizoma Zingiberis Officinalis, fresh ginger)

Standard daily dose: 3-9g

AH: Safe when used appropriately
BR: Reduces vomiting caused by chemotherapeutic drugs. Increases absorption of oral drugs.
PDR: Recommended safe dosage limit is six grams (6g). Avoid larger doses if being used to treat morning sickness or if used in patients taking anticoagulants.

Da Zao, Hong Zao
(Fructus Zizyphi Jujubae, red dates)

Standard daily dosage: 10-30g (3-12 pieces)
AH: Safe when used appropriately
PDR: No health risks or side effects are known in conjunction with the proper administration of designated therapeutic dosages.

COMMENTS

This is one of the most commonly prescribed Chinese medicinal formulas in Chinese medicine. It's scope of indication goes far beyond harmonizing the shao yang. It can be used in any situation where there is a liver-spleen disharmony with heat, dampness, and/or phlegm. Commonly, *Dang Shen* (Radix Codonopsitis Pilosulae) is substituted for *Ren Shen* (Radix Panacis Ginseng), and the form of *Gan Cao* (Radix Glycyrrhizae Uralensis) used is typically mix-fried.

XIAO QING LONG TANG
(Minor Blue-green Dragon Decoction, a.k.a. Minor Blue Dragon Combination)

Category: Exterior-resolving
Functions: Resolves the exterior and transforms fluids, warms the lungs and downbears counterflow
Chinese medical indications: Wind cold external contraction in a person with enduring lung-spleen vacuity and internal gathering of water fluids with fever and chills, although chills predominate, no sweating, coughing, panting and wheezing, profuse, white phlegm, chest oppression, generalized bodily heaviness and body aches, possible superficial edema and/or difficulty breathing lying down, moist, white tongue fur, and a floating, tight or bowstring pulse
Contraindications: Heat and/or yin vacuity
Western medical indications: Common cold, acute bronchitis, bronchial asthma, and influenza
Potential formula toxicities & interactions:
B&B: Should not be used long-term. Use with caution in hypertensive patients.

POTENTIAL MEDICINAL TOXICITIES & INTERACTIONS:

Ma Huang
(Herba Ephedrae, ephedra)

Standard daily dosage: 3-9g
AH: Not to be used during pregnancy. Contraindicated in anorexia, bulimia, and glaucoma. Not for long-term use.
BR: Increases thermogenesis when combined with methylxanthines in theophylline and caffeine. May induce toxicity with MAO-inhibitors. May reduce the effect of dexamethazone. Amytriptiline blocks its hypertensive effect. Antagonized by reserpine.
B&G: May raise blood pressure and cause tremors. As little as 15ml in a 1% solution may be toxic to some individuals. May cause arrhythmias if used in conjunction with cardiac glycosides. Antidote for poisoning is atropine.

All research sources concur that *Ma Huang* is a very powerful herb with many potential side effects and interactions and, therefore, must be administered with care. It enhances digitalis, antagonizes barbiturates,

and increases the effects of adrenergic agonists. It should only be prescribed by a properly trained practitioner and should not be given long-
term or during pregnancy.

GLW: Initially after poisoning, there are central nervous and sympathetic nervous system symptoms, such as vexation, agitation, and restlessness, extreme nerve reactivity, headache, dizziness, tinnitus, insomnia,
nausea, vomiting, upper abdominal discomfort, dry mouth, sweating,
increased blood pressure, dilated pupils, heart palpitations, shortness of
breath, and precordial pain. Graver reactions include difficulty urinating,
unclear vision, shock, syncope, difficulty breathing, fright reversal. If
critical, there may be respiratory failure and death.

The U.S. FDA has banned the inclusion of this medicinal in all dietary
supplements.

Gui Zhi
(Ramulus Cinnamomi Cassiae, cinnamon twigs)

Standard daily dosage: 3-15g
AH: Safe when used appropriately
B&G: Use with caution in the presence of fever, during pregnancy, or
during excessive menstruation.
PDR: Contraindicated during pregnancy.

Gan Jiang
(dry Rhizoma Zingiberis Officinalis, dry ginger)

Standard daily dosage: 3-12g
AH: Not to be used during pregnancy. Patients with gallstones should
consult a practitioner prior to use.
B&G: Use with caution during pregnancy.

Xi Xin
(Herba Asari Cum Radice)

Standard daily dosage: 1-3g
AH: Do not use during pregnancy. Contains aristolochic acid (AA). Do
not exceed recommended dose.
B&G: Nephrotoxic. Use with caution in patients with renal problems.
According to some traditional sources, may antagonize *Shan Zhu Yu*
(Fructus Corni Officinalis) and *Huang Qi* (Radix Astragali
Membranacei).
PDR: Not to be used during pregnancy.

GLW: Symptoms of adverse reaction include headache, vomiting, vexation and agitation, sweating, stiffness of the neck, oral thirst, a rapid pulse, increased body temperature and blood pressure, slightly dilated pupils, a red flushed face, twitching muscles, generalized tension which may become convulsions, clenched teeth, arched-back rigidity, unclear thinking, cramping of the four limbs, dimming of consciousness, urinary block, and, eventually, death due to respiratory paralysis.

Xi Xin is on the FDA's "B List" of herbs which may potentially contain aristolochic acid (AA). *Xi Xin* is harvested in China mostly from *Asarum sieboldi* and *Asarum heteropoides*, neither of which have conclusively been shown to contain AA. However, other species of *Asarum* are sometimes substituted, and these may contain AA. As of this writing, the FDA has set no acceptable limit to AA consumption by humans.

Wu Wei Zi
(Fructus Schisandrae Chinensis, schisandra)

Standard daily dosage: 1.5-9g
AH: Safe when used appropriately
B&G: Occasionally causes heartburn. In mice, toxic doses were 10-15g/kg. Symptoms of overdose included restlessness, insomnia, or dyspnea.
C&C: Contains potassium. Highly acidic. Could possibly cause crystalluria and hematuria. Could possibly cause hyperkalemia when used in large doses with potassium-sparing diuretics. Could possibly reduce the therapeutic effect of sodium bicarbonate, aluminum hydroxide, many antibiotics (especially aminoglycosides and sulfas), reserpine, caffeine, opiates, scopolamine, and berbamin.
PDR: No health risks or side effects are known in conjunction with the proper administration of designated therapeutic dosages.

Bai Shao, Shao Yao
(Radix Albus Paeoniae Lactiflorae, white peony root)

Standard daily dosage: 6-30g
AH: Safe when used appropriately
B&G: Use with caution in debilitated patients with diarrhea. According to some traditional sources, antagonizes *Shi Hu* (Herba Dendrobii) and *Mang Xiao* (Mirabilitum), counteracts *Bie Jia* (Carapax Amydae Sinensis) and *Xiao Ji* (Herba Cephalanopoloris Segeti), and is incompatible with *Li Lu* (Rhizoma Et Radix Veratri).
C&C: Contains calcium, tannic acid, potassium, and glycosides. Could possibly cause hyperkalemia when used with potassium-sparing diuret-

ics. Could possibly reduce the effect of most antibiotics, cause digitalis intoxication and heart arrhythmias, and Could possibly reduce the absorption and therapeutic effect of levadopa, isoniazid, chlorpromazine, calcium carbonate and gluconate, atropine, ephedrine, quinine, reserpine, vitamin B₁, trypsine, amylase, and pepsin. Vitamin C, nicotinic acid, glutamic acid, hydrochloric acid, and other highly acidic substances could possibly reduce the therapeutic effect of this medicinal.

Ban Xia
(Rhizoma Pinelliae Ternatae)

Standard daily dosage: 4.5-12g

AH: Do not use during pregnancy. (This medicinal is routinely used during pregnancy in China when indicated by disease and pattern discrimination.) Contraindicated in all hemorrhagic disorders.

B&G: Safe as long as it is properly prepared. Must be decocted with other herbs and not taken alone or uncooked. Toxic effects due to improper preparation or dosage include burning and numbness in throat and lips, nausea, and a feeling of pressure in the chest. Antidote is oral administration of raw ginger. Use with caution in patients with fever. According to some traditional sources, incompatible with *Wu Tou* (Radix Aconiti).

C&C: Contains alkaloids and glycosides. Could possibly reduce the absorption and therapeutic effect of potassium and sodium iodides, sodium bicarbonate, aluminum hydroxide, and magnesium sulfate. Vitamin C, nicotinic acid, glutamic acid, hydrochloric acid, and other highly acidic substances could possibly reduce the therapeutic effect of this medicinal.

GLW: Poisoning occurs within 15 minutes to three hours after ingestion of a suitable amount. Initially, there is burning pain in the mouth, tongue, and throat, and enlargement of the tongue. This is then followed by drooling, ulceration of the oral mucosa, unclear speech, difficulty swallowing, dizziness, low-grade fever, heart palpitations, numbness of the extremities, a somber white facial complexion, and a weak, forceless pulse. If severe, there may be convulsions and respiratory failure leading to death.

Gan Cao
(Radix Glycyrrhizae Uralensis, licorice root)

Standard daily dosage: 2-12g

AH: Do not use during pregnancy. (This medicinal is routinely used in Chinese medical gynecology during pregnancy as part of formulas appropriately prescribed on the basis of pattern discrimination.) As a single herb in high doses, it is contraindicated in diabetes, hypertension, and liver disorders. Not for long-term use.

BR: May increase toxicity of cardiac glycosides. May increase potassi-

um loss due to diuretics and laxatives. Possible additive effect to corticosteroids. May be synergistic with insulin in causing hypokalemia and
sodium retention.

B&G: According to some traditional sources, incompatible with *Gan Sui*
(Radix Euphorbiae Kansui), *Yuan Hua* (Flos Daphnes Genkwae), and
Yuan Zhi (Radix Polygalae Tenuifoliae). If taken long-term, it may cause
hypertension and/or edema. Contains glycyrrhetinic acid which could
possibly cause a reduction in thyroid activity and basal metabolic rate.

The research on *Gan Cao* concurs that this medicinal is generally safe
when used in small amounts as an envoy. It should not be taken long-term
or as a single herb during pregnancy. When used as a single medicinal or
in patients taking other potent Western pharmaceuticals, caution should be
exercised to guard against potential toxicity and drug interaction.

XIAO YAO SAN
(Rambling Powder, a.k.a. Bupleurum & Tang-kuei Formula)

Category: Harmonizing
Functions: Courses the liver and resolves depression, fortifies the spleen and harmonizes the constructive
Chinese medical indications: Liver-spleen disharmony complicated by blood vacuity and possible dampness with chest, breast, abdominal, and/or rib-side distention and pain, headache, dizziness, fatigue, reduced appetite, menstrual irregularities, a pale red tongue, and a bowstring pulse
Contraindications: None listed
Western medical indications: Depression, irregular menstruation, uterine bleeding, abnormal vaginal discharge, breast distention, premenstrual tension, climacteric disorders, chronic hepatitis, pleurisy, chronic gastritis, peptic ulcer, neurosis, anemia, insomnia, optic nerve atrophy, central retinitis
Potential formula toxicities & interactions: None listed

POTENTIAL MEDICINAL TOXICITIES & INTERACTIONS:

Chai Hu
(Radix Bupleuri)

Standard daily dosage: 3-12g
AH: Safe when used appropriately
B&G: May occasionally cause nausea and vomiting, in which case the dose should then be reduced significantly.
C&C: Vitamin C, nicotinic acid, glutamic acid, hydrochloric acid, and other highly acidic substances could possibly reduce the therapeutic effect of this medicinal.
PDR: Not to be administered during pregnancy. (This medicinal is routinely used in Chinese medical gynecology during pregnancy as part of formulas appropriately prescribed on the basis of pattern discrimination.) Overdose may lead to gastroenteritis, intestinal colic, and diarrhea due to saponin content.

Dang Gui
(Radix Angelicae Sinensis)

Standard daily dosage: 3-15g
AH: Do not use during pregnancy. (This medicinal is routinely used in Chinese medical gynecology during pregnancy as part of formulas appropriately prescribed on the basis of pattern discrimination.)

B&G: Use with caution in patients with diarrhea or abdominal distention.
C&C: Contains potassium. Could possibly cause hyperkalemia when used with potassium-sparing diuretics. May exaggerate the anticoagulative effect of warfarin (Coumadin).

Bai Shao, Shao Yao
(Radix Albus Paeoniae Lactiflorae, white peony root)

Standard daily dosage: 6-30g
AH: Safe when used appropriately
B&G: Use with caution in debilitated patients with diarrhea. According to some traditional sources, antagonizes *Shi Hu* (Herba Dendrobii) and *Mang Xiao* (Mirabilitum), counteracts *Bie Jia* (Carapax Amydae Sinensis) and *Xiao Ji* (Herba Cephalanopoloris Segeti), and is incompatible with *Li Lu* (Rhizoma Et Radix Veratri).
C&C: Contains calcium, tannic acid, potassium, and glycosides. Could possibly cause hyperkalemia when used with potassium-sparing diuretics. Could possibly reduce the effect of most antibiotics, cause digitalis intoxication and heart arrhythmias, and could possibly reduce the absorption and therapeutic effect of levadopa, isoniazid, chlorpromazine, calcium carbonate and gluconate, atropine, ephedrine, quinine, reserpine, vitamin B_1, trypsine, amylase, and pepsin. Vitamin C, nicotinic acid, glutamic acid, hydrochloric acid, and other highly acidic substances could possibly reduce the therapeutic effect of this medicinal.

Bai Zhu
(Rhizoma Atractylodis Macrocephalae)

Standard daily dosage: 4.5-9g
B&G: When rats were fed 0.5g/kg of this medicinal for two months, they developed a mild lymphopenia and anemia but suffered no damage to the brain, heart, or liver.

Fu Ling, Bai Fu Ling, Yun Ling
(Sclerotium Poriae Cocos)

Standard daily dosage: 9-15g
B&G: Large doses or long-term use is discouraged. Contraindicated in patients with frequent, copious urination. According to traditional sources, may counteract *Di Yu* (Radix Sanguisorbae Officinalis), *Qin Jiao* (Radix Gentianae Qinjiao), and *Bie Jia* (Carapax Amydae Sinensis).
C&C: Contains potassium. Could possibly cause hyperkalemia when used with potassium-sparing diuretics.

Gan Cao
(Radix Glycyrrhizae Uralensis, licorice root)

Standard daily dosage: 2-12g

AH: Do not use during pregnancy. (This medicinal is routinely used in Chinese medical gynecology during pregnancy as part of formulas appropriately prescribed on the basis of pattern discrimination.) As a single herb in high doses, it is contraindicated in diabetes, hypertension, and liver disorders. Not for long-term use.

BR: May increase toxicity of cardiac glycosides. May increase potassium loss due to diuretics and laxatives. Possible additive effect to corticosteroids. May be synergistic with insulin in causing hypokalemia and sodium retention.

B&G: According to some traditional sources, incompatible with *Gan Sui* (Radix Euphorbiae Kansui), *Yuan Hua* (Flos Daphnes Genkwae), and *Yuan Zhi* (Radix Polygalae Tenuifoliae). If taken long-term, it may cause hypertension and/or edema. Contains glycyrrhetinic acid which could possibly cause a reduction in thyroid activity and basal metabolic rate.

The research on *Gan Cao* concurs that this medicinal is generally safe when used in small amounts as an envoy. It should not be taken long-term or as a single herb during pregnancy. When used as a single medicinal or in patients taking other potent Western pharmaceuticals, caution should be exercised to guard against potential toxicity and drug interaction.

Bo He
(Herba Menthae Haplocalycis, field mint)

Standard daily dose: 1.5-6g

AH: Safe when used appropriately

B&G: Not recommended for nursing mothers as it may inhibit lactation.

Sheng Jiang
(uncooked Rhizoma Zingiberis Officinalis, fresh ginger)

Standard daily dose: 3-9g

AH: Safe when used appropriately

BR: Reduces vomiting caused by chemotherapeutic drugs. Increases absorption of oral drugs.

PDR: Recommended safe dosage limit is six grams (6g). Avoid larger doses if being used to treat morning sickness or if used in patients taking anticoagulants.

COMMENTS

When *Dan Pi* (Cortex Radicis Moutan) and *Zhi Zi* (Fructus Gardeniae Jasminoidis) are added to this formula, it is called either *Jia Wei Xiao Yao San* (Added Flavors Rambling Powder) or *Dan Zhi Xiao Yao San* (Moutan & Gardenia Rambling Powder). This modification treats a liver-spleen disharmony with depressive heat, especially depressive heat causing the blood to move frenetically outside its vessels. Most of the time, the form of *Gan Cao* (Radix Glycyrrhizae Uralensis) used in this formula is mix-fried.

Xing Su San
(Armeniaca & Perilla Powder, a.k.a. Apricot Seed & Perilla
Formula)

Category: Dryness-treating
Functions: Gently diffuses and cools dryness, diffuses the lungs
and transforms phlegm
Chinese medical indications: Externally contracted cool dryness with slight headache, chills but no sweating, cough with
watery phlegm, nasal congestion, dry throat, dry, white tongue
fur, and a floating bowstring pulse
Contraindications: None listed
Western medical indications: Common cold, chronic tracheitis,
acute and chronic bronchitis, bronchiectasis, and pulmonary edema
Potential formula toxicities & interactions: None listed

Potential Medicinal Toxicities & Interactions:

Zi Su Ye, Zi Su, Su Ye
(Folium Perillae Frutescentis, beefsteak leaves)

Standard daily dosage: 3-9g
PDR: Use during pregnancy is contraindicated because perillaldehyde
was demonstrated to have a mutagenic effect in some in vitro studies.
Studies showed that large doses can trigger pulmonary edema.

Qian Hu
(Radix Peucedani)

Standard daily dosage: 4.5-9g
B&G: According to traditional sources, may counteract *Li Lu* (Rhizoma
Et Radix Veratri).
C&C: Contains tannic acid. Could possibly reduce the absorption and
biologic effect of most antibiotics, isoniazid, chlorpromazine, calcium
carbonate and gluconate, atropine, ephedrine, quinine, reserpine, digitalis, vitamin B_1, trypsine, amylase, and pepsin.

Xing Ren, Ku Xing Ren
(Semen Pruni Armeniacae, apricot kernel)

Standard daily dosage: 3-9g

AH: To be used only under the supervision of an expert qualified in the appropriate use of this substance.

B&G: Use with caution when treating infants or patients with diarrhea. Contains amygdalin and amygdalase which break down to hydrocyanic acid in the digestive tract. Lethal dosage in adults is 50-60 uncooked kernels; children 10 kernels. Eating this medicinal uncooked or in large quantities could possibly cause dizziness, nausea, vomiting, and headache, which can progress to dyspnea, spasms, dilated pupils, arrhythmias, and coma. In the advent of overdosage activated charcoal and syrup of ipacec should be administered orally.

C&C: Contains potassium and glycosides (including cyanophoric glycoside). If taken with codeine, morphine, or other opiates, hydrocyanic acid is produced which can lead to respiratory failure and death. Could possibly cause hyperkalemia when used with potassium-sparing diuretics. Vitamin C, nicotinic acid, glutamic acid, hydrochloric acid, and other highly acidic substances will reduce the therapeutic effect of this medicinal.

GLW: In case of poisoning, typically, 1-2 hours after ingestion there is a bitter taste and astringent feeling within the mouth, drooling, headache, dizziness, nausea, vomiting accompanied by watery diarrhea, heart palpitations, and lack of strength. In more serious cases, there is difficulty breathing. Sometimes one can smell cyanide on the person's breath. Eventually, breathing becomes weak, consciousness becomes unclear, and the pupils of the eye dilate widely with loss of reactivity to light. The teeth become clenched, blood pressure drops, there are generalized convulsions, and respiratory paralysis leads to death.

The maximum concentration of toxins in this medicinal are in the skin and the tip. When used in Chinese medicine, the kernels are blanched to remove the skin and the tips are broken off.

Jie Geng
(Radix Platycodi Grandiflori, bellflower root)

Standard daily dosage: 3-9g

AH: Not to be used during pregnancy. As a single herb in high doses, it is contraindicated in diabetes, hypertension, and liver disorders. Not for long-term use.

B&G: Contraindicated in patients with hemoptysis. According to some traditional sources, counteracts *Long Dan Cao* (Radix Gentianae Longdancao) and *Long Yan Rou* (Arillus Euphoriae Longanae).

C&C: Contains calcium and glycosides. Could possibly reduce the effect of most antibiotics, cause digitalis intoxication and heart arrhythmias, hinder the absorption of isoniazid, and reduce the biological effect of levadopa. Vitamin C, nicotinic acid, glutamic acid, hydrochloric acid, and other highly acidic substances could possibly reduce the therapeutic effect of this medicinal.

Zhi Ke, Zhi Qiao
(Fructus Citri Aurantii, bitter orange)

Standard daily dose: 3-9g
AH: Safe when used appropriately
B&G: Use with caution during pregnancy
C&C: Contains tannic acid. Highly acidic. Could possibly cause crystalluria and hematuria. Could possibly reduce the absorption and biologic effect of most antibiotics, isoniazid, chlorpromazine, calcium carbonate and gluconate, atropine, ephedrine, quinine, reserpine, digitalis, vitamin B1, trypsine, amylase, and pepsin, sodium bicarbonate, aluminum hydroxide, caffeine, opiates, scopolamine, and berbamin.
PDR: May cause UV-sensitivity in light-skinned individuals. Otherwise no health hazards are known in conjunction with the proper administration of designated therapeutic dosages.

Chen Pi, Ju Pi, Ju Hong
(Pericarpium Citri Reticulatae, tangerine peel)

Standard daily dosage: 3-9g
AH: Safe when used appropriately
C&C: Contains potassium. Could possibly cause hyperkalemia when used with potassium-sparing diuretics.

Fu Ling, Bai Fu Ling, Yun Ling
(Sclerotium Poriae Cocos)

Standard daily dosage: 9-15g
B&G: Large doses or long-term use is discouraged. Contraindicated in patients with frequent, copious urination. According to traditional sources, may counteract *Di Yu* (Radix Sanguisorbae Officinalis), *Qin Jiao* (Radix Gentianae Qinjiao), and *Bie Jia* (Carapax Amydae Sinensis).
C&C: Contains potassium. Could possibly cause hyperkalemia when used with potassium-sparing diuretics.

Ban Xia
(Rhizoma Pinelliae Ternatae)

Standard daily dosage: 4.5-12g

AH: Do not use during pregnancy. (This medicinal is routinely used during pregnancy in China when indicated by disease and pattern discrimination.) Contraindicated in all hemorrhagic disorders.

B&G: Safe as long as it is properly prepared. Must be decocted with other herbs and not taken alone or uncooked. Toxic effects due to improper preparation or dosage include burning and numbness in throat and lips, nausea, and a feeling of pressure in the chest. Antidote is oral administration of raw ginger. Use with caution in patients with fever. According to some traditional sources, incompatible with *Wu Tou* (Radix Aconiti).

C&C: Contains alkaloids and glycosides. Could possibly reduce the absorption and therapeutic effect of potassium and sodium iodides, sodium bicarbonate, aluminum hydroxide, and magnesium sulfate. Vitamin C, nicotinic acid, glutamic acid, hydrochloric acid, and other highly acidic substances could possibly reduce the therapeutic effect of this medicinal.

GLW: Poisoning occurs within 15 minutes to three hours after ingestion of a suitable amount. Initially, there is burning pain in the mouth, tongue, and throat, and enlargement of the tongue. This is then followed by drooling, ulceration of the oral mucosa, unclear speech, difficulty swallowing, dizziness, low-grade fever, heart palpitations, numbness of the extremities, a somber white facial complexion, and a weak, forceless pulse. If severe, there may be convulsions and respiratory failure leading to death.

Sheng Jiang
(uncooked Rhizoma Zingiberis Officinalis, fresh ginger)

Standard daily dose: 3-9g
AH: Safe when used appropriately
BR: Reduces vomiting caused by chemotherapeutic drugs. Increases absorption of oral drugs.
PDR: Recommended safe dosage limit is six grams (6g). Avoid larger doses if being used to treat morning sickness or if used in patients taking anticoagulants.

Da Zao, Hong Zao
(Fructus Zizyphi Jujubae, red dates)

Standard daily dosage: 10-30g (3-12 pieces)
AH: Safe when used appropriately
PDR: No health risks or side effects are known in conjunction with the proper administration of designated therapeutic dosages.

Gan Cao
(Radix Glycyrrhizae Uralensis, licorice root)

Standard daily dosage: 2-12g

AH: Do not use during pregnancy. (This medicinal is routinely used in Chinese medical gynecology during pregnancy as part of formulas appropriately prescribed on the basis of pattern discrimination.) As a single herb in high doses, it is contraindicated in diabetes, hypertension, and liver disorders. Not for long-term use.

BR: May increase toxicity of cardiac glycosides. May increase potassium loss due to diuretics and laxatives. Possible additive effect to corticosteroids. May be synergistic with insulin in causing hypokalemia and sodium retention.

B&G: According to some traditional sources, incompatible with *Gan Sui* (Radix Euphorbiae Kansui), *Yuan Hua* (Flos Daphnes Genkwae), and *Yuan Zhi* (Radix Polygalae Tenuifoliae). If taken long-term, it may cause hypertension and/or edema. Contains glycyrrhetinic acid which could possibly cause a reduction in thyroid activity and basal metabolic rate.

The research on *Gan Cao* concurs that this medicinal is generally safe when used in small amounts as an envoy. It should not be taken long-term or as a single herb during pregnancy. When used as a single medicinal or in patients taking other potent Western pharmaceuticals, caution should be exercised to guard against potential toxicity and drug interaction.

XUE FU ZHU YU TANG
(Blood Mansion Dispel Stasis Decoction)

Category: Blood-quickening
Functions: Quickens the blood and dispels stasis, moves the qi and stops pain
Chinese medical indications: Blood stasis in the chest with pain in the chest and rib-side, enduring, recalcitrant headache with fixed, piercing pain, enduring, incessant hiccup, a choking sensation when drinking, dry heaves, depression accompanied by vexatious heat in the chest, heart palpitations, insomnia, easy anger, evening tidal fever, purple lips, a sooty facial complexion, a dark red or purple tongue or possible static macules or speckles, and a bowstring, tight, deep, choppy, or intermittent pulse
Contraindications: Bleeding conditions or pregnancy
Western medical indications: Coronary artery disease, angina pectoris, cor pulmonale, rheumatic heart disease, intercostal neuralgia, costochondritis, functional neurosis, postconcussion syndrome, migraine, trigeminal neuralgia, external injury to chest, irregular menstruation, dysmenorrhea, menopausal syndrome, cerebral hemorrhage, and urticaria
Potential formula toxicities & interactions: None listed

POTENTIAL MEDICINAL TOXICITIES & INTERACTIONS:

Tao Ren
(Semen Pruni Persicae, peach kernel)

Standard daily dosage: 4.5-9g
AH: Not to be used during pregnancy.
B&G: Contraindicated during pregnancy.
C&C: Contains potassium and glycosides (including cyanophoric glycosides). If taken with codeine, morphine, or other opiates, hydrocyanic acid is produced which can lead to respiratory failure and death. Could possibly cause hyperkalemia when used with potassium-sparing diuretics. Vitamin C, nicotinic acid, glutamic acid, hydrochloric acid, and other highly acidic substances could possibly reduce the therapeutic effect of this medicinal.
GLW: In case of poisoning, typically, 1-2 hours after ingestion there is a bitter taste and astringent feeling within the mouth, drooling, headache, dizziness, nausea, vomiting accompanied by watery diarrhea, heart palpitations, and lack of strength. In more serious cases, there is difficulty breathing. Sometimes one can smell cyanide on the person's breath.

Eventually, breathing becomes weak, consciousness becomes unclear, and the pupils of the eye dilate widely with loss of reactivity to light. The teeth become clenched, blood pressure drops, there are generalized convulsions, and respiratory paralysis leads to death.

Most of the toxins in this medicinal reside in the skin and tip. Therefore, this medicinal is blanched before using and its tip is broken off in order to make it less or non-toxic.

Hong Hua
(Flos Carthami Tinctorii, safflower flowers)

Standard daily dosage: 3-9g
AH: Not to be used during pregnancy. Contraindicated in hemorrhagic diseases or patients with peptic ulcers.
B&G: Contraindicated during pregnancy. In several studies, animals fed the medicinal often experienced weight loss.
C&C: Contains potassium and glycosides. Could possibly cause hyperkalemia when used with potassium-sparing diuretics. Vitamin C, nicotinic acid, glutamic acid, hydrochloric acid, and other highly acidic substances could possibly reduce the therapeutic effect of this medicinal.
PDR: Not for use during pregnancy.

Dang Gui
(Radix Angelicae Sinensis)

Standard daily dosage: 3-15g
AH: Do not use during pregnancy. (This medicinal is routinely used in Chinese medical gynecology during pregnancy as part of formulas appropriately prescribed on the basis of pattern discrimination.)
B&G: Use with caution in patients with diarrhea or abdominal distention.
C&C: Contains potassium. Could possibly cause hyperkalemia when used with potassium-sparing diuretics. May exaggerate the anticoagulative effect of warfarin (Coumadin).

Chuan Xiong
(Radix Ligustici Wallichii)

Standard daily dosage: 3-9g (In China today, it is not uncommon for this medicinal to be prescribed up to 15 grams per day in decoction.)
AH: Do not use during pregnancy. (This medicinal is routinely used in Chinese medical gynecology during pregnancy as part of formulas appropriately prescribed on the basis of pattern discrimination.)
B&G: Not for patients with migraine headache or excessive menstrual bleeding. Overdosage causes vomiting and dizziness. According to some

traditional texts, antagonizes *Shan Zhu Yu* (Fructus Corni Officinalis) and *Huang Qi* (Radix Astragali Membranacei), counteracts *Hua Shi* (Talcum) and *Huang Lian* (Rhizoma Coptidis Chinensis), and is incompatible with *Li Lu* (Rhizoma Et Radix Veratri).

C&C: Contains alkaloids and potassium. Could possibly cause hyperkalemia when used with potassium-sparing diuretics. Could possibly reduce the absorption and therapeutic effect of potassium and sodium iodides, sodium bicarbonate, aluminum hydroxide, and magnesium sulfate.

Chi Shao
(Radix Rubrus Paeoniae Lactiflorae, red peony root)

Standard daily dosage: 4.5-9g
C&C: Contains tannic acid, potassium, and glycosides. Could possibly cause hyperkalemia when used with potassium-sparing diuretics. Could possibly reduce the absorption and biologic effect of most antibiotics, isoniazid, chlorpromazine, calcium carbonate and gluconate, atropine, ephedrine, quinine, reserpine, digitalis, vitamin B$_1$, trypsine, amylase, and pepsin. Vitamin C, nicotinic acid, glutamic acid, hydrochloric acid, and other highly acidic substances could possibly reduce the therapeutic effect of this medicinal.

Chuan Niu Xi
(Radix Cyathulae)

Standard daily dosage: 9-15g
AH: Not to be used during pregnancy. Contraindicated in menorrhagia.
B&G: Contraindicated during pregnancy, in debilitated patients with diarrhea, and in patients with excessive menstruation. According to some traditional sources, should not be used with *Bai Qian* (Radix Et Rhizoma Cynanchi Baiqian).
C&C: Contains alkaloids, potassium, and glycosides. Could possibly cause hyperkalemia when used with potassium-sparing diuretics. Could possibly reduce the absorption and therapeutic effect of potassium and sodium iodides, sodium bicarbonate, aluminum hydroxide, and magnesium sulfate. Vitamin C, nicotinic acid, glutamic acid, hydrochloric acid, and other highly acidic substances could possibly reduce the therapeutic effect of this medicinal.

Chai Hu
(Radix Bupleuri)

Standard daily dosage: 3-12g
AH: Safe when used appropriately
B&G: May occasionally cause nausea and vomiting, in which case the dose should then be reduced significantly.

C&C: Vitamin C, nicotinic acid, glutamic acid, hydrochloric acid, and other highly acidic substances could possibly reduce the therapeutic effect of this medicinal.

PDR: Not to be administered during pregnancy. (This medicinal is routinely used in Chinese medical gynecology during pregnancy as part of formulas appropriately prescribed on the basis of pattern discrimination.) Overdose may lead to gastroenteritis, intestinal colic, and diarrhea due to saponin content.

Jie Geng
(Radix Platycodi Grandiflori, bellflower root)

Standard daily dosage: 3-9g

AH: Contraindicated in hemoptysis, especially in cases of tuberculosis. Use with caution in bleeding peptic ulcer.

B&G: Contraindicated in patients with hemoptysis. According to some traditional sources, counteracts *Long Dan Cao* (Gentiana Longdancao) and *Long Yan Rou* (Arillus Euphoriae Longanae).

C&C: Contains calcium and glycosides. Could possibly reduce the effect of most antibiotics, cause digitalis intoxication and heart arrhythmias, hinder the absorption of isoniazid, and reduce the biological effect of levadopa. Vitamin C, nicotinic acid, glutamic acid, hydrochloric acid, and other highly acidic substances could possibly reduce the therapeutic effect of this medicinal.

Zhi Ke, Zhi Qiao
(Fructus Citri Aurantii, bitter orange)

Standard daily dose: 3-9g

AH: Safe when used appropriately

B&G: Use with caution during pregnancy

C&C: Contains tannic acid. Highly acidic. Could possibly cause crystalluria and hematuria. Could possibly reduce the absorption and biologic effect of most antibiotics, isoniazid, chlorpromazine, calcium carbonate and gluconate, atropine, ephedrine, quinine, reserpine, digitalis, vitamin B_1, trypsine, amylase, and pepsin, sodium bicarbonate, aluminum hydroxide, caffeine, opiates, scopolamine, and berbamin.

PDR: May cause UV-sensitivity in light-skinned individuals. Otherwise no health hazards are known in conjunction with the proper administration of designated therapeutic dosages.

Sheng Di, Sheng Di Huang
(uncooked Radix Rehmanniae Glutinosae)

Standard daily dosage: 9-30g

AH: Contraindicated in patients with diarrhea or lack of appetite

B&G: Contraindicated in pregnant women with anemias or digestive weakness

C&C: Contains potassium. Could possibly cause hyperkalemia when used with potassium-sparing diuretics.

PDR: No health risks or side effects are known in conjunction with the proper administration of designated therapeutic dosages.

Gan Cao
(Radix Glycyrrhizae Uralensis, licorice root)

Standard daily dosage: 2-12g

AH: Do not use during pregnancy. (This medicinal is routinely used in Chinese medical gynecology during pregnancy as part of formulas appropriately prescribed on the basis of pattern discrimination.) As a single herb in high doses, it is contraindicated in diabetes, hypertension, and liver disorders. Not for long-term use.

BR: May increase toxicity of cardiac glycosides. May increase potassium loss due to diuretics and laxatives. Possible additive effect to corticosteroids. May be synergistic with insulin in causing hypokalemia and sodium retention.

B&G: According to some traditional sources, incompatible with *Gan Sui* (Radix Euphorbiae Kansui), *Yuan Hua* (Flos Daphnes Genkwae), and *Yuan Zhi* (Radix Polygalae Tenuifoliae). If taken long-term, it may cause hypertension and/or edema. Contains glycyrrhetinic acid which could possibly cause a reduction in thyroid activity and basal metabolic rate.

The research on *Gan Cao* concurs that this medicinal is generally safe when used in small amounts as an envoy. It should not be taken long-term or as a single herb during pregnancy. When used as a single medicinal or in patients taking other potent Western pharmaceuticals, caution should be exercised to guard against potential toxicity and drug interaction.

COMMENTS

Xue Fu Zhu Yu Tang is part of a family of *Zhu Yu Tang* (Dispel Stasis Decoction) formulas created by Wang Qing-ren for the treatment of blood stasis in various parts of the body. In this case, the *xue fu* or blood mansion is the chest. Therefore, this formula is particularly indicated for blood stasis in the chest. However, it has also come to be used for mental-emotional problems due to blood stasis based on the Chinese medical fact that the spirit resides in the heart which is located in the center of the chest.

YI GUAN JIAN
(One Link Brew, a.k.a.
All-The-Way-Through Brew, Linking Decoction)

Category: Yin-supplementing
Functions: Nourishes and enriches the liver and kidneys, courses the liver and rectifies the qi
Chinese medical indications: Liver blood-kidney yin vacuity with liver depression qi stagnation manifesting as chest and rib-side pain, stomach duct distention, dry mouth and parched throat, acid regurgitation, a dry, red tongue, and a fine, bowstring pulse
Contraindications: Pain due to phlegm and/or dampness
Western medical indications: Chronic active hepatitis, cirrhosis, costochondritis, peptic ulcer, essential hypertension, hypertension during pregnancy, Addison's disease, thrombocytopenic purpura, pulmonary tuberculosis, diabetes mellitus, chronic orchiditis, and neurasthenia
Potential formula toxicities & interactions: None listed

POTENTIAL MEDICINAL TOXICITIES & INTERACTIONS:

Sheng Di, Sheng Di Huang
(uncooked Radix Rehmanniae Glutinosae)

Standard daily dosage: 9-30g
AH: Contraindicated in patients with diarrhea or lack of appetite
B&G: Contraindicated in pregnant women with anemias or digestive weakness
C&C: Contains potassium. Could possibly cause hyperkalemia when used with potassium-sparing diuretics.
PDR: No health risks or side effects are known in conjunction with the proper administration of designated therapeutic dosages.

Gou Qi Zi, Qi Zi
(Fructus Lycii Chinensis, lycium berries)

Standard daily dosage: 6-18g
AH: Not to be used during pregnancy. (No such prohibition exists with traditional Chinese medicine regarding this medicinal.)
C&C: Contains tannic acid and potassium. Could possibly cause hyperkalemia when used with potassium-sparing diuretics. Could possibly reduce the absorption and biologic effect of most antibiotics, isoniazid,

chlorpromazine, calcium carbonate and gluconate, atropine, ephedrine, quinine, reserpine, digitalis, vitamin B1, trypsine, amylase, and pepsin.
PDR: Not for use during pregnancy.

Sha Shen
(Radix Glehniae Littoralis)

Standard daily dosage: 9-15g
AH: Safe when used appropriately
B&G: According to some traditional sources, antagonizes *Fang Ji* (Radix Aristolochiae Fangchi) and is incompatible with *Li Lu* (Rhizoma Et Radix Veratri).

Mai Men Dong, Mai Dong
(Tuber Ophiopogoni Japonici)

Standard daily dosage: 6-15g
AH: Safe when used appropriately
B&G: According to some traditional sources, antagonizes *Kuan Dong Hua* (Flos Tussilaginis Farfarae) and counteracts *Ku Shen* (Radix Sophorae Flavescentis) and *Bai Mu Er* (Fructificatio Tremellae Fuciformis).
C&C: Contains glycosides. Vitamin C, nicotinic acid, glutamic acid, hydrochloric acid, and other highly acidic substances could possibly reduce the therapeutic effect of this medicinal.

Dang Gui
(Radix Angelicae Sinensis)

Standard daily dosage: 3-15g
AH: Do not use during pregnancy. (This medicinal is routinely used in Chinese medical gynecology during pregnancy as part of formulas appropriately prescribed on the basis of pattern discrimination.)
B&G: Use with caution in patients with diarrhea or abdominal distention.
C&C: Contains potassium. Could possibly cause hyperkalemia when used with potassium-sparing diuretics. May exaggerate the anticoagulative effect of warfarin (Coumadin).

Chuan Lian Zi, Jin Ling Zi
(Fructus Meliae Toosendan)

Standard daily dosage: 3-9g
AH: Safe when used appropriately
GLW: Symptoms of adverse reaction include abdominal distention, abdominal pain, vomiting, diarrhea, poor appetite, dizziness, headache, a

red facial complexion, blurred vision, inhibited speech, uneasy respiration, epistaxis, hemorrhage of the liver, kidney, and/or intestines, mania and agitation, convulsions, numbness of the four extremities, heart arrhythmia, shrunken pupils. Poisoning can lead to toxic hepatitis and red blood cells in the urine. In grave conditions, there may be atrial fibrillation, frequent premature beats, and atrioventricular conduction block, low blood pressure, syncope, shock, and even death.

YIN CHEN HAO TANG
(Artemisia Yinchenhao Decoction, a.k.a. Capillaris Combination)

Category: Dampness-dispelling
Functions: Clears heat, disinhibits dampness, and recedes yellowing (*i.e.*, jaundice)
Chinese medical indications: Liver-gallbladder damp heat jaundice with abdominal distention, difficult urination, thirst but the ability to only take sips, a bitter taste in the mouth, slimy, yellow tongue fur, and a slippery, rapid, possibly bowstring pulse
Contraindications: Yang jaundice
Western medical indications: Acute hepatitis, hepatic necrosis, cirrhosis, cholecystitis, cholelithiasis, favism, malarial diseases, typhoid fever, leukemia, leptospirosis, nephritis, edema, beriberi, stomatitis, urticaria, pruritis, gingivitis, eye diseases, and uterine bleeding
Potential formula toxicities & interactions:
FL/B&B: Use with caution during pregnancy due to the inclusion of *Da Huang* (Radix Et Rhizoma Rhei).

POTENTIAL MEDICINAL TOXICITIES & INTERACTIONS:

Yin Chen Hao
(Herba Artemisiae Yinchenhao)

Standard daily dosage: 9-30g
AH: Not to be used during pregnancy.
B&G: One study showed that using this medicinal along with *Da Zao* (Fructus Zizyphi Jujubae) to treat infectious hepatitis caused heart block in two patients.
C&C: Contains potassium. Could possibly cause hyperkalemia when used with potassium-sparing diuretics.

Zhi Zi, Shan Zhi, Shan Zhi Zi
(Fructus Gardeniae Jasminoidis, dried gardenia fruit pods)

Standard daily dosage: 3-12g
AH: Safe when used appropriately
B&G: Contains geniposide which caused diarrhea in mice.
C&C: Contains potassium and glycosides. Could possibly cause hyper-

kalemia when used with potassium-sparing diuretics. Vitamin C, nicotinic acid, glutamic acid, hydrochloric acid, and other highly acidic substances could possibly reduce the therapeutic effect of this medicinal.

Da Huang, Dai Huang, Chuan Jun, Jun
(Radix Et Rhizoma Rhei, rhubarb root)

Standard daily dosage: 3-12g
AH: Do not use during pregnancy. Not to be used while nursing.
Contraindicated in intestinal obstruction, abdominal pain of unknown
origin, or any inflammatory condition of the intestines.
BR: Reduces absorption of oral drugs. Overuse may cause hypokalemia
and increased toxicity of cardiac glycosides. May aggravate potassium
loss from diuretics.
B&G: Use with extreme caution during pregnancy, menstruation, or
postpartum. Contraindicated for nursing mothers since active ingredients
enter the milk.
C&C: Contains alkaloids, tannic acid, potassium, and glycosides. Could
possibly cause hyperkalemia when used with potassium-sparing diuretics. Vitamin C, nicotinic acid, glutamic acid, hydrochloric acid, and
other highly acidic substances could possibly reduce the therapeutic
effect of this medicinal.
PDR: Consult a physician before using this medicinal during pregnancy
or while nursing. Contraindicated in cases of intestinal obstruction,
acute inflammatory intestinal disease, appendicitis and abdominal pain
of unknown origin.

COMMENTS

In Chinese medicine, jaundice (due to any underlying reason) is divided
into two types. Yin jaundice and yang jaundice. Yin jaundice is due to
spleen vacuity resulting in damp heat, whereas yang jaundice is due to
replete damp heat evils. This formula is specifically for the treatment of
yin jaundice.

YIN QIAO SAN
(Lonicera & Forsythia Powder, a.k.a. Lonicera & Forsythia Formula)

Category: Exterior-resolving
Functions: Acridly and cooly penetrates the exterior, clears heat and resolves toxins
Chinese medical indications: Externally contracted wind heat evils resulting in fever, slight or no chills, headache, thirst, cough, sore throat, a red-tipped tongue with thin, white or thin, yellow fur, and a floating, rapid pulse
Contraindications: Externally contracted wind dampness
Western medical indications: Common cold, flu, acute tonsillitis, mumps, measles, scarlet fever, epidemic meningitis, encephalitis B, acute suppurative infections, and early stage sores
Potential formula toxicities & interactions: None listed

POTENTIAL MEDICINAL TOXICITIES & INTERACTIONS:

Jin Yin Hua
(Flos Lonicerae Japonicae, honeysuckle flowers)

Standard daily dosage: 9-15g
AH: Safe when used appropriately
C&C: Contains potassium and glycosides. Could possibly cause hyperkalemia when used with potassium-sparing diuretics. Vitamin C, nicotinic acid, glutamic acid, hydrochloric acid, and other highly acidic substances could possibly reduce the therapeutic effect of this medicinal.
PDR: No health risks or side effects are known in conjunction with the proper administration of designated therapeutic dosages.

Lian Qiao
(Fructus Forsythiae Suspensae, dried forsythia fruit pods)

Standard daily dosage: 6-15g
AH: Not to be used during pregnancy. (This medicinal is commonly used in China during pregnancy for the treatment of wind heat external contractions and heat toxins.)
B&G: Contraindicated in patients with diarrhea, carbuncles that have already ulcerated, and skin ulcers.
C&C: Contains potassium and glycosides. Could possibly cause hyperkalemia when used with potassium-sparing diuretics. Vitamin C, nico-

tinic acid, glutamic acid, hydrochloric acid, and other highly acidic substances could possibly reduce the therapeutic effect of this medicinal.

Jie Geng
(Radix Platycodi Grandiflori, bellflower root)

Standard daily dosage: 3-9g
AH: Contraindicated in hemoptysis, especially in cases of tuberculosis. Use with caution in bleeding peptic ulcer.
B&G: Contraindicated in patients with hemoptysis. According to some traditional sources, counteracts *Long Dan Cao* (Radix Gentianae Longdancao) and *Long Yan Rou* (Arillus Euphoriae Longanae).
C&C: Contains calcium and glycosides. Could possibly reduce the effect of most antibiotics, cause digitalis intoxication and heart arrhythmias, hinder the absorption of isoniazid, and reduce the biological effect of levadopa. Vitamin C, nicotinic acid, glutamic acid, hydrochloric acid, and other highly acidic substances could possibly reduce the therapeutic effect of this medicinal.

Niu Bang Zi, Niu Bang, Niu Zi
(Fructus Arctii Lappae, burdock seeds)

Standard daily dosage: 3-9g
C&C: Vitamin C, nicotinic acid, glutamic acid, hydrochloric acid, and other highly acidic substances could possibly reduce the therapeutic effect of this medicinal.
PDR: No health hazards are known in conjunction with the proper administration of designated therapeutic dosages.

Bo He
(Herba Menthae Haplocalycis, field mint)

Standard daily dose: 1.5-6g
AH: Safe when used appropriately
B&G: Not recommended for nursing mothers as it may inhibit lactation.

Dan Dou Chi
(Semen Praeparatum Sojae, prepared soybeans)

Standard daily dosage: 6-15g
B&G: Not for nursing mothers. Inhibits lactation.
C&C: Contains amylase. Tetracyclines, sulphanomides, and aspirin could possibly reduce the therapeutic effect of this medicinal.

PDR: Minor side effects include occasional gastrointestinal effects, such as stomach pain, loose stools, and diarrhea.

Jing Jie Sui, Jing Jie
(Herba Seu Flos Schizonepetae Tenuifoliae)

Standard daily dosage: 3-9g

No toxicity or interaction information listed in the sources

Dan Zhu Ye
(Herba Lophatheri Gracilis)

Standard daily dosage: 6-9g
B&G: Use with caution in pregnancy.
C&C: Contains potassium. Could possibly cause hyperkalemia when used with potassium-sparing diuretics.

Lu Gen
(Rhizoma Phragmitis Communis)

Standard daily dosage: 15-30g
PDR: No health risks or side effects are known in conjunction with the proper administration of designated therapeutic dosages.

Gan Cao
(Radix Glycyrrhizae Uralensis, licorice root)

Standard daily dosage: 2-12g
AH: Do not use during pregnancy. (This medicinal is routinely used in Chinese medical gynecology during pregnancy as part of formulas appropriately prescribed on the basis of pattern discrimination.) As a single herb in high doses, it is contraindicated in diabetes, hypertension, and liver disorders. Not for long-term use.
BR: May increase toxicity of cardiac glycosides. May increase potassium loss due to diuretics and laxatives. Possible additive effect to corticosteroids. May be synergistic with insulin in causing hypokalemia and sodium retention.
B&G: According to some traditional sources, incompatible with *Gan Sui* (Radix Euphorbiae Kansui), *Yuan Hua* (Flos Daphnes Genkwae), and *Yuan Zhi* (Radix Polygalae Tenuifoliae). If taken long-term, it may cause hypertension and/or edema. Contains glycyrrhetinic acid which could possibly cause a reduction in thyroid activity and basal metabolic rate.

The research on *Gan Cao* concurs that this medicinal is generally safe when used in small amounts as an envoy. It should not be taken long-term or as a single herb during pregnancy. When used as a single medicinal or in patients taking other potent Western pharmaceuticals, caution should be exercised to guard against potential toxicity and drug interaction.

COMMENTS

This is the most commonly prescribed formula for the treatment of common colds associated primarily with sore throat and fever, and many ready-made versions of it exist in the marketplace. However, to be effective, these ready-made versions typically need to be taken at several times the dose recommended on the packaging. In addition, if one discontinues this medication as soon as the symptoms abate, the cold may immediately return.

YU NU JIAN
(Jade Lady Brew, a.k.a.
Jade Woman Decoction, Rehmannia & Gypsum Combination)

Category: Heat-clearing
Functions: Drains heat from the stomach and nourishes yin
Chinese medical indications: Stomach heat with yin vacuity
due to vigorous stomach fire damaging kidney yin manifesting
as toothache, loose teeth, bleeding gums, frontal headache, easy
anger, possible fever, thirst with a liking for chilled drinks, a dry,
red tongue with yellow fur, and a slippery, vacuous pulse
Contraindications: Diarrhea
Western medical indications: Toothache, gingivitis, stomatitis,
and glossitis
Potential formula toxicities & interactions: None listed

POTENTIAL MEDICINAL TOXICITIES & INTERACTIONS:

Shi Gao
(Gypsum Fibrosum)

Standard daily dosage: 9-30g
B&G: Can cause gastric upset in some patients.
C&C: Contains calcium. Could possibly reduce the effect of most
antibiotics and levadopa, cause digitalis intoxication and heart arrhythmias, and hinder the absorption of isoniazid.

Shu Di, Shu Di Huang
(cooked Radix Rehmanniae Glutinosae)

Standard daily dosage: 9-30g
AH: Contraindicated in patients with diarrhea or indigestion
B&G: Overuse can lead to abdominal distention and loose stools. Side
effects include diarrhea, abdominal pain, dizziness, lethargy, and heart
palpitations which often disappear upon continued administration of the
herb.
PDR: No health risks or side effects are known in conjunction with the
proper administration of designated therapeutic dosages.

Zhi Mu
(Rhizoma Anemarrhenae Aspheloidis)

Standard daily dosage: 6-12g
AH: Safe when used appropriately
B&G: May cause diarrhea in some patients.
C&C: Contains potassium and glycosides. Could possibly cause hyper-kalemia when used with potassium-sparing diuretics. Vitamin C, nico-tinic acid, glutamic acid, hydrochloric acid, and other highly acidic sub-stances could possibly reduce the therapeutic effect of this medicinal.
PDR: No health hazards are known in conjunction with the proper administration of designated therapeutic dosages.

Mai Men Dong, Mai Dong
(Tuber Ophiopogoni Japonici)

Standard daily dosage: 6-15g
AH: Safe when used appropriately
B&G: According to some traditional sources, antagonizes *Kuan Dong Hua* (Flos Tussilaginis Farfarae) and counteracts *Ku Shen* (Radix Sophorae Flavescentis) and *Bai Mu Er* (Fructificatio Tremellae Fuciformis).
C&C: Contains glycosides. Vitamin C, nicotinic acid, glutamic acid, hydrochloric acid, and other highly acidic substances could possibly reduce the therapeutic effect of this medicinal.

Niu Xi, Huai Niu Xi, Tu Niu Xi
(Radix Achyranthis Bidentatae)

Standard daily dosage: 9-15g
AH: Not to be used during pregnancy. Contraindicated in menorrhagia.
B&G: Contraindicated during pregnancy, in debilitated patients with diarrhea, and in patients with excessive menstruation. According to some traditional sources, should not be used with *Bai Qian* (Radix Et Rhizoma Cynanchi Baiqian).
C&C: Contains alkaloids, potassium, and glycosides. Could possibly cause hyperkalemia when used with potassium-sparing diuretics. Could possibly reduce the absorption and therapeutic effect of potassium and sodium iodides, sodium bicarbonate, aluminum hydroxide, and magne-sium sulfate. Vitamin C, nicotinic acid, glutamic acid, hydrochloric acid, and other highly acidic substances could possibly reduce the therapeutic effect of this medicinal.

YU PING FENG SAN
(Jade Windscreen Powder)

Category: Securing and astringing
Functions: Boosts the qi, secures the exterior, and stops sweating
Chinese medical indications: External defensive insecurity resulting in easy contraction of external evils, aversion to wind, spontaneous perspiration, a pale facial complexion, a pale tongue with white fur, and a vacuous or soggy pulse
Contraindications: None listed
Western medical indications: Allergic rhinitis, sweating due to autonomic dystonia, upper respiratory infection, mild bronchitis, exacerbation of chronic bronchitis, and hyperthyroid condition
Potential formula toxicities & interactions: None listed

POTENTIAL MEDICINAL TOXICITIES & INTERACTIONS:

Huang Qi, Bei Qi
(Radix Astragali Membranacei, astragalus root)

Standard daily dosage: 9-60g
AH: Safe when used appropriately
C&C: Contains alkaloids and potassium. Could possibly cause hyperkalemia when used with potassium-sparing diuretics. Could possibly reduce the absorption and therapeutic effect of potassium and sodium iodides, sodium bicarbonate, aluminum hydroxide, and magnesium sulfate.
PDR: Caution should be taken with patients receiving immunosuppressive therapy, such as transplant patients or patients with autoimmune disorders. May cause neurological dysfunction in high doses. May potentiate the risk of bleeding when used concomitantly with anticoagulants, antiplatelets, or antithrombotic agents.

Bai Zhu
(Rhizoma Atractylodis Macrocephalae)

Standard daily dosage: 4.5-9g
AH: Safe when used appropriately
B&G: When rats were fed 0.5g/kg of this medicinal for two months, they developed a mild lymphopenia and anemia but suffered no damage to the brain, heart, or liver.

Fang Feng
(Radix Ledebouriellae Divaricatae)

Standard daily dosage: 3-9g
AH: Safe when used appropriately
B&G: According to some traditional sources, may antagonize *Gan Jiang* (dry Rhizoma Zingiberis Officinalis), *Li Lu* (Rhizoma Et Radix Veratri) and counteracts *Bei Xie* (Rhizoma Dioscoreae Hypoglaucae).
C&C: Contains glycosides. Vitamin C, nicotinic acid, glutamic acid, hydrochloric acid, and other highly acidic substances could possibly reduce the therapeutic effect of this medicinal.

Sheng Jiang
(uncooked Rhizoma Zingiberis Officinalis, fresh ginger)

Standard daily dose: 3-9g
AH: Safe when used appropriately
BR: Reduces vomiting caused by chemotherapeutic drugs. Increases absorption of oral drugs.
PDR: Recommended safe dosage limit is six grams (6g). Avoid larger doses if being used to treat morning sickness or if used in patients taking anticoagulants.

COMMENTS

The ingredients in this formula are commonly added to other formulas whenever an element of defensive qi vacuity complicates a patient's overall condition.

YUE JU WAN
(Escape Restraint Pills)

Category: Qi-rectifying
Functions: Moves the qi and resolves depression
Chinese medical indications: Qi, blood, dampness, phlegm, food, and heat depressions manifesting as chest oppression, abdominal glomus, rib-side pain, burping/belching, vomiting, acid regurgitation, mild cough with profuse phlegm, scanty appetite, and indigestion
Contraindications: Stasis and stagnation due to vacuity
Western medical indications: Gastrointestinal neurosis, gastric or duodenal ulcer, chronic gastritis, infectious hepatitis, chronic cholecystitis, cholelithiasis, intercostal neuralgia, irregular menstruation, and dysmenorrhea
Potential formula toxicities & interactions: None listed

POTENTIAL MEDICINAL TOXICITIES & INTERACTIONS:

Cang Zhu
(Rhizoma Atractylodis)

Standard daily dosage: 4.5-9g
AH: Safe when used appropriately
B&G: Use with caution in patients with loose, watery stools.
PDR: No health risks or side effects are known in conjunction with the proper administration of designated therapeutic dosages.

Chuan Xiong
(Radix Ligustici Wallichii)

Standard daily dosage: 3-9g (In China today, it is not uncommon for this medicinal to be prescribed up to 15 grams per day in decoction.)
AH: Do not use during pregnancy. (This medicinal is routinely used in Chinese medical gynecology during pregnancy as part of formulas appropriately prescribed on the basis of pattern discrimination.)
B&G: Not for patients with migraine headache or excessive menstrual bleeding. Overdosage causes vomiting and dizziness. According to some traditional texts, antagonizes *Shan Zhu Yu* (Fructus Corni Officinalis) and *Huang Qi* (Radix Astragali Membranacei), counteracts *Hua Shi* (Talcum) and *Huang Lian* (Rhizoma Coptidis Chinensis), and is incompatible with *Li Lu* (Rhizoma Et Radix Veratri).
C&C: Contains alkaloids and potassium. Could possibly cause hyperkalemia when used with potassium-sparing diuretics. Could possibly reduce the absorption and therapeutic effect of potassium and sodium

iodides, sodium bicarbonate, aluminum hydroxide, and magnesium sulfate.

Xiang Fu
(Rhizoma Cyperi Rotundi)

Standard daily dosage: 4.5-12g
AH: Safe when used appropriately

Zhi Zi, Shan Zhi, Shan Zhi Zi
(Fructus Gardeniae Jasminoidis, dried gardenia fruit pods)

Standard daily dosage: 3-12g
B&G: Contains geniposide which caused diarrhea in mice.
C&C: Contains potassium and glycosides. Could possibly cause hyper-kalemia when used with potassium-sparing diuretics. Vitamin C, nicotinic acid, glutamic acid, hydrochloric acid, and other highly acidic substances could possibly reduce the therapeutic effect of this medicinal.

Shen Qu
(Massa Medica Fermentata)

Standard daily dosage: 6-15g
B&G: Use with caution during pregnancy.
C&C: Contains amylase. Tetracyclines, sulphanomides, and aspirin could possibly reduce the therapeutic effect of this medicinal.

COMMENTS

This formula is not commonly used in clinical practice. It is important more as a theoretical model for teaching purposes than as a clinically useful formula.

ZHEN GAN XI FENG TANG
(Settle the Liver & Extinguish Wind Decoction)

Category: Wind-treating
Functions: Settles the liver and extinguishes wind, enriches yin and subdues yang
Chinese medical indications: Liver-kidney yin vacuity with ascendant liver yang hyperactivity or internal stirring of liver wind manifesting as dizziness, vertigo, distended eyes, tinnitus, a feverish sensation in the head, headache, easy anger, a flushed face as if intoxicated, and a bowstring, forceful pulse
Contraindications: Spleen qi or yang vacuity
Western medical indications: Wind stroke, convulsion, epilepsy, cerebrovascular accident, aphasia, apraxia, renal hypertension, essential hypertension, hypertensive encephelopathy, cerebral arteriorsclerosis, arteriorsclerotic heart disease, hyperthyroidism, premenstrual tension, postpartum fever with spasms and convulsions
Potential formula toxicities & interactions: None listed

POTENTIAL MEDICINAL TOXICITIES & INTERACTIONS:

Niu Xi, Huai Niu Xi, Tu Niu Xi
(Radix Achyranthis Bidentatae)

Standard daily dosage: 9-15g
AH: Not to be used during pregnancy. Contraindicated in menorrhagia.
B&G: Contraindicated during pregnancy, in debilitated patients with diarrhea, and in patients with excessive menstruation. According to some traditional sources, should not be used with *Bai Qian* (Radix Et Rhizoma Cynanchi Baiqian).
C&C: Contains alkaloids, potassium, and glycosides. Could possibly cause hyperkalemia when used with potassium-sparing diuretics. Could possibly reduce the absorption and therapeutic effect of potassium and sodium iodides, sodium bicarbonate, aluminum hydroxide, and magnesium sulfate. Vitamin C, nicotinic acid, glutamic acid, hydrochloric acid, and other highly acidic substances will reduce the therapeutic effect of this medicinal.

Dai Zhe Shi
(Haemititum, hematite)

Standard daily dosage: 9-30g
B&G: Use with caution during pregnancy. Signs of toxicity include weakness, slowness of movement, and paroxysmal spasms leading to paralysis and death. Two grams per day for seven days caused death in mice. Researchers have found small amounts of arsenic salts in some samples, thus accounting for its toxicity. According to some traditional sources, counteracts *Fu Zi* (Radix Lateralis Praeparatus Aconiti Carmichaeli).
C&C: Contains iron. Could possibly reduce the effect of most antibiotics, levadopa, and prednisolone and hinder the absorption of isoniazid.

Long Gu
(Os Draconis, fossilized bone)

Standard daily dosage: 15-30g
B&G: According to some traditional sources, counteracts *Shi Gao* (Gypsum Fibrosum) and should not be mixed with fish.
C&C: Contains calcium, iron, magnesium, aluminum, and potassium. Could possibly cause hyperkalemia when used with potassium-sparing diuretics. Could possibly reduce the effect of most antibiotics, levadopa, and prednisolone, cause digitalis intoxication and heart arrhythmias, and hinder the absorption of isoniazid.

Mu Li
(Concha Ostreae, oyster shell)

Standard daily dosage: 15-30g
AH: Not to be used during pregnancy.
B&G: Contraindicated when the patient has high fever without sweating. Overdose may lead to indigestion or constipation. According to some traditional sources, works synergistically with *Bei Mu* (Bulbus Fritillariae), *Gan Cao* (Radix Glycyrrizae Uralensis), *Niu Xi* (Radix Achyranthis Bidentatae), and *Yuan Zhi* (Radix Polygalae Tenuifoliae) and has adverse effects when combined with *Ma Huang* (Herba Ephedrae), *Wu Zhu Yu* (Fructus Evodiae Rutecarpae), and *Xi Xin* (Herba Asari Cum Radice).
C&C: Contains calcium, iron, magnesium, and aluminum. Could possibly reduce the effects of most antibiotics, levadopa, and prednisolone, cause digitalis intoxication and heart arrhythmias, and hinder the absorption of isoniazid.

Gui Ban
(Plastrum Testudinis, tortoise plastron)

Standard daily dosage: 9-30g
B&G: Contraindicated in pregnancy. According to some traditional sources, antagonizes *Sha Shen* (Radix Glehniae Littoralis) and *Ren Shen* (Radix Panacis Ginseng).

Xuan Shen, Yuan Shen
(Radix Scrophulariae Ningpoensis)

Standard daily dosage: 9-30g
C&C: Contains alkaloids, potassium, and glycosides. Could possibly cause hyperkalemia when used with potassium-sparing diuretics. Could possibly reduce the absorption and therapeutic effect of potassium and sodium iodides, sodium bicarbonate, aluminum hydroxide, and magnesium sulfate. Vitamin C, nicotinic acid, glutamic acid, hydrochloric acid, and other highly acidic substances could possibly reduce the therapeutic effect of this medicinal.

Tian Men Dong, Tian Dong
(Tuber Asparagi Cochinensis)

Standard daily dosage: 6-15g
AH: Safe when used appropriately
B&G: Contraindicated in patients with loss of appetite and diarrhea or cough from the common cold.
PDR: Contains steroid saponins, and flavinoids. Should not be administered in the presence of kidney diseases due to the irritating effect of the saponins. Otherwise considered safe with the proper administration of designated therapeutic dosages.

Bai Shao, Shao Yao
(Radix Albus Paeoniae Lactiflorae, white peony root)

Standard daily dosage: 6-30g
AH: Safe when used appropriately
B&G: Use with caution in debilitated patients with diarrhea. According to some traditional sources, antagonizes *Shi Hu* (Herba Dendrobii) and *Mang Xiao* (Mirabilitum), counteracts *Bie Jia* (Carapax Amydae Sinensis) and *Xiao Ji* (Herba Cephalanopoloris Segeti), and is incompatible with *Li Lu* (Rhizoma Et Radix Veratri).
C&C: Contains calcium, tannic acid, potassium, and glycosides. Could

possibly cause hyperkalemia when used with potassium-sparing diuretics. Could possibly reduce the effect of most antibiotics, cause digitalis intoxication and heart arrhythmias, and could possibly reduce the absorption and therapeutic effect of levadopa, isoniazid, chlorpromazine, calcium carbonate and gluconate, atropine, ephedrine, quinine, reserpine, vitamin B_1, trypsine, amylase, and pepsin. Vitamin C, nicotinic acid, glutamic acid, hydrochloric acid, and other highly acidic substances could possibly reduce the therapeutic effect of this medicinal.

Yin Chen Hao
(Herba Artemisiae Yinchenhao)

Standard daily dosage: 9-30g
AH: Not to be used during pregnancy.
B&G: One study showed that using this medicinal along with *Da Zao* (Fructus Zizyphi Jujubae) to treat infectious hepatitis caused heart block in two patients.
C&C: Contains potassium. Could possibly cause hyperkalemia when used with potassium-sparing diuretics.

Chuan Lian Zi, Jin Ling Zi
(Fructus Meliae Toosendan)

Standard daily dosage: 3-9g
AH: Safe when used appropriately
GLW: Symptoms of adverse reaction include abdominal distention, abdominal pain, vomiting, diarrhea, poor appetite, dizziness, headache, a red facial complexion, blurred vision, inhibited speech, uneasy respiration, epistaxis, hemorrhage of the liver, kidney, and/or intestines, mania and agitation, convulsions, numbness of the four extremities, heart arrhythmia, shrunken pupils. Poisoning can lead to toxic hepatitis and red blood cells in the urine. In grave conditions, there may be atrial fibrillation, frequent premature beats, and atrioventricular conduction block, low blood pressure, syncope, shock, and even death.

Mai Ya
(Fructus Germinatus Hordei Vulgaris, malted barley)

Standard daily dosage: 12-30g
AH: Not to be used during pregnancy.
B&G: According to one traditional source, long-term use may damage the kidneys.
C&C: Contains amylase. Tetracyclines, sulphanomides, and aspirin could possibly reduce the therapeutic effect of this medicinal.

Gan Cao
(Radix Glycyrrhizae Uralensis, licorice root)

Standard daily dosage: 2-12g

AH: Do not use during pregnancy. (This medicinal is routinely used in Chinese medical gynecology during pregnancy as part of formulas appropriately prescribed on the basis of pattern discrimination.) As a single herb in high doses, it is contraindicated in diabetes, hypertension, and liver disorders. Not for long-term use.

BR: May increase toxicity of cardiac glycosides. May increase potassium loss due to diuretics and laxatives. Possible additive effect to corticosteroids. May be synergistic with insulin in causing hypokalemia and sodium retention.

B&G: According to some traditional sources, incompatible with *Gan Sui* (Radix Euphorbiae Kansui), *Yuan Hua* (Flos Daphnes Genkwae), and *Yuan Zhi* (Radix Polygalae Tenuifoliae). If taken long-term, it may cause hypertension and/or edema. Contains glycyrrhetinic acid which could possibly cause a reduction in thyroid activity and basal metabolic rate.

The research on *Gan Cao* concurs that this medicinal is generally safe when used in small amounts as an envoy. It should not be taken long-term or as a single herb during pregnancy. When used as a single medicinal or in patients taking other potent Western pharmaceuticals, caution should be exercised to guard against potential toxicity and drug interaction.

ZHEN WU TANG
(True Warrior Decoction, a.k.a. Vitality Combination)

Category: Dampness-dispelling
Functions: Warms the yang and disinhibits urination
Chinese medical indications: Spleen-kidney yang vacuity with internal gathering of water evils manifesting as abdominal pain which is aggravated by cold, difficult urination, deep aching and heaviness of the extremities, generalized edema, loose stools, dizziness, heavy head, heart palpitations, coughing, vomiting, a pale or dry, swollen tongue with teeth-marks on its edges and white, slimy fur, and a deep, fine, forceless pulse
Contraindications: None listed
Western medical indications: Chronic nephritis, rheumatic valvular heart disease, congestive heart failure, liver cirrhosis and other hepatic disorders leading to edema and ascites, chronic enteritis, chronic diarrhea, Meniere's disease, primary hypertension, primary hyperaldosteronism, hypothyroidism, rheumatoid arthritis, and chronic bronchitis
Potential formula toxicities & interactions: None listed

POTENTIAL MEDICINAL TOXICITIES & INTERACTIONS:

Fu Zi, Shu Fu Zi, Fu Pian
(Radix Lateralis Praeparatus Aconiti Carmichaeli, wolfsbane, monkshood)

Standard daily dosage: 1.5-15g
AH: To be used only under the supervision of an expert qualified in the appropriate use of this substance.
B&G: Contraindicated during pregnancy. A very toxic medicinal which can be fatal if ingested in its uncooked form or in an inappropriate dose. It is generally combined with *Gan Cao* (Radix Glycyrhizae Uralensis) and *Gan Jiang* (dry Rhizoma Zingiberis Officinalis) in decoctions to reduce its toxicity. Symptoms of toxicity include drooling, gastric upset, light-headedness, blurred vision, and numbness and tingling of the extremities. More severe symptoms include premature atrial contractions, dyspnea, and reduced temperature and blood pressure. Emergency measures include the administration of atropine.
C&C: Contains alkaloids. Could possibly reduce the absorption and therapeutic effect of potassium and sodium iodides, sodium bicarbonate, aluminum hydroxide, and magnesium sulfate.

PDR: Contains nor-diterpene alkaloids, including aconitine. Highly toxic; small doses can be fatal.

GLW: If mild poisoning, there is a burning hot sensation in the mouth and on the tongue, numbness, and pain which gradually spreads to the four limbs and then to the whole body, nausea, vomiting, dizziness, heart palpitations, rapid breathing, vexation, agitation, restlessness, drooling. If more severe poisoning, there may be generalized sweating, paralysis, convulsions, urinary incontinence, dilated pupils, slowed reaction to light, slow heartbeat, arrhythmia, low blood pressure, a somber white facial complexion, reversal chilling of the four limbs, lowered body temperature, and circulatory collapse leading to death.

Bai Zhu
(Rhizoma Atractylodis Macrocephalae)

Standard daily dosage: 4.5-9g
AH: Safe when used appropriately
B&G: When rats were fed 0.5g/kg of this medicinal for two months, they developed a mild lymphopenia and anemia but suffered no damage to to the brain, heart, or liver.

Fu Ling, Bai Fu Ling, Yun Ling
(Sclerotium Poriae Cocos)

Standard daily dosage: 9-15g
B&G: Large doses or long-term use is discouraged. Contraindicated in patients with frequent, copious urination. According to traditional sources, may counteract *Di Yu* (Radix Sanguisorbae Officinalis), *Qin Jiao* (Radix Gentianae Qinjiao), and *Bie Jia* (Carapax Amydae Sinensis).
C&C: Contains potassium. Could possibly cause hyperkalemia when used with potassium-sparing diuretics.

Sheng Jiang
(uncooked Rhizoma Zingiberis Officinalis, fresh ginger)

Standard daily dose: 3-9g
AH: Safe when used appropriately
BR: Reduces vomiting caused by chemotherapeutic drugs. Increases absorption of oral drugs.
PDR: Recommended safe dosage limit is six grams (6g). Avoid larger doses if being used to treat morning sickness or if used in patients taking anticoagulants.

Bai Shao, Shao Yao
(Radix Albus Paeoniae Lactiflorae, white peony root)

Standard daily dosage: 6-30g

AH: Safe when used appropriately

B&G: Use with caution in debilitated patients with diarrhea. According to some traditional sources, antagonizes *Shi Hu* (Herba Dendrobii) and *Mang Xiao* (Mirabilitum), counteracts *Bie Jia* (Carapax Amydae Sinensis) and *Xiao Ji* (Herba Cephalanopoloris Segeti), and is incompatible with *Li Lu* (Rhizoma Et Radix Veratri).

C&C: Contains calcium, tannic acid, potassium, and glycosides. Could possibly cause hyperkalemia when used with potassium-sparing diuretics. Could possibly reduce the effect of most antibiotics, cause digitalis intoxication and heart arrhythmias, and could possibly reduce the absorption and therapeutic effect of levadopa, isoniazid, chlorpromazine, calcium carbonate and gluconate, atropine, ephedrine, quinine, reserpine, vitamin B_1, trypsine, amylase, and pepsin. Vitamin C, nicotinic acid, glutamic acid, hydrochloric acid, and other highly acidic substances could possibly reduce the therapeutic effect of this medicinal.

COMMENTS

This formula is a first aid formula meant to rescue seriously ill patients. It is not meant for long-term administration.

ZHI BAI DI HUANG WAN
(Anemarrhena & Phellodendron Rehmannia Pills)

Category: Yin-supplementing
Functions: Supplements the kidneys and enriches yin, drains fire as well as clears and eliminates dampness and heat
Chinese medical indications: Kidney yin vacuity with either fire flaming internally or damp heat manifesting as dizziness, tinnitus, low back and knee soreness and limpness, nocturia, hot flashes, night sweats, steaming bones, tidal heat, a dry mouth and tongue, strangury, a red tongue with either scanty, yellow or slimy, yellow fur at the root, and a fine, rapid, surging, rapid, or fine, slippery, and rapid pulse
Contraindications: Absence of fire flaring or damp heat
Western medical indications: Chronic prostatitis, benign prostatic hypertrophy, senile vaginitis, hyperthyroidism, chronic nephritis, chronic glomerulonephritis, hypertension, pulmonary tuberculosis, functional uterine bleeding, and perimenopausal syndrome
Potential formula toxicities & interactions: None listed

POTENTIAL MEDICINAL TOXICITIES & INTERACTIONS:

Shu Di, Shu Di Huang
(cooked Radix Rehmanniae Glutinosae)

Standard daily dosage: 9-30g
AH: Contraindicated in patients with diarrhea or indigestion
B&G: Overuse can lead to abdominal distention and loose stools. Side effects include diarrhea, abdominal pain, dizziness, lethargy, and heart palpitations which often disappear upon continued administration of the herb.
PDR: No health risks or side effects are known in conjunction with the proper administration of designated therapeutic dosages.

Shan Zhu Yu, Shan Zhu Rou
(Fructus Corni Officinalis)

Standard daily dosage: 3-60g
AH: Contraindicated in patients with difficult or painful urination.
B&G: Contraindicated in patients with difficult or painful urination. According to some traditional sources, antagonizes *Jie Geng* (Radix

Platycodi Grandiflori), *Fang Feng* (Radix Lebouriellae Divaricatae), and *Fang Ji* (Radix Aristolochiae Fangchi).

C&C: Contains tannic acid and glycosides. Could possibly reduce the absorption and biologic effect of most antibiotics, isoniazid, chlorpromazine, calcium carbonate and gluconate, atropine, ephedrine, quinine, reserpine, digitalis, vitamin B_1, trypsine, amylase, and pepsin. Vitamin C, nicotinic acid, glutamic acid, hydrochloric acid, and other highly acidic substances could possibly reduce the therapeutic effect of this medicinal.

PDR: No health hazards are known in conjunction with proper administration of designated therapeutic dosages.

Shan Yao
(Radix Dioscoreae Oppositae)

Standard daily dosage: 9-30g

AH: Safe when used appropriately

B&G: According to some traditional sources, antagonizes *Gan Sui* (Radix Euphorbiae Kansui).

C&C: Contains alkaloids, potassium, amylase, and glycosides. Could possibly cause hyperkalemia when used with potassium-sparing diuretics. Could possibly reduce the absorption and therapeutic effect of potassium and sodium iodides, sodium bicarbonate, aluminum hydroxide, magnesium sulfate, tetracyclines, sulphanomides, and aspirin. Vitamin C, nicotinic acid, glutamic acid, hydrochloric acid, and other highly acidic substances could possibly reduce the therapeutic effect of this medicinal.

PDR: Use of this medicinal may reduce the antiinflammatory effect of indomethacin. May have an additive estrogenic effect when administered with estrogen-containing drugs. Poisoning in overdosages may occur from the picrotoxin-like effect of dioscorin.

Fu Ling, Bai Fu Ling, Yun Ling
(Sclerotium Poriae Cocos)

Standard daily dosage: 9-15g

B&G: Large doses or long-term use is discouraged. Contraindicated in patients with frequent, copious urination. According to traditional sources, may counteract *Di Yu* (Radix Sanguisorbae Officinalis), *Qin Jiao* (Radix Gentianae Qinjiao), and *Bie Jia* (Carapax Amydae Sinensis).

C&C: Contains potassium. Could possibly cause hyperkalemia when used with potassium-sparing diuretics.

Dan Pi, Mu Dan Pi
(Cortex Radicis Moutan, tree peony root bark)

Standard daily dosage: 6-12g
AH: Not to be used during pregnancy (This ingredient is commonly used in China during pregnancy to treat heat in the blood and/or blood stasis.)
B&G: Should not be used during pregnancy or in patients with excessive sweating or profuse menstruation. Avoid using with garlic. According to some traditional sources, may counteract the effect of *Tu Si Zi* (Semen Cuscutae Chinensis), *Bei Mu* (Bulbus Fritillariae), and *Da Huang* (Radix Et Rhizoma Rhei).
C&C: Contains tannic acid, potassium, and glycosides. Could possibly cause hyperkalemia when used with potassium-sparing diuretics. Could possibly reduce the absorption and biologic effect of most antibiotics, isoniazid, chlorpromazine, calcium carbonate and gluconate, atropine, ephedrine, quinine, reserpine, digitalis, vitamin B_1B_1, trypsine, amylase, and pepsin. Vitamin C, nicotinic acid, glutamic acid, hydrochloric acid, and other highly acidic substances could possibly reduce the therapeutic effect of this medicinal.

Ze Xie
(Rhizoma Alismatis Orientalis)

Standard daily dosage: 6-15g
AH: Prolonged use may cause gastrointestinal irritation.
B&G: Although considered safe, prolonged usage may irritate the intestinal tract and could possibly cause gastroenteritis.
C&C: Contains alkaloids and potassium. Could possibly cause hyperkalemia when used with potassium-sparing diuretics and reduce the absorption and therapeutic effect of potassium and sodium iodides, sodium bicarbonate, aluminum hydroxide, magnesium sulfate.
PDR: Contains triterpenes, sesquiterpenes, flavone sulfate, and caffeic acid derivatives. No health hazards or side effects with proper administration of designated therapeutic dosages.

Zhi Mu
(Rhizoma Anemarrhenae Aspheloidis)

Standard daily dosage: 6-12g
AH: Safe when used appropriately
B&G: May cause diarrhea in some patients.
C&C: Contains potassium and glycosides. Could possibly cause hyperkalemia when used with potassium-sparing diuretics. Vitamin C, nico-

tinic acid, glutamic acid, hydrochloric acid, and other highly acidic substances could possibly reduce the therapeutic effect of this medicinal.

PDR: No health hazards are known in conjunction with the proper administration of designated therapeutic dosages.

Huang Bai, Huang Bo
(Cortex Phellodendri)

Standard daily dosage: 3-12g

AH: Not to be used during pregnancy (This medicinal is commonly used during pregnancy in China.)

B&G: Chinese literature reports one case of a patient who developed a skin rash after ingestion.

C&C: Contains alkaloids and quercetin. Could possibly reduce the absorption and therapeutic effect of potassium and sodium iodides, sodium bicarbonate, calcium gluconate, carbonate, and lactate, aluminum hydroxide, magnesium and ferrous sulfates, and bismuth subcarbonate.

ZHI GAN CAO TANG
(Mix-fried Licorice Decoction)

Category: Qi and blood supplementing
Functions: Supplements the qi and nourishes the blood, enriches the yin and restores the pulse
Chinese medical indications: Heart qi and blood vacuity resulting in heart palpitations, easy anger, insomnia, emaciation, shortness of breath, constipation, a dry mouth and parched throat, a pale, shiny tongue, and a bound and/or faint pulse
Contraindications: Yin vacuity heat
Western medical indications: Superventricular arrythmia, rheumatic heart disease, mitral stenosis, mitral valve prolapse, hyperthyroidism, pulmonary tuberculosis, emphysema, and neurasthenia
Potential formula toxicities & interactions:
B&B: Use with caution in patients with severe diarrhea.

POTENTIAL MEDICINAL TOXICITIES & INTERACTIONS:

Gan Cao
(Radix Glycyrrhizae Uralensis, licorice root)

Standard daily dosage: 2-12g
AH: Do not use during pregnancy. (This medicinal is routinely used in Chinese medical gynecology during pregnancy as part of formulas appropriately prescribed on the basis of pattern discrimination.) As a single herb in high doses, it is contraindicated in diabetes, hypertension, and liver disorders. Not for long-term use.
BR: May increase toxicity of cardiac glycosides. May increase potassium loss due to diuretics and laxatives. Possible additive effect to corticosteroids. May be synergistic with insulin in causing hypokalemia and sodium retention.
B&G: According to some traditional sources, incompatible with *Gan Sui* (Radix Euphorbiae Kansui), *Yuan Hua* (Flos Daphnes Genkwae), and *Yuan Zhi* (Radix Polygalae Tenuifoliae). If taken long-term, it may cause hypertension and/or edema. Contains glycyrrhetinic acid which could possibly cause a reduction in thyroid activity and basal metabolic rate.

The research on *Gan Cao* concurs that this medicinal is generally safe when used in small amounts as an envoy. It should not be taken long-term or as a single herb during pregnancy. When used as a single medicinal or in patients taking other potent Western pharmaceuticals, caution should be exercised to guard against potential toxicity and drug interaction.

Ren Shen
(Radix Panacis Ginseng, ginseng)

Standard daily dosage: 1-30g
AH: Contraindicated in hypertension
BR: May cause manic episodes in patients on MAO-inhibitors. May cause hypertension if consumed with caffeine. Possible additive effects to insulin. May reduce the anticoagulative effect of warfarin (Coumadin).
B&G: Contraindicated for hypertensive patients. Overdose can lead to headache, insomnia, heart palpitations, and a rise in blood pressure. A traditional antidote is mung bean soup.
C&C: Vitamin C, nicotinic acid, glutamic acid, hydrochloric acid, and other highly acidic substances could possibly reduce the therapeutic effect of this medicinal.
PDR: Contraindicated in patients with hypertension. Not recommended in large doses during pregnancy or lactation due to potential neonatal androgenization. Enhances the effect of insulin and other antidiabetic agents. Use with MAO-inhibitors may cause headaches, tremors, and manias.

Gui Zhi
(Ramulus Cinnamomi Cassiae, cinnamon twigs)

Standard daily dosage: 3-15g
AH: Safe when used appropriately
B&G: Use with caution in the presence of fever, during pregnancy, or during excessive menstruation.
PDR: Contraindicated during pregnancy.

Sheng Di, Sheng Di Huang
(uncooked Radix Rehmanniae Glutinosae)

Standard daily dosage: 9-30g
AH: Contraindicated in patients with diarrhea or lack of appetite
B&G: Contraindicated in pregnant women with anemias or digestive weakness
C&C: Contains potassium. Could possibly cause hyperkalemia when used with potassium-sparing diuretics.
PDR: No health risks or side effects are known in conjunction with the proper administration of designated therapeutic dosages.

Mai Men Dong, Mai Dong
(Tuber Ophiopogoni Japonici)

Standard daily dosage: 6-15g

AH: Safe when used appropriately

B&G: According to some traditional sources, antagonizes *Kuan Dong Hua* (Flos Tussilaginis Farfarae) and counteracts *Ku Shen* (Radix Sophorae Flavescentis) and *Bai Mu Er* (Fructificatio Tremellae Fuciformis).

C&C: Contains glycosides. Vitamin C, nicotinic acid, glutamic acid, hydrochloric acid, and other highly acidic substances could possibly reduce the therapeutic effect of this medicinal.

E Jiao
(Gelatinum Corii Asini, donkey skin glue)

Standard daily dosage: 3-15g

B&G: According to some traditional sources, counteracts *Da Huang* (Radix Et Rhizoma Rhei).

Huo Ma Ren
(Semen Cannabis Sativae, cannabis seeds, marijuana seeds)

Standard daily dosage: 9-45g

B&G: Symptoms of overdose may include nausea, vomiting, diarrhea, numbness of the extremities, irritability, chorea, miosis, and in severe cases coma and death. Treatment is based on gastric lavage, fluids, and symptomatic therapy.

C&C: Contains alkaloids. Could possibly reduce the absorption and therapeutic effect of potassium and sodium iodides, sodium bicarbonate, aluminum hydroxide, and magnesium sulfate.

PDR: No health risks or side effects are known in conjunction with the proper administration of designated therapeutic dosages.

Sheng Jiang
(uncooked Rhizoma Zingiberis Officinalis, fresh ginger)

Standard daily dose: 3-9g

AH: Safe when used appropriately

BR: Reduces vomiting caused by chemotherapeutic drugs. Increases absorption of oral drugs.

PDR: Recommended safe dosage limit is six grams (6g). Avoid larger doses if being used to treat morning sickness or if used in patients taking anticoagulants.

Da Zao, Hong Zao
(Fructus Zizyphi Jujubae, red dates)

Standard daily dosage: 10-30g (3-12 pieces)

AH: Safe when used appropriately

PDR: No health risks or side effects are known in conjunction with the proper administration of designated therapeutic dosages.

ZHI SOU SAN
(Stop Coughing Powder, a.k.a.
Platycodon & Schizonpeta Formula)

Category: Phlegm-transforming
Functions: Stops cough and transform phlegm, resolves the exterior and diffuses the lungs
Chinese medical indications: Retained wind evils in the lungs causing cough with or without slight chills and fever, an itchy throat, thin, white tongue fur, and a floating, moderate (*i.e.,* slightly slow) pulse
Contraindications: Yin vacuity or lung heat coughs
Western medical indications: Coughing due to respiratory tract infection, acute bronchitis, pertussis, and early stages of viral or mycoplasm pneumonia
Potential formula toxicities & interactions: None listed

POTENTIAL MEDICINAL TOXICITIES & INTERACTIONS:

Jie Geng
(Radix Platycodi Grandiflori, bellflower root)

Standard daily dosage: 3-9g
AH: Contraindicated in hemoptysis, especially in cases of tuberculosis. Use with caution in bleeding peptic ulcer.
B&G: Contraindicated in patients with hemoptysis. According to some traditional sources, counteracts *Long Dan Cao* (Radix Gentianae Longdancao) and *Long Yan Rou* (Arillus Euphoriae Longanae).
C&C: Contains calcium and glycosides. Could possibly reduce the effect of most antibiotics, cause digitalis intoxication and heart arrhythmias, hinder the absorption of isoniazid, and reduce the biological effect of levadopa. Vitamin C, nicotinic acid, glutamic acid, hydrochloric acid, and other highly acidic substances could possibly reduce the therapeutic effect of this medicinal.

Jing Jie Sui, Jing Jie
(Herba Seu Flos Schizonepetae Tenuifoliae)

Standard daily dosage: 3-9g

No toxicity or interaction information listed in the sources

Zi Wan
(Radix Asteris Tatarici)

Standard daily dosage: 3-9g
B&G: Large dosages and long-term usage not recommended. According to traditional sources, counteracts *Yin Chen Hao* (Herba Artemesiae Capillaris).
C&C: Contains quercetin and glycosides. Could possibly reduce the absorption of calcium gluconate, carbonate, and lactate, aluminum hydroxide, magnesium and ferrous sulfates, and bismuth subcarbonate. Vitamin C, nicotinic acid, glutamic acid, hydrochloric acid, and other highly acidic substances could possibly reduce the therapeutic effect of this medicinal.

Bai Bu
(Radix Stemonae)

Standard daily dosage: 3-9g
C&C: Contains alkaloids. Could possibly reduce the absorption and therapeutic effect of potassium and sodium iodides, sodium bicarbonate, aluminum hydroxide, and magnesium sulfate.
GLW: Symptoms of adverse reaction, if mild, include a burning hot, dry sensation in the mouth and nose reaching the throat, dizziness, chest oppression, rapid breathing, indigestion. More rarely, there is abdominal pain, diarrhea, and epistaxis. Extreme overdose leading to poisoning can result in respiratory paralysis, syncope, and convulsions.

Bai Qian
(Radix Et Rhizoma Cynanchii Baiqian)

Standard daily dosage: 3-9g

No toxicity or interaction information listed in the sources

Gan Cao
(Radix Glycyrrhizae Uralensis, licorice root)

Standard daily dosage: 2-12g
AH: Do not use during pregnancy. (This medicinal is routinely used in Chinese medical gynecology during pregnancy as part of formulas appropriately prescribed on the basis of pattern discrimination.) As a single herb in high doses, it is contraindicated in diabetes, hypertension, and liver disorders. Not for long-term use.
BR: May increase toxicity of cardiac glycosides. May increase potassium loss due to diuretics and laxatives. Possible additive effect to corti-

costeroids. May be synergistic with insulin in causing hypokalemia and sodium retention.

B&G: According to some traditional sources, incompatible with *Gan Sui* (Radix Euphorbiae Kansui), *Yuan Hua* (Flos Daphnes Genkwae), and *Yuan Zhi* (Radix Polygalae Tenuifoliae). If taken long-term, it may cause hypertension and/or edema. Contains glycyrrhetinic acid which could possibly cause a reduction in thyroid activity and basal metabolic rate.

The research on *Gan Cao* concurs that this medicinal is generally safe when used in small amounts as an envoy. It should not be taken long-term or as a single herb during pregnancy. When used as a single medicinal or in patients taking other potent Western pharmaceuticals, caution should be exercised to guard against potential toxicity and drug interaction.

Chen Pi, Ju Pi, Ju Hong
(Pericarpium Citri Reticulatae, tangerine peel)

Standard daily dosage: 3-9g
AH: Safe when used appropriately
C&C: Contains potassium. Could possibly cause hyperkalemia when used with potassium-sparing diuretics.

ZHU SHA AN SHEN WAN
(Cinnabar Quiet the Spirit Pills, a.k.a. Cinnabar Formula)

Category: Heavy, settling, spirit-quieting
Functions: Settles the heart and quiets the spirit, drains fire and nourishes yin
Chinese medical indications: Heart fire harassing the spirit and damaging the blood and yin resulting in insomnia, continuous heart palpitations, vexatious heat in the chest, a desire to vomit with inability to do so, profuse dreams, a red tongue, especially the tip, and a fine, rapid pulse
Contraindications: None listed
Western medical indications: Mood disorders, depression, anxiety disorders, psychosis, insomnia, palpitations, and mitral valve prolapse syndrome
Potential formula toxicities & interactions:
FL/B&B: To avoid mercury poisoning, *Zhu Sha* (Cinnabaris) should not be taken in large doses or long-term.

POTENTIAL MEDICINAL TOXICITIES & INTERACTIONS:

Zhu Sha
(Cinnabaris, cinnabar)

Standard daily dosage: 0.2-2.7g in pills and powders
B&G: Contains mercuric sulfide which is highly toxic. Should not be used in large amounts or long-term. To prevent mercury poisoning, do not heat.
GLW: Symptoms of adverse reaction include burning pain in the oral cavity and throat, swelling and distention of the mucosa, bleeding, ulceration, and a metallic taste in the mouth, nausea, vomiting, abdominal pain, diarrhea, mucus in the stools or hemafecia. If severe, there is hemorrhagic enteritis, clenched teeth, fright reversal, and trembling. If the kidneys are poisoned, there is edema, scanty urination, albuminuria, and acute kidney failure, syncope, convulsions, low blood pressure, shock, and eventual respiratory failure.

Huang Lian
(Rhizoma Coptidis Chinensis)

Standard daily dosage: 1.5-9g
AH: Not to be used during pregnancy. (This medicinal is commonly used during pregnancy in China when indicated by disease and pattern discrimination.)

B&G: Contains berberine. Long-term use may damage the digestive system. According to some traditional sources, antagonizes *Ju Hua* (Flos Chrysanthemi Morifolii), *Xuan Shen* (Radix Scrophulariae Ningpoensis), *Bai Xian Pi* (Cortex Radicis Dictamni Dasycarpi), and *Jiang Can* (Bombyx Batryticatus). According to some traditional sources, counteracts *Kuan Dong Hua* (Flos Tussilaginis Farfarae) and *Niu Xi* (Radix Achyranthis Bidentatae), Some traditional sources say it should not be taken with pork.

C&C: Contains alkaloids, quercetin, and potassium. Could possibly cause hyperkalemia when used with potassium-sparing diuretics. Could possibly reduce the absorption and therapeutic effect of potassium and sodium iodides, sodium bicarbonate, calcium gluconate, carbonate, and lactate, aluminum hydroxide, magnesium and ferrous sulfates, and bismuth subcarbonate.

Dang Gui
(Radix Angelicae Sinensis)

Standard daily dosage: 3-15g
AH: Do not use during pregnancy. (This medicinal is routinely used in Chinese medical gynecology during pregnancy as part of formulas appropriately prescribed on the basis of pattern discrimination.)
B&G: Use with caution in patients with diarrhea or abdominal distention.
C&C: Contains potassium. Could possibly cause hyperkalemia when used with potassium-sparing diuretics. May exaggerate the anticoagulative effect of warfarin (Coumadin).

Sheng Di, Sheng Di Huang
(uncooked Radix Rehmanniae Glutinosae)

Standard daily dosage: 9-30g
AH: Contraindicated in patients with diarrhea or lack of appetite
B&G: Contraindicated in pregnant women with anemias or digestive weakness
C&C: Contains potassium. Could possibly cause hyperkalemia when used with potassium-sparing diuretics.
PDR: No health risks or side effects are known in conjunction with the proper administration of designated therapeutic dosages.

Gan Cao
(Radix Glycyrrhizae Uralensis, licorice root)

Standard daily dosage: 2-12g
AH: Do not use during pregnancy. (This medicinal is routinely used in Chinese medical gynecology during pregnancy as part of formulas appropriately prescribed on the basis of pattern discrimination.) As a single herb in high doses, it is contraindicated in diabetes, hypertension, and liver disorders. Not for long-term use.

BR: May increase toxicity of cardiac glycosides. May increase potassium loss due to diuretics and laxatives. Possible additive effect to corticosteroids. May be synergistic with insulin in causing hypokalemia and sodium retention.

B&G: According to some traditional sources, incompatible with *Gan Sui* (Radix Euphorbiae Kansui), *Yuan Hua* (Flos Daphnes Genkwae), and *Yuan Zhi* (Radix Polygalae Tenuifoliae). If taken long-term, it may cause hypertension and/or edema. Contains glycyrrhetinic acid which could possibly cause a reduction in thyroid activity and basal metabolic rate.

The research on *Gan Cao* concurs that this medicinal is generally safe when used in small amounts as an envoy. It should not be taken long-term or as a single herb during pregnancy. When used as a single medicinal or in patients taking other potent Western pharmaceuticals, caution should be exercised to guard against potential toxicity and drug interaction.

COMMENTS

Hu Po (Succinum) is commonly substituted for *Zhu Sha* in this formula due to *Zhu Sha*'s toxicity.

Contents

APPENDIX 1

AMERICAN HERBAL PRODUCTS ASSOCIATION (AHPA)

HERBAL CLASSIFICATION SYSTEM

Class 1   Herbs which can be safely consumed when used appropriately

Class 2   Herbs for which restrictions apply unless directed by a qualified expert

2a   For external use only
2b   Not to be used during pregnancy
2c   Not to be used while nursing
2d   Other specific use restrictions

Class 3   Herbs which require the following labeling, "To be used only under the supervision of an expert qualified in the appropriate use of this substance"

Class 4   Herbs for which insufficient data are available for classification

CLASS 1 CHINESE MEDICINALS
ACCORDING TO *BOTANICAL SAFETY HANDBOOK*

Class 1   Herbs which can be safely consumed when used appropriately

Nan Sha Shen (Radix Adenophorae Strictae)
Huo Xiang (Herba Agastachis Seu Pogostemi)
He Huan Hua (Flos Albizziae Julibrissinis)
Gao Liang Jiang (Rhizoma Alpiniae Officinari)
Cao Guo (Fructus Amomi Tsao-kuo)
Zhi Mu (Rhizoma Anemarrhenae Aspheloidis)
Bai Zhi (Radix Angelicae Dahuricae)
Niu Bang Zi (Fructus Arctii Lappae)
Tian Men Dong (Tuber Asparagi Cochinensis)
Huang Qi (Radix Astragali Membranacei)
Cang Zhu (Rhizoma Atractylodis)
Bai Zhu (Rhizoma Atractylodis Macrocephalae)
Mu Xiang (Radix Auklandiae Lappae)
Dong Gua Pi (Pericarpium Benincasae Hispidae)
Chai Hu (Radix Bupleuri)
Mu Gua (Fructus Chaenomelis Lagenariae)
Gou Ji (Rhizoma Cibotii Barometsis)
Gui Zhi (Ramulus Cinnamomi Cassiae)
Rou Cong Rong (Herba Cistanchis Deserticolae Seu Salsae)
Zhi Ke (Fructus Citri Aurantii)
Chen Pi (Pericarpium Citri Reticulatae)
Qing Pi (Fructus Citri Reticulatae Viride)
Wei Ling Xian (Radix Clematidis Chinensis)
She Chuang Zi (Fructus Cnidii Monnieri)
Dang Shen (Radix Codonopsitis Pilosulae)
Dong Chong Xia Cao (Cordyceps Sinensis)
Shan Zha (Fructus Crataegi)
Tu Si Zi (Semen Cuscutae Chinensis)
Bai Wei (Radix Cynanchi Atrati)
Xiang Fu (Rhizoma Cyperi Rotundi)
Xue Jie (Sanguis Draconis)
Shi Hu (Herba Dendrobii)
Shan Yao (Radix Dioscoreae Oppositae)
Xu Duan (Radix Dipsaci)
Gu Sui Bu (Rhizoma Drynariae)
Han Lian Cao (Herba Ecliptae Prostratae)
Bai Dou Kou (Fructus Cardamomi)
Da Qing Ye (Folium Daqingye)
Ci Wu Jia (Radix Eleuthrococci Senticosi)
Hai Tong Pi (Cortex Erythiniae)
Du Zhong (Cortex Eucommiae Ulmoidis)
Qian Shi (Semen Euryalis Ferocis)

Xiao Hui Xiang (Fructus Foeniculi Vulgaris)
Ling Zhi (Fructificatio Ganodermae Lucidi)
Zhi Zi (Fructus Gardeniae Jasminoidis)
Tian Ma (Rhizoma Gastrodiae Elatae)
Qin Jiao (Radix Gentianae Qinjiao)
Long Dan Cao (Radix Gentianae Longdancao)
Sha Shen (Radix Glehniae Littoralis)
Bai Mao Gen (Rhizoma Imperatae Cylindricae)
Xuan Fu Hua (Flos Inulae Racemosae)
Ban Lan Gen (Radix Isatidis Seu Baphicacanthi)
Fang Feng (Radix Ledebouriellae Divaricatae)
Gao Ben (Radix Et Rhizoma Ligustici Chinensis)
Nu Zhen Zi (Fructus Ligustri Lucidi)
Bai He (Bulbus Lilii)
Ren Dong Teng (Caulis Lonicerae Japonicae)
Jin Yin Hua (Flos Lonicerae Japonicae)
Xin Yi Hua (Flos Magnoliae Liliflorae)
Chuan Lian Zi (Fructus Meliae Toosendan)
Bo He (Herba Menthae Haplocalycis)
Ba Ji Tian (Radix Morindae Officinalis)
Sang Bai Pi (Cortex Radicis Mori Albi)
Sang Ye (Folium Mori Albi)
Sang Shen (Fructus Mori Albi)
Sang Zhi (Ramulus Mori Albi)
Lian Zi Xin (Embryo Nelumbinis Nuciferae)
He Ye (Folium Nelumbinis Nuciferae)
Ou Jie (Nodus Rhizomatis Nelumbinis Nuciferae)
Lian Xu (Stamen Nelumbinis Nuciferae)
Qiang Huo (Radix Et Rhizoma Notopterygii)
Ru Xiang (Resina Olibani)
Mai Men Dong (Tuber Ophiopogonis Japonici)
Bai Shao (Radix Albus Paeoniae Lactiflorae)
Xi Yang Shen (Radix Panacis Quinquefolii)
Ying Su Ke (Pericarpium Papaveris Somniferi)
Yu Zhu (Rhizoma Polygoni Odorati)
Huang Jing (Rhizoma Polygonati)
Zhu Ling (Sclerotium Polypori Umbellati)
Xia Ku Cao (Spica Prunellae Vulgaris)
Wu Mei (Fructus Pruni Mume)
Ge Gen (Radix Puerariae Lobatae)
Mei Gui Hua (Flos Rosae Rugosae)
Dan Shen (Radix Salviae Miltiorrhizae)
Wu Wei Zi (Fructus Schisandrae Chinensis)
Huang Qin (Radix Scutellariae Baicalensis)
Hei Zhi Ma (Semen Sesami Indici)
Bai Jie Zi (Semen Sinapis Albae)
Ku Shen (Radix Sophorae Flavescentis)
Fang Ji (Radix Stephania Tetrandrae)

Ding Xiang (Flos Caryophylli)
Pu Gong Ying (Herba Taraxaci Mongolici)
Gua Lou (Fructus Trichosanthis Kirlowii)
Gua Lou Ren (Semen Trichosanthis Kirlowii)
Gou Teng (Ramulus Uncariae Cum Uncis)
Yu Mi Xu (Stigma Zeae Maydis)
Sheng Jiang (uncooked Rhizoma Zingiberis Officinalis)
Da Zao (Fructus Zizyphi Jujubae)

CLASS 2 CHINESE MEDICINALS ACCORDING TO *BOTANICAL SAFETY HANDBOOK*

Class 2 Herbs for which restrictions apply unless directed by a qualified expert
2a For external use only
2b Not to be used during pregnancy
2c Not to be used while nursing
2d Other specific use restrictions

Niu Xi (Radix Achyranthis Bidentatae), 2b, 2d, contraindicated in menorrhagia
Shi Chang Pu (Rhizoma Acori Graminei), 2b
He Huan Pi (Cortex Albizziae Julibrissinis), 2b
Ze Xie (Rhizoma Alismatis), 2d, prolonged use may cause gastrointestinal irritation
Da Suan (Bulbus Allii Sativi), 2c
Lu Hui (Herba Aloes), 2b, 2d, contraindicated in intestinal obstruction, colitis, hemorrhoids, during menstruation
Chuan Xin Lian (Herba Andrographidis Paniculatae), 2b
Du Huo (Radix Angelicae Pubescentis), 2d, avoid prolonged exposure to sunlight
Dang Gui (Radix Angelicae Sinensis), 2b
Tian Nan Xing (Rhizoma Arisaematis), 2b
Qing Hao (Herba Artemisiae Annuae Seu Apiaceae), 2b
Yin Chen Hao (Herba Artemisiae Yinchenhao), 2b
Ai Ye (Folium Artemisiae Argyi), 2b
Xi Xin (Herba Asari Cum Radice), 2b, 2d, not for long-term use
Hong Hua (Flos Carthami Tinctorii), 2b, 2d, contraindicated in hemorrhagic diseases
Sheng Ma (Rhizoma Cimicifugae), 2b, 2c
Zhang Nao (Camphora), 2b, 2d, not for long-term use
Rou Gui (Cortex Cinnamomi Cassiae), 2b
Yi Yi Ren (Semen Coicis Lachryma-jobi), 2b
Huang Lian (Rhizoma Coptidis Chinensis), 2b
Shan Zhu Yu (Fructus Corni Officinalis), 2d, contraindicated in difficult or painful urination
Yan Hu Suo (Rhizoma Corydalis Yanhusuo), 2b
Jiang Huang (Rhizoma Curcumae Longae), 2b, 2d, contraindicated in bile duct obstruction

E Zhu (Rhizoma Curcumae Zedoariae), 2b

Chuan Niu Xi (Radix Cyathulae), 2b

Suo Yang (Herba Cynomorii Songarici), 2d, contraindicated in diarrhea

Ma Huang (Radix Ephedrae), 2b, 2d, contraindicated in anorexia, bulimia, glaucoma; not for long-term use

Yin Yang Huo (Herba Epimedii), 2d, not for long-term use

Mu Zei Cao (Herba Equiseti Hiemalis), 2b

Pi Pa Ye (Folium Eriobotryae Japonicae), 2d, not for long-term use

Wu Zhu Yu (Fructus Evodiae Rutecarpae), 2d, do not exceed dose

Lian Qiao (Fructus Forsythiae Suspensae), 2b

Chuan Bei Mu (Bulbus Fritillariae Cirrhosae), 2b

Zhe Bei Mu (Bulbus Fritillariae Thunbergii), 2b

Bai Guo Ye (Folium Ginkgonis Bilobae), 2d, may potentiate MAO-inhibitors

Gan Cao (Radix Glycyrrhizae Uralensis), 2b, 2d, not for prolonged use; contraindicated in diabetes, hypertension, liver disorders, etc.

Mai Ya (Fructus Germinatus Hordei Vulgaris), 2b

Yi Mu Cao (Herba Leonuri Heterophylli), 2b

Chuan Xiong (Radix Ligustici Wallichii), 2b

Di Gu Pi (Cortex Radicis Lycii Chinensis), 2b

Gou Qi Zi (Fructus Lycii Chinensis), 2b

Hou Po (Cortex Magnoliae Officinalis), 2b

Dan Pi (Cortex Radicis Moutan), 2b

Rou Dou Kou (Fructus Myristicae Fragrantis), 2b

Mo Yao (Resina Myrrhae), 2b, 2d, contraindicated in excessive uterine bleeding

Song Qi (Rhizoma Nardostachydis), 2b

Lian Zi (Semen Nelumbinis Nuciferae), 2d, contraindicated in constipation & stomach distention

Ren Shen (Radix Panacis Ginseng), 2d, contraindicated in hypertension

Huang Bai (Cortex Phellodendri), 2b

Ban Xia (Rhizoma Pinelliae Ternatae), 2b, 2d, contraindicated in all hemorrhagic disorders

Jie Geng (Radix Platycodi Grandiflori), 2d, contraindicated in spitting blood & TB

Yuan Zhi (Radix Polygalae Tenuifoliae), 2d, contraindicated in ulcers & gastritis

He Shou Wu (Radix Polygoni Multiflori), 2d, contraindicated in diarrhea

Tao Ren (Semen Pruni Persicae), 2b

San Qi (Radix Notoginseng), 2b

Sheng Di (uncooked Radix Rehmanniae Glutinosae), 2d, contraindicated in diarrhea

Shu Di (cooked Radix Rehmanniae Glutinosae), 2d, contraindicated in diarrhea

Da Huang (Radix Et Rhizoma Rhei), 2b, 2d, contraindicated in intestinal obstruction, etc.

Fu Pen Zi (Fructus Rubi Chingii), 2d, contraindicated in difficult urination

Tan Xiang (Lignum Santali Albi), 2d, contraindicated in diseases involving the parenchyma of the kidney

Pu Gong Ying (Radix Taraxaci Mongolici Cum Radice), 2d, contraindicated
in blockage of the bile duct, etc.
He Zi (Fructus Terminaliae Chebulae), 2d, contraindicated in acute cough,
acute diarrhea, early stage dysentery
Tian Hua Fen (Radix Trichosanthis Kirlowii), 2b
Hu Lu Ba (Semen Trigonellae Foeni-graeci), 2b
Kuan Dong Hua (Flos Tussilaginis Farfarae), 2b, 2d, not for long-term use
Chuan Jiao (Pericarpium Zanthoxyli Bungeani), 2b
Suan Zao Ren (Semen Zizyphi Spinosae), 2b

CLASS 3 CHINESE MEDICINALS
ACCORDING TO *BOTANICAL SAFETY HANDBOOK*

Class 3 Herbs which require the following labeling, "To be used only under the supervision of an expert qualified in the appropriate use of this substance"

Fu Zi (Radix Lateralis Praeparatus Aconiti Carmichaeli)
Ku Lian Pi (Cortex Radicis Meliae Azerdachis)
Xing Ren (Semen Pruni Armeniacae)
Shi Liu Pi (Pericarpium Punicae Granati)

CLASS 4 CHINESE MEDICINALS
ACCORDING TO *BOTANICAL SAFETY HANDBOOK*

Class 4 Herbs for which insufficient data are available for classification

Jin Qian Cao (Herba Desmodii Seu Lysimachiae)

APPENDIX 2
WESTERN DRUGS

NEPHROTOXIC DRUGS

acetazolamide
aminoglycosides
aminopyrine
aminosalicylate
amphotericin
ampicillin
cephalothin
cisplatin
colistin
cotrimoxazole
cyclophosphamide
dextran (LMW)
erythromycin
fenoprofen
furosemide
ibuprofen
indomethacin
mannitol
methicillin
methoxyflurane
mithramycin
naproxen
oxacillin
penicillamine
pentamide
phenacetin
phenindione
phenylbutazone
polymixin B
quinine
rifampin
salicylates
sulfonamides
tetracyclines

thiazides
vancomycin
zoxazolamine

DRUGS KNOWN TO CAUSE CHOLESTASIS

aminosalicylic acid
androgens
azathioprine
benzodiazepines
carbamazepine
carbarsone
chlorpropamide
propoxyphene
estrogens
penicillin
imipramine
meprobamate
methimazole
nicotinic acid
progestins
penicillin
phenothiazines
oral contraceptives
sulfonamides
sulfones
erythromycin estolate

DRUGS KNOWN TO CAUSE HEPATOCELLULAR DAMAGE

acetaminophen
allopurinol
aminosalicylic acid

amitriptyline
androgens
asparaginase
aspirin
azathioprine
carbamazepine
chlorambucil
chloramphenicol
chlorpropamide
dantrolene
disulfiram
estrogens
ethanol
ethionamide
halothane
ibuprofen
indomethacin
iron salts
isoniazid
MAO-inhibitors
mercaptopurine
methotrexate
methoxyflurane
methyldopa
mithramycin
nicotinic acid
nitrofurantoin
oral contraceptives
papaverine
paramethadione
penicillin
phenobarbital
phenazopyridine
phenylbutazone
phenytoin
probenecid
procainamide
propylthiouracil
pyrazinamide
quinidine
sulfonamides
tetracyclines
trimethadione
valproic acid

DRUGS THAT HAVE CAUSED APLASTIC ANEMIA

acetazolamide
amphotericin
arsenicals
aspirin
bismuth
carbamazepine
carbimazole
carbutamide
chloramphenicol
chlordiazepoxide
chlorothiazide
chlorpheniramine
chlorpromazine
chlorpropamide
colchicine
dinitrophenol
indomethacin
mephenytoin
meprobamate
methimazole
oxyphenbutazone
penicillin
perchlorate
phenacetin
phenylbutazone
phenytoin
primidone
promazine
pyrimethamine
quinacrine
ristocetin
streptomycin
sulfonamides
tetracycline
thiocyanate
thiouracil
tolbutamide
trifluoperazine
trimethadione
tripelennamine

POSSIBLE HERB-DRUG INTERACTIONS

Medicinal	May interact with	Potential effects
Sheng Ma (*Rhizoma Cimicifugae*)	Estrogens OCs	May decrease response to estrogen
	Antihyperlipidemics	Possible additive effect
Dang Gui (*Radix Angelicae Sinensis*)	Anticoagulants Antiplatelet agents	Possible additive effect
	Estrogens	May result in estrogen excess
Sheng Jiang (uncooked *Rhizoma Zingiberis Officinalis*)	Anticoagulants Antiplatelet agents	Possible additive effect
Ren Shen (*Radix Panacis Ginseng*)	Hypoglycemic drugs	Possible additive effect
	Furosemide	Decreased diuretic effect
	Digoxin	Increased serum concentration
	MAO-inhibitors	Headache, visual hallucinations, tremor, manic episodes
	Anticoagulants Antiplatelet agents	Decreased warfarin effect

Medicinal	May interact with	Potential effects
	Estrogens Corticosteroids	Possible additive effect
Shan Zha (*Fructus Crataegi*)	Antihypertensives	Increased risk of bleeding
	Digoxin	Possible additive effect
Kun Bu (*Thallus Algae*)	Thyroid hormones	May interfere with thyroid hormone replacement
Gan Cao (*Radix Glycyrrhizae Uralensis*)	Spironolactone	Decreased diuretic effect
	Cardiac glycosides	Possible digoxin toxicity
	Thiazide diuretics	May cause hypokalemia
	Corticosteroids Cyclosporine	May decrease response to these drugs
	MAO-inhibitors	May increase risk of hypertensive crisis
Ma Huang (*Herba Ephedrae*)	Oxytocin Methyldopa Beta-blockers MAO-inhibitors Theophylline Cardiac glycosides	May cause hypertension, CNS stimulation
Che Qian Zi (*Semen Plantaginis*)	Antihyperlipidemics	Possible additive effects
	Anticoagulants	May interfere with anti-coagulant therapy
Ci Wu Jia (*Radix Eleuthrococci Senticosi*)	Digitalis	May interfere with drug level assay
Jiang Huang (*Tuber Curcumae Longae*)	Antiplatelet agents	Possible additive effects

Tyler, Varro, E. 2003. *Physicians' Desk Reference for Herbal Medicines*, 2nd ed., Montvale, NJ: Thomson Medical Economics

A recent addition to the PDR family. Mostly Western in focus, but contains many Oriental medicinals along with actions and pharmacology, contraindications, precautions and adverse reactions, dosages, and literature references. Based on many German "E" Commission findings.

Bensky, Dan, & Barolet, Randall. 1990. *Chinese Herbal Medicine: Formulas and Strategies*. Seattle: Eastland Press

Currently the "gold standard" reference for Chinese medicinal formula prescriptions. Well-researched and clearly written. Used in many colleges of Oriental medicine for training herbal practitioners. Almost 300 primary formulas are listed along with their ingredients, indications for their use, analysis of their medicinals, and cautions and contraindications.

Bensky, Dan, & Gamble, Andrew. 1993. *Chinese Herbal Medicine: Materia Medica*, Seattle: Eastland Press

The most widely used English language reference for Chinese herbal medicinals. Each entry contains illustrations of the medicinal's wild appearance, where it is grown and harvested, information on its proper preparation and prescription, popular combinations with other medicinals, as well as cautions and contraindications. A must for the library of any serious herbalist.

Blackwell, Richard. 1996. "Cases of Herb Toxicity: Adverse Events Involving Certain Chinese Herbal Medicines and the Response of the Profession." http://acupuncture.com/Herbology/Toxic.htm

A very concise and well-documented discussion of the most well-known cases of Chinese medicinal toxicity and interaction. Contains an extensive bibliography with links to many Websites related to herbal medicinals.

Brinker, Francis. 1998. *Herb Contraindications and Drug Interactions*, 2nd ed., Sandy: Eclectic Medical Publications

An easy-to-consult listing of both Western and Oriental medicinal herbs written by a naturopathic physician. Appendix section lists medicinal advisories by condition and Western orthodox drug interactions.

Chan, Kelvin, & Cheung, Lily. 2003. *Interactions Between Chinese Herbal Medicinal Products and Orthodox Drugs*. London: Taylor & Francis

A very readable and informative guide to interactions between Eastern and Western medicinal substances. Many tables showing the interactions and their consequences. Also lists many ready-made medicine interactions. A must for the pharmacology scholar interested in this topic.

Chen, John. 2001. "Aristolochic Acid and Chinese Herbs." http://acupuncture.com/Herbology/aristo.htm

A brief but informative article written shortly after the FDA sent out its advisory letter. Good list of references plus links to several Websites.

Dharmananda, Subhuti, Ph.D. Undated. "Safety Issues Affecting Chinese Herbs: The Case of Asarum." *www.itmonline.org/arts/asarum.htm*

An excellent on-line discussion of *Xi Xin* (Herba Asari Cum Radice) in particular and toxicity issues in Chinese medicine in general. Underscores that many of the current concerns about Chinese medicinal toxicity are overblown. Contains many useful footnotes for finding further information on these issues.

Flaws, Bob. 2001. *70 Essential Chinese Herbal Formulas*, 2nd ed., Boulder: Blue Poppy Press

An excellent reference or textbook for both the beginning and advanced herbalist. Highlights and thoroughly analyzes the core formulas comprising the Chinese herbal medicinal pharmacy. Uses Wiseman and Ye's Chinese medical terminology throughout.

Gao, Lu-wen. 2003. *You Du Zhong Yao Lin Chuang Jing Yao (Essentials of the Clinical Use of Toxic Chinese Medicinals)*. Beijing: Study Center Press

A Chinese language text on the toxicity of many Chinese medicinals. If this were available in English, it would be a useful reference for poison control centers and Western physicians who treat toxicology cases.

Huang, Kee Chang. 1998. *The Pharmacology of Chinese Herbs*, 2nd ed. New York: CRC Press

A must for the pharmacologist who is studying this subject. Chemistry, actions, pharmacokinetics, adverse effects, and therapeutic uses are all covered for individual medicinals. Many molecular diagrams.

McGuffin, Michael *et al*. eds. 1997. *American Herbal Products Association's Botanical Safety Handbook*. New York: CRC Press

A relatively complete guide supported and endorsed by AHPA which lists and categorizes the safety of both Western and Oriental individual medicinals. Herbs are classed in four categories with conditions for their safe prescription and consumption.

Samenuk, David, M.D., *et al*. 2002. "Adverse Cardiovascular Events Temporally Associated With Ma Huang, an Herbal Source of Ephedrine." *Mayo Clinic Proceedings, #77*

One of the better articles highlighting the dangers of *Ma Huang* (Herba Ephedrae) intoxication. An excellent compendium of research from the FDA and other sources. http://mayo.edu/proceedings/2002/jan/7701a1

Varner, John S., LAc. Undated. "Green Medicine, Muddy Water." http://www.craneherb.com/PDFs/GreenMedicine2.pdf

An on-line essay about toxicity in Chinese medicine. In general, cautions that the current concern is largely overblown and based on false assumptions and concerns.

Wiseman, Nigel, ed. 1996. *English-Chinese Chinese-English Dictionary of Chinese Medicine*. Changhsa: Hunan Science & Technology Press

The standard for precise terminology in Chinese medicine. The first choice for herbalists worldwide.

Wiseman, Nigel & Ye, Feng. 1999. *A Practical Dictionary of Chinese Medicine*, Brookline: Paradigm Publications

A relatively complete Chinese medical dictionary using Wiseman *et al*.'s excellent standard translational terminology. Another must for all serious English language speaking practitioners of Chinese medicine.

GENERAL INDEX

A

A-V block, 67
abdominal migraine, 290
abnormal vaginal discharge, 46, 271, 305
acute abdominal pain, 77
acute bacillary dysentery, 46
acute bronchitis, 139, 218, 300, 350
acute cervical myositis, 122
acute conjunctivitis, 46, 149
acute cystitis, 91, 180
acute enteritis, 46, 149
acute hemorrhagic esophagitis, 237
acute hepatitis, 27, 322
acute icteric hepatitis, 149, 180
acute leukemia, 292
acute nephritis, 31
acute pancreatitis, 55
acute prostatitis, 31
acute pyelonephritis, 31
acute suppurative infections, 324
acute tonsillitis, 218, 324
acute transverse myelitis, 94
Addison's disease, 159, 319
adrenal insufficiency, 248
agalactia, 61
AHPA, 23-24, 357, 359, 369
albuminuria, 30, 159, 257, 268, 353
allergic colitis, 245, 250
allergic purpura, 129
allergic rhinitis, 65, 122, 330

D

H

habitual constipation, 77, 191

habitual miscarriage, 61

hangover, 114

heart arrhythmias, 30, 32, 37, 42-44, 55, 60, 70, 83, 88, 112, 123, 126-127, 134, 137, 148, 189, 192, 198, 220, 222-223, 231, 247, 253, 261, 268-269, 280, 293, 303, 306, 317, 325, 328, 335, 337, 341, 350

heart disease, 129, 235, 264, 314, 334, 339, 346

heart failure, 248, 283, 339

heart palpitations, 31, 38, 41, 49, 51-52, 56, 62, 67-69, 80, 94, 96, 102, 104, 106-107, 112, 114-115, 117, 123, 125, 129, 135-136, 139, 142, 147, 149, 153, 159, 161, 164, 169, 175, 177, 186-187, 189-190, 194, 196-198, 209-210, 216, 219, 223, 225-226, 228, 234-235, 242, 249, 252, 258, 264-265, 272, 275-276, 281-282, 288, 291, 297-298, 301, 303, 310, 312, 314, 328, 339-340, 342, 346-347, 353

hemafecia, 30, 151, 252, 257, 268, 353

hematuria, 16, 32, 36, 78, 91, 95, 98, 116, 118, 146, 157, 166, 182, 192, 211, 217, 236, 238, 246, 251, 267, 273, 275, 285, 302, 311, 317

hemiplegia, 108, 260

hemophilus vaginitis, 271

hemoptysis, 37, 40, 42, 59, 149, 151, 220, 231, 237, 268, 310, 317, 325, 350

hemorrhagic enteritis, 30, 257, 268, 353

hemorrhoids, 61, 77, 145-146, 191, 360

hepatic coma, 27, 254, 292

hepatic necrosis, 322

hepatitis, 15, 27, 51, 55, 61, 85, 149, 163, 180, 228, 245, 275, 283, 296, 305, 319, 321-322, 332, 337

hepatoxicity, 13-15, 65, 257

hernia, 61, 79, 87, 167, 200, 202, 245

hernia pain, 79

herpes infections, 180

hiccup, 168, 314

high fever, 27-28, 35, 44, 70, 127, 136, 149, 198, 242, 254, 256, 292, 335

hydrocele, 200, 283

hydrochloric acid, 29, 32-33, 35, 37-38, 41-44, 46-48, 51-52, 55-60, 62-65, 67-69, 71, 75, 77, 79, 83, 88, 95-97, 103, 105-107, 109-110, 112, 114, 118-119, 123, 126, 129, 132, 134-135, 137, 139-140, 142, 144-145, 148, 150, 153, 155, 157-158, 160, 162, 164, 169, 175, 178-182, 186, 189, 192-193, 195-197, 207, 209-210, 213, 215, 219-220, 223-225, 228, 230-231, 234-239, 242, 246-247, 253, 259-261, 263, 265-268, 270, 272-273, 276, 280-282, 288, 291, 293, 296-298, 303, 305-306, 310-312, 314-317, 320, 323-325, 329, 331, 333-334, 336-337, 341, 343-345, 347-348, 350-351

hyperkalemia, 28-31, 33, 36-37, 40-42, 44, 47, 49, 52-53, 56-57, 59, 61, 63, 68, 70-71, 73, 77-79, 82-85, 87-89, 91-92, 97-100, 106-107, 110-113, 115, 118-119, 123, 125-127, 130, 132, 134-135, 137, 139-141, 143-144, 147-151, 153-154, 156-157, 160-162, 164-166, 168, 172-173, 178-179, 181-183, 186, 189, 192-193, 198, 200-

M

N

O

P

T

U

PIN YIN FORMULA INDEX

ENGLISH FORMULA INDEX

PIN YIN HERB INDEX

R

OTHER BOOKS ON CHINESE MEDICINE AVAILABLE FROM:
BLUE POPPY PRESS

5441 Western, Suite 2, Boulder, CO 80301

For ordering 1-800-487-9296 PH. 303\447-8372 FAX 303\245-8362

Email: info@bluepoppy.com Website: www.bluepoppy.com

ACUPOINT POCKET REFERENCE by Bob Flaws
ISBN 0-936185-93-7
ISBN 978-0-936185-93-4

ACUPUNCTURE & IVF by Lifang Liang
ISBN 0-891845-24-1
ISBN 978-0-891845-24-6

ACUPUNCTURE FOR STROKE REHABILITATION
Three Decades of Information from China
by Hoy Ping Yee Chan, et al.
ISBN 1-891845-35-7
ISBN 978-1-891845-35-2

ACUPUNCTURE PHYSICAL MEDICINE: An
Acupuncture Touchpoint Approach to the Treatment
of Chronic Pain, Fatigue, and Stress Disorders
by Mark Seem
ISBN 1-891845-13-6
ISBN 978-1-891845-13-0

AGING & BLOOD STASIS: A New Approach to
TCM Geriatrics by Yan De-xin
ISBN 0-936185-63-6
ISBN 978-0-936185-63-7

A NEW AMERICAN ACUPUNTURE By Mark Seem
ISBN 0-936185-44-9
ISBN 978-0-936185-44-6

BETTER BREAST HEALTH NATURALLY
with CHINESE MEDICINE
by Honora Lee Wolfe & Bob Flaws
ISBN 0-936185-90-2
ISBN 978-0-936185-90-3

BIOMEDICINE: A Textbook for Practitioners of
Acupuncture and Oriental Medicine
by Bruce H. Robinson, MD
ISBN 1-891845-38-1
ISBN 978-1-891845-38-3

THE BOOK OF JOOK:
Chinese Medicinal Porridges
by B. Flaws
ISBN 0-936185-60-6
ISBN 978-0-936185-60-0

CHANNEL DIVERGENCES
Deeper Pathways of the Web
by Miki Shima and Charles Chase
ISBN 1-891845-15-2
ISBN 978-1-891845-15-4

CHINESE MEDICAL OBSTETRICS
by Bob Flaws
ISBN 1-891845-30-6
ISBN 978-1-891845-30-7

CHINESE MEDICAL PALMISTRY:
Your Health in Your Hand
by Zong Xiao-fan & Gary Liscum
ISBN 0-936185-64-3
ISBN 978-0-936185-64-4

CHINESE MEDICAL PSYCHIATRY
A Textbook and Clinical Manual
by Bob Flaws and James Lake, MD
ISBN 1-845891-17-9
ISBN 978-1-845891-17-8

CHINESE MEDICINAL TEAS: Simple, Proven, Folk
Formulas for Common Diseases & Promoting Health
by Zong Xiao-fan & Gary Liscum
ISBN 0-936185-76-7
ISBN 978-0-936185-76-7

CHINESE MEDICINAL WINES & ELIXIRS
by Bob Flaws
ISBN 0-936185-58-9
ISBN 978-0-936185-58-3

CHINESE MEDICINE & HEALTHY WEIGHT
MANAGEMENT: An Evidence-based Integrated
Approach by Juliette Aiyana, L. Ac.
ISBN 1-891845-44-6
ISBN 978-1-891845-44-4

CHINESE PEDIATRIC MASSAGE THERAPY: A
Parent's & Practitioner's Guide to the Prevention &
Treatment of Childhood Illness
by Fan Ya-li
ISBN 0-936185-54-6
ISBN 978-0-936185-54-5

CHINESE SELF-MASSAGE THERAPY:
The Easy Way to Health
by Fan Ya-li
ISBN 0-936185-74-0
ISBN 978-0-936185-74-3

THE CLASSIC OF DIFFICULTIES:
A Translation of the Nan Jing
translation by Bob Flaws
ISBN 1-891845-07-1
ISBN 978-1-891845-07-9

A COMPENDIUM OF CHINESE MEDICAL
MENSTRUAL DISEASES
by Bob Flaws
ISBN 1-891845-31-4
ISBN 978-1-891845-31-4

CONTROLLING DIABETES NATURALLY WITH
CHINESE MEDICINE
by Lynn Kuchinski
ISBN 0-936185-06-3
ISBN 978-0-936185-06-2

CURING ARTHRITIS NATURALLY WITH
CHINESE MEDICINE
by Douglas Frank & Bob Flaws
ISBN 0-936185-87-2
ISBN 978-0-936185-87-3

CURING DEPRESSION NATURALLY WITH
CHINESE MEDICINE
by Rosa Schnyer & Bob Flaws
ISBN 0-936185-94-5
ISBN 978-0-936185-94-1

CURING FIBROMYALGIA NATURALLY WITH
CHINESE MEDICINE
by Bob Flaws
ISBN 1-891845-09-8
ISBN 978-1-891845-09-3

CURING HAY FEVER NATURALLY WITH
CHINESE MEDICINE
by Bob Flaws
ISBN 0-936185-91-0
ISBN 978-0-936185-91-0

CURING HEADACHES NATURALLY WITH
CHINESE MEDICINE
by Bob Flaws
ISBN 0-936185-95-3
ISBN 978-0-936185-95-8

CURING IBS NATURALLY WITH CHINESE
MEDICINE
by Jane Bean Oberski
ISBN 1-891845-11-X
ISBN 978-1-891845-11-6

CURING INSOMNIA NATURALLY WITH
CHINESE MEDICINE
by Bob Flaws
ISBN 0-936185-86-4
ISBN 978-0-936185-86-6

CURING PMS NATURALLY WITH CHINESE
MEDICINE
by Bob Flaws
ISBN 0-936185-85-6
ISBN 978-0-936185-85-9

DISEASES OF THE KIDNEY & BLADDER
by Hoy Ping Yee Chan, et al.
ISBN 1-891845-37-3
ISBN 978-1-891845-35-6

THE DIVINE FARMER'S MATERIA MEDICA
A Translation of the Shen Nong Ben Cao
translation by Yang Shouz-zhong
ISBN 0-936185-96-1
ISBN 978-0-936185-96-5

DUI YAO: THE ART OF COMBINING
CHINESE HERBAL MEDICINALS
by Philippe Sionneau
ISBN 0-936185-81-3
ISBN 978-0-936185-81-1

ENDOMETRIOSIS, INFERTILITY AND
TRADITIONAL CHINESE MEDICINE:
A Laywoman's Guide
by Bob Flaws
ISBN 0-936185-14-7
ISBN 978-0-936185-14-9

THE ESSENCE OF LIU FENG-WU'S
GYNECOLOGY
by Liu Feng-wu, translated by Yang Shou-zhong
ISBN 0-936185-88-0
ISBN 978-0-936185-88-0

EXTRA TREATISES BASED ON INVESTIGATION
& INQUIRY:
A Translation of Zhu Dan-xi's Ge Zhi Yu Lun
translation by Yang Shou-zhong
ISBN 0-936185-53-8
ISBN 978-0-936185-53-8

FIRE IN THE VALLEY: TCM Diagnosis & Treatment
of Vaginal Diseases
by Bob Flaws
ISBN 0-936185-25-2
ISBN 978-0-936185-25-5

FU QING-ZHU'S GYNECOLOGY
trans. by Yang Shou-zhong and Liu Da-wei
ISBN 0-936185-35-X
ISBN 978-0-936185-35-4

FULFILLING THE ESSENCE:
A Handbook of Traditional & Contemporary
Treatments for Female Infertility
by Bob Flaws
ISBN 0-936185-48-1
ISBN 978-0-936185-48-4

GOLDEN NEEDLE WANG LE-TING: A 20th
Century Master's Approach to Acupuncture
by Yu Hui-chan and Han Fu-ru, trans. by Shuai Xue-zhong
ISBN 0-936185-78-3
ISBN 978-0-936185-78-1

A HANDBOOK OF TCM PATTERNS
& THEIR TREATMENTS
by Bob Flaws & Daniel Finney
ISBN 0-936185-70-8
ISBN 978-0-936185-70-5

A HANDBOOK OF TRADITIONAL
CHINESE DERMATOLOGY
by Liang Jian-hui, trans. by Zhang Ting-liang
& Bob Flaws
ISBN 0-936185-46-5
ISBN 978-0-936185-46-0

A HANDBOOK OF TRADITIONAL
CHINESE GYNECOLOGY
by Zhejiang College of TCM, trans. by Zhang Ting-liang
& Bob Flaws
ISBN 0-936185-06-6 (4th edit.)
ISBN 978-0-936185-06-4

A HANDBOOK OF CHINESE HEMATOLOGY
by Simon Becker
ISBN 1-891845-16-0
ISBN 978-1-891845-16-1

A HANDBOOK of TCM PEDIATRICS
by Bob Flaws
ISBN 0-936185-72-4
ISBN 978-0-936185-72-9

THE HEART & ESSENCE OF DAN-XI'S
METHODS OF TREATMENT
by Xu Dan-xi, trans. by Yang Shou-zhong
ISBN 0-926185-50-3
ISBN 978-0-936185-50-7

HERB TOXICITIES & DRUG INTERACTIONS:
A Formula Approach by Fred Jennes with Bob Flaws
ISBN 1-891845-26-8
ISBN 978-1-891845-26-0

IMPERIAL SECRETS OF HEALTH & LONGEVITY
by Bob Flaws
ISBN 0-936185-51-1
ISBN 978-0-936185-51-4

INSIGHTS OF A SENIOR ACUPUNCTURIST
by Miriam Lee
ISBN 0-936185-33-3
ISBN 978-0-936185-33-0

INTEGRATED PHARMACOLOGY: Combining Modern
Pharmacology with Chinese Medicine
by Dr. Greg Sperber with Bob Flaws
ISBN 1-891845-41-1
ISBN 978-0-936185-41-3

INTRODUCTION TO THE USE OF
PROCESSED CHINESE MEDICINALS
by Philippe Sionneau
ISBN 0-936185-62-7
ISBN 978-0-936185-62-0

KEEPING YOUR CHILD HEALTHY WITH
CHINESE MEDICINE
by Bob Flaws
ISBN 0-936185-71-6
ISBN 978-0-936185-71-2

THE LAKESIDE MASTER'S STUDY OF THE
PULSE
by Li Shi-zhen, trans. by Bob Flaws
ISBN 1-891845-01-2
ISBN 978-1-891845-01-7

MANAGING MENOPAUSE NATURALLY WITH
CHINESE MEDICINE
by Honora Lee Wolfe
ISBN 0-936185-98-8
ISBN 978-0-936185-98-9

MASTER HUA'S CLASSIC OF THE
CENTRAL VISCERA
by Hua Tuo, trans. by Yang Shou-zhong
ISBN 0-936185-43-0
ISBN 978-0-936185-43-9

THE MEDICAL I CHING: Oracle of the
Healer Within
by Miki Shima
ISBN 0-936185-38-4
ISBN 978-0-936185-38-5

MENOPAIUSE & CHINESE MEDICINE
by Bob Flaws
ISBN 1-891845-40-3
ISBN 978-1-891845-40-6

MOXIBUSTION: The Power of Mugwort Fire
by Lorraine Wilcox
ISBN 1-891845-46-2
ISBN 978-1-891845-46-8

TEST PREP WORKBOOK FOR THE NCCAOM BIO-
MEDICINE MODULE: Exam Preparation & Study
Guide
by Zhong Bai-song
ISBN 1-891845-34-9
ISBN 978-1-891845-34-5

POINTS FOR PROFIT: The Essential Guide to
Practice Success for Acupuncturists 3rd Edition
by Honora Wolfe, Eric Strand & Marilyn Allen
ISBN 1-891845-25-X
ISBN 978-1-891845-25-3

PRINCIPLES OF CHINESE MEDICAL ANDROLOGY:
An Integrated Approach to Male Reproductive and
Urological Health by Bob Damone
ISBN 1-891845-45-4
ISBN 978-1-891845-45-1

PRINCE WEN HUI's COOK: Chinese Dietary
Therapy
By Bob Flaws & Honora Wolfe
ISBN 0-912111-05-4
ISBN 978-0-912111-05-6

THE PULSE CLASSIC:
A Translation of the Mai Jing
by Wang Shu-he, trans. by Yang Shou-zhong
ISBN 0-936185-75-9
ISBN 978-0-936185-75-0

THE SECRET OF CHINESE PULSE DIAGNOSIS
by Bob Flaws
ISBN 0-936185-67-8
ISBN 978-0-936185-67-5

SECRET SHAOLIN FORMULAS for the Treatment
of External Injury
by De Chan, trans. by Zhang Ting-liang & Bob Flaws
ISBN 0-936185-08-2
ISBN 978-0-936185-08-8

STATEMENTS OF FACT IN TRADITIONAL
CHINESE MEDICINE   Revised & Expanded
by Bob Flaws
ISBN 0-936185-52-X
ISBN 978-0-936185-52-1

STICKING TO THE POINT 1:
A Rational Methodology for the Step by Step
Formulation & Administration of an Acupuncture
Treatment
by Bob Flaws
ISBN 0-936185-17-1
ISBN 978-0-936185-17-0

STICKING TO THE POINT 2:
A Study of Acupuncture & Moxibustion Formulas
and Strategies
by Bob Flaws
ISBN 0-936185-97-X
ISBN 978-0-936185-97-2

A STUDY OF DAOIST ACUPUNCTURE &
MOXIBUSTION
by Liu Zheng-cai
ISBN 1-891845-08-X
ISBN 978-1-891845-08-6

THE SUCCESSFUL CHINESE HERBALIST
by Bob Flaws and Honora Lee Wolfe
ISBN 1-891845-29-2
ISBN 978-1-891845-29-1

THE SYSTEMATIC CLASSIC OF ACUPUNCTURE
& MOXIBUSTION
A translation of the Jia Yi Jing
by Huang-fu Mi, trans. by Yang Shou-zhong &
Charles Chace
ISBN 0-936185-29-5
ISBN 978-0-936185-29-3

THE TAO OF HEALTHY EATING ACCORDING TO
CHINESE MEDICINE
by Bob Flaws
ISBN 0-936185-92-9
ISBN 978-0-936185-92-7

TEACH YOURSELF TO READ MODERN
MEDICAL CHINESE
by Bob Flaws
ISBN 0-936185-99-6
ISBN 978-0-936185-99-6

TEST PREP WORKBOOK FOR BASIC TCM THEORY
by Zhong Bai-song
ISBN 1-891845-43-8
ISBN 978-1-891845-43-7

TREATING PEDIATRIC BED-WETTING WITH
ACUPUNCTURE & CHINESE MEDICINE
by Robert Helmer
ISBN 1-891845-33-0
ISBN 978-1-891845-33-8

TREATISE on the SPLEEN & STOMACH: A
Translation and annotation of Li Dong-yuan's
Pi Wei Lun
by Bob Flaws
ISBN 0-936185-41-4
ISBN 978-0-936185-41-5

THE TREATMENT OF CARDIOVASCULAR
DISEASES WITH CHINESE MEDICINE
by Simon Becker, Bob Flaws &
Robert Casañas, MD
ISBN 1-891845-27-6
ISBN 978-1-891845-27-7

THE TREATMENT OF DIABETES MELLITUS
WITH CHINESE MEDICINE
by Bob Flaws, Lynn Kuchinski &
Robert Casañas, M.D.
ISBN 1-891845-21-7
ISBN 978-1-891845-21-5

THE TREATMENT OF DISEASE IN TCM, Vol. 1:
Diseases of the Head & Face, Including Mental &
Emotional Disorders
by Philippe Sionneau & Lü Gang
ISBN 0-936185-69-4
ISBN 978-0-936185-69-9

THE TREATMENT OF DISEASE IN TCM, Vol. II:
Diseases of the Eyes, Ears, Nose, & Throat
by Sionneau & Lü
ISBN 0-936185-73-2
ISBN 978-0-936185-73-6

THE TREATMENT OF DISEASE IN TCM, Vol. III:
Diseases of the Mouth, Lips, Tongue, Teeth & Gums
by Sionneau & Lü
ISBN 0-936185-79-1
ISBN 978-0-936185-79-8

THE TREATMENT OF DISEASE IN TCM, Vol IV:
Diseases of the Neck, Shoulders, Back, & Limbs
by Philippe Sionneau & Lü Gang
ISBN 0-936185-89-9
ISBN 978-0-936185-89-7

THE TREATMENT OF DISEASE IN TCM, Vol V:
Diseases of the Chest & Abdomen
by Philippe Sionneau & Lü Gang
ISBN 1-891845-02-0
ISBN 978-1-891845-02-4

THE TREATMENT OF DISEASE IN TCM, Vol VI:
Diseases of the Urogential System & Proctology
by Philippe Sionneau & Lü Gang
ISBN 1-891845-05-5
ISBN 978-1-891845-05-5

THE TREATMENT OF DISEASE IN TCM, Vol VII:
General Symptoms
by Philippe Sionneau & Lü Gang
ISBN 1-891845-14-4
ISBN 978-1-891845-14-7

THE TREATMENT OF EXTERNAL DISEASES
WITH ACUPUNCTURE & MOXIBUSTION
by Yan Cui-lan and Zhu Yun-long, trans. by Yang Shou-zhong
ISBN 0-936185-80-5
ISBN 978-0-936185-80-4

THE TREATMENT OF MODERN WESTERN
MEDICAL DISEASES WITH CHINESE MEDICINE
by Bob Flaws & Philippe Sionneau
ISBN 1-891845-20-9
ISBN 978-1-891845-20-8

UNDERSTANDING THE DIFFICULT PATIENT: A
Guide for Practitioners of Oriental Medicine
by Nancy Bilello, RN, L.ac.
ISBN 1-891845-32-2
ISBN 978-1-891845-32-1

YI LIN GAI CUO (Correcting the Errors in the Forest
of Medicine)
by Wang Qing-ren
ISBN 1-891845-39-X
ISBN 978-1-891845-39-0

70 ESSENTIAL CHINESE HERBAL FORMULAS
by Bob Flaws
ISBN 0-936185-59-7
ISBN 978-0-936185-59-0

160 ESSENTIAL CHINESE READY-MADE
MEDICINES
by Bob Flaws
ISBN 1-891945-12-8
ISBN 978-1-891945-12-3

630 QUESTIONS & ANSWERS ABOUT CHINESE
HERBAL MEDICINE:
A Workbook & Study Guide
by Bob Flaws
ISBN 1-891845-04-7
ISBN 978-1-891845-04-8

260 ESSENTIAL CHINESE MEDICINALS
by Bob Flaws
ISBN 1-891845-03-9
ISBN 978-1-891845-03-1

750 QUESTIONS & ANSWERS ABOUT
ACUPUNCTURE
Exam Preparation & Study Guide
by Fred Jennes
ISBN 1-891845-22-5
ISBN 978-1-891845-22-2